'Often we assume that recognising and dealing with trauma is primarily an issue for psychology. Psychology is important, but it is not the only voice that can speak powerfully into this deeply troubling human experience. In this excellent collection of essays, the voice of practical theology and biblical studies is given entry into the complexities of trauma. The result is a powerful, interdisciplinary perspective that offers both understanding and healing. This book makes an important contribution to the conversation.'

Professor John Swinton, Chair in Divinity and Religious Studies at the School of Divinity, History, and Philosophy, University of Aberdeen

'This is a timely, challenging and profoundly hopeful book: for all those who want to go deeper in understanding the impact of trauma and how we hold those individuals and communities at times when the world seems to have fallen apart. It is an extraordinary work of deep pastoral theology which makes a significant contribution to the church's practice and understanding, and points us towards hope even as it discusses the most hopeless situations we may face.'

The Most Revd and Rt Hon Justin Welby, Archbishop of Canterbury

'This book is the outcome of sincere, critical, and inspiring conversations about the depth of human suffering on the one hand and of spiritual reflection on the other. I had the privilege of participating in one of these conversations and these pages reflect the authors' wise and gentle mixture of critical theology, victim advocacy, and pastoral and liturgical advice. A rich resource for every congregation encountering tragedies, in other words: for every congregation, period.'

Professor R. Ruard Ganzevoort, Professor of Practical Theology, Free University, Amsterdam

Tragedies and Christian Congregations

When tragedy strikes a community, it is often unexpected with long-lasting effects on the people left in its wake. Too often, adequate systems are not in place to aid those affected in processing what has happened. This study uniquely combines practical theology, pastoral insight and scientific data to demonstrate how Christian congregations can be helped to be resilient in the face of sudden devastating events.

Beginning by identifying the characteristics of trauma in individuals and communities, this collection of essays from practitioners and academics locates sudden trauma-inducing tragedies as a problem in practical theology. A range of biblical and theological responses are presented, but contemporary scientific understanding is also included in order to challenge and stretch some of these traditional theological resources. The pastoral section of the book examines the ethics of response to tragedy, locating the role of the minister in relation to other helping agencies and exploring the all-too-topical issue of ministerial abuse.

Developing a nuanced rationale for good practical, pastoral, liturgical and theological responses to major traumas, this book will be of significant value to scholars of practical theology as well as practitioners counselling in and around church congregations.

Megan Warner is Postdoctoral Researcher to the Tragedies and Congregations Project at the University of Exeter and Visiting Fellow of King's College London's Department of Theology and Religious Studies. Her primary field of scholarship is Biblical Studies, specialising in Old Testament/Hebrew Bible. Megan is a Licensed Lay Minister and a member of the General Synod of the Church England. She is the author of SPCK's 2016 Lent Book, *Abraham: A Journey through Lent* and *Re-Imagining Abraham: A Re-Assessment of the Influence of Deuteronomism in Genesis* (Brill, 2018).

Christopher Southgate is Professor of Christian Theodicy at the University of Exeter and Director of the Tragedy and Congregations project. In the past he has been a biochemist, a bookseller, a house-husband and a lay chaplain in university and mental health settings. He trained ordinands for the South West Ministry Training Course for 16 years, serving as Principal from 2013 to 2017. His theological monographs include *Theology in a Suffering World: Glory and Longing* (Cambridge University Press) and *The Groaning of Creation* (Westminster John Knox Press). He is also the author of eight collections of poetry.

Carla A. Grosch-Miller has spent more than 20 years in parish ministry in the United States and the United Kingdom and 15 years as a staff or short-course theological educator in diverse ministerial training institutions including the South West Ministry Training Course, the Southern Theological Education and Training Scheme and the Cambridge Theological Federation. As Senior Minister of a Chicago area United Church of Christ between 1996 and 2003, she led the church through responses to the Columbine High School shooting, the 9/11 terrorist attack and the disappearance of a teenaged member, as well as less extraordinary church family crises. She is the author of *Psalms Redux: Psalms and Prayers* (Canterbury, 2015).

Hilary Ison has been a parish priest, hospice chaplain, adviser for women in ministry and member of a bishop's senior staff team, a theological educator and, latterly, a member of the team of Selection Secretaries overseeing the national selection panels for those offering for ordained ministry in the Church of England. Her recent training is in Systems Constellations, a method of exploring traumatic events and difficult personal and organisational issues in individual or group settings. Her freelance work has included individual supervision, facilitation of reflective practice groups and practical theology research projects as an associate member of the Oxford Centre for Ecclesiology and Practical Theology, Ripon College, Cuddesdon.

Explorations in Practical, Pastoral and Empirical Theology
Series Editors: Leslie J. Francis, Jeff Astley, Martyn Percy and Nicola Slee

Theological reflection on the church's practice is now recognised as a significant element in theological studies in the academy and seminary. Routledge's series in practical, pastoral and empirical theology seeks to foster this resurgence of interest and encourage new developments in practical and applied aspects of theology worldwide. This timely series draws together a wide range of disciplinary approaches and empirical studies to embrace contemporary developments including the expansion of research in empirical theology, psychological theology, ministry studies, public theology, Christian education and faith development; key issues of contemporary society such as health, ethics and the environment; and more traditional areas of concern such as pastoral care and counselling.

Reimagining Theologies of Marriage in Contexts of Domestic Violence
When Salvation is Survival
Rachel Starr

Women Choosing Silence
Relationality and Transformation in Spiritual Practice
Alison Woolley

Ecclesial Leadership as Friendship
Chloe Lynch

Poetry, Practical Theology, and Reflective Practice
Mark Pryce

Tragedies and Christian Congregations
The Practical Theology of Trauma
Megan Warner, Christopher Southgate, Carla A. Grosch-Miller and Hilary Ison

For more information and a full list of titles in the series, please visit: www.routledge.com/religion/series/APPETHEO

Tragedies and Christian Congregations

The Practical Theology of Trauma

Edited by Megan Warner, Christopher Southgate, Carla A. Grosch-Miller and Hilary Ison

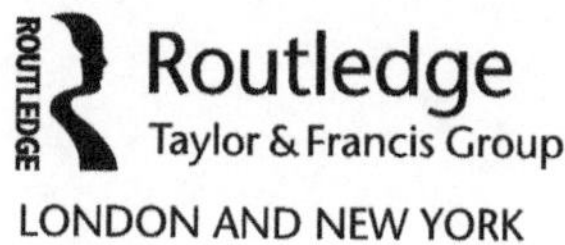

LONDON AND NEW YORK

First published 2020
by Routledge
2 Park Square, Milton Park, Abingdon, Oxon OX14 4RN

and by Routledge
605 Third Avenue, New York, NY 10017

First issued in paperback 2021

Routledge is an imprint of the Taylor & Francis Group, an informa business

Publisher's Note
The publisher has gone to great lengths to ensure the quality of this reprint but points out that some imperfections in the original copies may be apparent.

British Library Cataloguing-in-Publication Data
A catalogue record for this book is available from the British Library

Library of Congress Cataloging-in-Publication Data
A catalog record for this book has been requested

Typeset in Sabon
by Apex CoVantage, LLC

ISBN 13: 978-1-03-208862-4 (pbk)
ISBN 13: 978-1-138-48140-4 (hbk)

Contents

Figures

Foreword

James Jones

This is an extremely important book.

Tragedy and trauma are facts of life and death. 'Sufferance is the badge of all our tribe', Shakespeare said. To be human is to suffer and to know what it means to be broken-hearted. How we then live and relate to each other in such a world is the subject of this book. It goes well beyond wrestling about the inevitable theological and philosophical questions posed by suffering and serves almost as a primer for those who want to reflect on and learn from the tragedies and traumas in which we are invariably immersed and even baptized.

I chaired the Hillsborough Independent Panel which reported, first to the families, in 2012 in Liverpool's Anglican Cathedral. It led to fresh inquests and to the determination that the 96 Liverpool fans who had died in the Hillsborough Stadium in Sheffield on 15 April 1989 had been 'unlawfully killed'. The bereaved families have fought for three decades to establish the truth, accountability and justice. Throughout that period, they have experienced both tragedy and trauma in all the mental, emotional, physical and social dimensions.

I also chaired the Gosport Independent Panel in Hampshire which reported in 2018 and revealed that at the Gosport War Memorial Hospital, there was an institutionalised practice of shortening at least 456 lives by excessive prescribing and administering of opioids without clinical indication. The situation is currently subject to police assessment. Hundreds of families have experienced tragedy and trauma which continue to this day.

As I have read this book every chapter has spoken to me and resonated with me. In accepting the invitation to chair these panels I have responded consciously, believing that my calling as a Christian and as a deacon, priest and bishop has been to serve in the mission of healing the broken-hearted.

In his Nazareth manifesto, Jesus described his own mission in terms of releasing and healing those whose lives had been shattered and broken into pieces – traumatised. What I had not anticipated was how my own heart would be broken in the process literally physically, emotionally and spiritually, because in the middle of chairing the Hillsborough Panel I had a triple heart bypass, and at the end of the day when we reported to the Gosport families in Portsmouth Cathedral after we had delivered our report, I found myself unexpectedly shuddering with tears. I have always been reluctant to refer to this because the trauma absorbed by association compares not one jot with what the families have had to endure. But reading this book to write this Foreword also makes me want to confess the connection and acknowledge the contagion of human sorrow.

With both panels, I sensed the appropriateness of gathering the families in the local cathedral to hear, before anyone else, what the panels had found. Colleagues on both panels wanted a place where the families could learn what had happened to their relatives with dignity, a space where they could honour their love for those they had lost and somewhere where they could remember them with respect and cherish their memory. We also needed a building big enough to cater for all the needs of the families and to protect them from the media whom we housed in a separate place until the families were ready to meet them. On both occasions, although unspoken by me at the time, I felt that here in the House of God, with the presentation of our reports, Truth was calling out to Justice: Truth and Justice, two foundational pillars of the Kingdom of God, which deeply resonated with the aspirations of the Families.

Place, space, symbol and ritual are the stuff of religion. Each plays its part in response to tragedy and trauma as the chapters of this book reveal: the Church of St Clements in the Grenfell Tower tragedy, Southwark Cathedral in response to the Borough Market terrorist attack and Christchurch Cathedral in New Zealand in the aftermath of the massacre at the two mosques.

Symbols also have a role to play in the aftermath of tragedy. Flowers, candles, ribbons and slogans, such as 'Je suis Charlie', become a means of dealing with trauma as the liturgies examined in this book powerfully demonstrate. But they also have a powerful role pastorally. This came home to me personally after presenting the Hillsborough Report. Three episodes stand out.

The actual Report was taken by one survivor of the tragedy to his mother's grave. She, like other bereaved relatives, had been heart-broken and traumatised not just by the death of her son but by the falsehood that the fans themselves were the architects of their own deaths through hooliganism. 'Look, Mum, he was not a hooligan. The Panel found out the truth'. The Report assumed a sacramental nature in the cemetery.

The other two episodes relate to two women who have been leading figures in the Hillsborough campaign for truth and accountability. Margaret Aspinall, whose son James died at Hillsborough, is the chair of the Hillsborough Family Support Group; Anne Williams was the mother of Kevin, who also died, and founded Hope for Hillsborough and campaigned for fresh inquests which were denied three times.

I wanted to give each of them a personal gift to mark the conclusion of the Panel's work. On the mantlepiece of my study at Bishop's Lodge, I had a number of ornaments, of which one was a marble Pieta given to me some

20 years earlier by my mother and another was a cross of nails. By the time the Panel reported, Anne Williams had been diagnosed with terminal cancer. Before she died, I was asked to visit her.

As I stood in front of the ornaments, I knew deep within myself that I had to take the Pieta to Anne. The sight of Mary holding Jesus taken down from the Cross must have spoken to me of the bond between Anne and Kevin.

We talked together, and just before I offered to say a prayer, I presented her with the Pieta. As I placed it into her hands she said, 'How did you know?' 'How did I know what?' I replied. 'How did you know that the last gift that Kevin gave me before he died was a miniature Pieta?' The Pieta, I gather, now sits on the mantlepiece in her daughter's home, a symbol of the bond between Anne and Kevin and of the faith that gave Anne 'a sure and certain hope of the resurrection to eternal life', for both her and Kevin.

To Margaret Aspinall, I gave the cross of nails. It was not until seven years later that I discovered that Margaret takes the cross with her everywhere. On the day the jury returned in April 2019, the families that were waiting in Liverpool to hear the verdict relayed from the court in Preston passed the cross to each other. To them it was a symbol of the Truth and Justice to which they had given three decades of their lives. What is significant to me is that the context for each of these two religious symbols was not the church but the wider world of the Kingdom beyond the ecclesial walls.

During the course of chairing the Gosport Independent Panel, I met quarterly with the families. For more than 20 years, they had questioned how their loved ones had been treated at the Gosport War Memorial Hospital. The Panel's report, published on 20 June 2018 and presented to them first, revealed how there had been an 'institutionalised shortening' of hundreds of lives through the prescription and administration of excessive doses of diamorphine without clinical indication. In addition to chairing the regular Family Liaison Meetings, I would also stand at the door to welcome relatives and at the end to say farewell. Towards the end of our work and as I left the Family Liaison Meeting, I sensed rising within me all the emotions I used to feel as a vicar at the end of a service.

Here was a people being bound together by tragedy. What I became aware of in these encounters is that tragedy and trauma were binding these individual families into a community. Attendance was consistently high and the families found mutual support in their loss and continuing grief.

It felt to me like a church. Just as the first Christians were bound together by the trauma of the death of Christ so those bereaved through public tragedy find a common bond. And just as the memory of Christ has been sustained and handed down from generation to generation through annual remembrance of Holy Week, Good Friday and Easter Sunday, so those who are the bereaved and the survivors of major disasters keep alive the memory through anniversaries and memorials. These events nourish grief.

Observers and commentators of tragedy and trauma talk too loosely about closure. There can never be, nor should there ever be, closure to love.

Grief is a journey without destination, full of thoughts of what should have been and what might have been. Religious remembrance positively resists closure as it keeps alive the memory. The essential function of the service of Holy Communion, the Eucharist, is to remember, which is the antithesis of closure. Indeed, 'anamnesis' is a remembering that re-creates the past to relive it in the present so as to take it into the future and hand it down to the next generation.

From a Christian's point of view the journey of grief without destination is one that God himself has travelled. At the Cross and in the silence, God the Father was as bereft as Christ's own mother and his beloved friend. Jesus died a traumatic death in a trinity of grief and love of which there never should be closure.

When St Paul wrote about 'seeing through a glass darkly' to describe the limits of our understanding he used the word *enigma*, which is popularly translated as *darkly*. He was hinting at the truth that when it comes to comprehending the unfathomable we have only enigmas, stories, parables, allegories, similes and metaphors. So here is a story to show that far from being a distant spectator of our tragedies and traumas, God has passed this way too:

> There was an earthquake. A school was destroyed. Teachers and children were killed. A badly injured child was rescued from the rubble. Rushed to the hospital he was taken into the operating theatre. While his mother waited outside a surgeon spent hours trying to save his life. After 7 hours of painstaking surgery the child died. Instead of asking the nurse to tell the child's mother the surgeon took it upon himself. At first the mother would not believe it, then she cried hysterically, throwing herself at the surgeon and pummelling his chest in her angry grief. Instead of pushing her away he held her until she rested sobbing and cradled in his arms. At which point tears fell from his eyes onto her head as he too began to weep – he had come to the hospital when hearing that in that same earthquake he too had lost his own child.

I recall in the aftermath of the Zeebrugge disaster, in which 193 lost their lives as the *Herald of Free Enterprise* capsized, a seaman who'd escaped the disaster through a last-minute change to the rota, saying, 'God was on my side'. I could understand his feeling of good fortune but was left wondering where God was for those who drowned. It is a question that bereaved families have wrestled with ever since. A question that has added to the gravity of doubt and dragged them down deeper into despair. It is the question that turns agnostics into atheists. The truth explored in these pages lies somewhere in the thought that God was with them and by their side as they died.

W. H. Vanstone, in his book *Love's Endeavour, Love's Expense*, offers a meditation on the plight of the primary schoolchildren of Aberfan who were smothered to death by a collapsing slag heap from a disused coal mine.

Where was God that morning? Did he have his finger on the heap waiting until the children were unsafely inside before he let go and allowed the heap to sweep away their little lives? No. God was with the children, crying and dying.

Colin Parry, whose son Tim was murdered by the Irish Republican Army when they planted a bomb in the garrison town of Warrington, writes about being with him in the last moments of his son's life. Colin asks the nurse to remove all the tubes and to leave the room. He climbs on to the bed to lie side by side with Tim. The father holding his son, his child. It is a perfect picture of the bond between Creator and Creature in the valley of the shadow of death.

Jesus captured this thought in his saying, 'Are not two sparrows sold for a penny but not one of them falls to the ground without the Father'. Maybe he was speaking with insight into his own fate. But we don't always see or feel these positive images through the veil of our tears. In the trauma of our grief it may take years, if ever, before we have any sense of God sharing our distress. When it happens, it often takes us by surprise. If grief is a journey without destination very often the milestones appear out of nowhere and unexpectedly.

At the 30th anniversary of the Zeebrugge disaster in a service in the parish church of St Mary's Dover, they ceremonially brought in the ship's bell. The bereaved were invited to gather around it. For many who had lost loved ones, it became the token of their loss. Afterwards, I was with a mother and her two daughters. The one a widow and the others two fatherless daughters whose mother had never in the 30 years shed a tear. She tried to explain to me why seeing the ship's bell meant so much to her after all these years. She was struggling for words to explain her emotions.

I sought very tentatively to help her find the words to express her feelings about the ship's bell and suggested, 'Was it like this was the soul of the ship?'. I had hardly finished the sentence when she suddenly cried and tears flowed. She wept, cradled in the arms of her daughters. We returned to the church and to the soul of the ship. We prayed. It was the ship's bell that had become an unexpected milestone in the journey of grief without destination.

The Christian faith is rooted in the conviction that God himself is immersed and baptised in the experience of bereavement and grief. When Jesus contemplated his own destiny, he confessed to his soul being like a shipwreck. The prospect of the spiritual as well as the physical torment made him feel his soul was on the rocks. Even so he moved forward trusting that this was part of a greater purpose that would culminate in the salvation of the human family. He had a sense of timing about the events that led to his Crucifixion expressing with the phrases 'the time is not yet' or 'the time is fulfilled'. And even though these events were the responsibility of others, such as the betrayal by Judas or the trial by Pilate, nevertheless they fell under and into the sovereign purposes of God. It is difficult to hold these two concepts – human freedom and divine sovereignty – together. But the following picture, although not perfect, has helped me hold them in tension. I would go so far as to describe it as a parable of an evangelical theology of providence in the light of disaster, as explored in this book by Roger P. Abbott.

Imagine a master painter at work. The vision in his mind transfers through brush and paint onto the canvas. Not only is he a painter; he is also a grandfather and surrounding his easel are lots of adorable but mischievous grandchildren each with their own designs on the canvas. While he is at work the children are dabbing their fingers in the palette of paints and daubing the canvas. Yet so patient a grandfather and so brilliant an artist, instead of shooing the grandchildren away, he painstakingly incorporates all their smudging into the image that he is creating so that, in the end, their actions freely chosen add depth and texture of the vision.

Therefore, even the betrayal by Judas and the sentence of death by Pilate which were actions freely chosen were woven into the greater tapestry.

Yet, of course, we are still left with many imponderables.

When during the course of Chairing the Hillsborough Independent Panel, I was diagnosed as needing a triple heart bypass. I asked the doctor if I would be able to complete my work on the Panel. I recall recuperating after the operation and praying that God would speed my recovery so that I could complete the work. But it was not lost on me that here I was praying for healing to the very God to whom the 96 and their families had appealed. Why should he help me and have been apparently indifferent to them? I have no answer to that. It is impenetrable.

Yet as I have reflected on the divine image in people of different abilities (inadequately described as disabled) I have wondered if it is too fanciful to believe in a God of different abilities.

Indeed, you could argue that the Trinity is an expression of different abilities exercised by the three different persons of the Trinity. And the Cross itself is a picture of both God the Father and God the Son limiting their own ability to express their power in and towards some greater purpose.

Those who are differently able ('disabled') wear and manifest the marks of the differently-able-God and reflect his image in the world. Those marks might even include wounds of rejection.

In my years as Bishop of Liverpool I was constantly learning from the black community whose history in the city went back hundreds of years, not least because, in 2004, we commemorated the bicentenary of the abolition of the slave trade. They helped me to identify the signs of racism and to see that the overturning of the tables in the Temple by Jesus was a statement not against commercialism but against racism. The Temple hierarchy had given over to the traders the sacred space reserved for non-Jewish peoples who wanted to come close to God. It was called the Court of the Gentiles.

Jesus emphasised the point by quoting from the Old Testament prophets of Jeremiah and Isaiah: 'My House shall be a House of Prayer for all races but you . . .'.

As I researched the history of slavery and its trade, I remember feeling physically sick by some of the evidence. If only such racism were historic. Tragically in my time in Liverpool, we witnessed the brutal murder of Anthony Walker, a promising young black student. There is a sense in which every racist crime makes the black community relive the trauma of the past – the rejection, the dehumanisation, the degradation. What I find so amazing, and I do not use the word lightly, is the way that black slaves not only embraced the Christian faith of their oppressors but musicalised it with the most soulful songs. It is as if out of their trauma they sang their Gospel songs back in the faces of their owners, showing them the true meaning of the faith that they were traducing by their oppression.

In the recent history of Liverpool, the black community ministered to the city in a remarkable way. The black and white Gospel choir under the leadership of Tani Omideyi led the worship each year at the Hillsborough Memorial Service at Anfield stadium. The event fell into two parts. The first part involved singing, prayers and the lighting of 96 candles in remembrance. The second part became something of a rally as speakers called for truth, accountability and justice.

At the 20th anniversary after the act of remembrance, a Government minister spoke and was interrupted by a lone voice in the stand shouting, 'Justice for the 96'. In that moment, the whole stadium of more than 30,000 people rose and chanted, 'Justice for the 96'. If you had rehearsed the members of the crowd, they could not have chanted in greater unison and harmony. It was electrifying. It was a religious experience binding together thousands of people in a just cause for the truth in solidarity with their loved ones for whom two decades on they continued to grieve. Flowing from this protest the Government minister, Andy Burnham, persuaded the Prime Minister to set up the Hillsborough Independent Panel which I was then asked to chair.

Every day for the three months before publishing the report of the Hillsborough Independent Panel, I had read Jesus's parable of the widow and the unjust judge. It felt to me as if it could have been written for the Hillsborough families:

> Then Jesus told them a parable about their need to pray always and not to lose heart. He said 'In a certain city there was a judge who neither feared God nor had respect for people. In that city there was a widow who kept coming to him and saying 'Grant me justice against my opponents'. For a while he refused but later he said to himself, 'Though I have no fear of God and no respect for anybody, yet because the widow kept bothering me, I will grant her justice so that she may not wear me out by constantly coming.'
>
> And the Lord said 'Listen to what the unjust judge says and will not God grant justice to his chosen ones who cry to him day and night. Will he delay long in helping them. I tell you, he will quickly grant justice to them and yet when the Son of Man comes will he find faith on earth.'
>
> (Luke 18: 1–8)

I used to think that this parable was just about prayer. In the Hillsborough context, it came through to me as also a parable about justice – justice delayed and denied and justice (eventually) granted. It made me search for a definition of justice. I found it in the Institutes of Lactantius: 'The whole point of justice consists precisely in providing for others through humanity what we provide for our own family out of affection'.

I was later asked to give the address at the 27th and last commemoration of the Hillsborough disaster at Anfield. I told the crowd of some 20,000 that I had read that parable every day for three months before the Report. I said how the widow had pleaded for Justice but that the Judge couldn't give a damn about her, the people or God. Then, when I added emphatically, 'But she wouldn't give up', the crowd applauded and stood. On the train home that night, I could not help thinking that 2000 years on, people were cheering one of Jesus's parables. Perhaps we do not live in such a post-Christian society after all. If only people of faith would connect more with the issues of tragedy and trauma in which ordinary people are immersed then there would be a broader bridge between the Church and the world over which we could travel. This book broadens that bridge. I wish I had been able to read it at the outset of my ministry.

The Right Reverend James Jones KBE
Easter 2019

Contributors

Roger P. Abbott is Senior Research Associate in 'Natural' Disasters at the Faraday Institute, University of Cambridge (although he is persuaded there are no disasters that are actually natural, just human). Following over thirty years of pastoral experience, Roger gained his PhD in a practical theology of disaster response, from the University of Wales, Trinity & St. David. He has taught in the field of pastoral response to trauma, has run a consultancy on pastoral care of trauma and has been an active responder to traumatic incidents in the United Kingdom since 1989. He is a member of the British and Irish Association for Practical Theologians and of the Society for the Study of Theology. He is the author of *Sit on our Hands, or Stand on our Feet?* (2013).

Deanne Gardner is a qualified psychotherapist with a specialisation in Humanistic Person-Centred Psychotherapy. She works creatively with adult survivors of incest and sexual abuse, offering long-term therapy. Her work is based around dealing with trauma and the myriad issues linked to abuse and has included working with clients within the prison system, counselling young people in a secondary school setting and working with issues based around multicultural experiences. She is currently undertaking doctoral studies exploring the experience of clergy spouses in the New Testament Church of God.

Elaine Graham is Grosvenor Research Professor of Practical Theology at the University of Chester, a position she has held since 2009. In March 2014, she was installed as Canon Theologian at Chester Cathedral. She is the author of several major books, including *Transforming Practice* (1996), *Representations of the Post-Human* (2002) and *Words Made Flesh* (2009); with Heather Walton and Frances Ward, *Theological Reflection: Methods* (2005; 2nd edition, 2019); and with Zoe Bennett, Stephen Pattison and Heather Walton, *Invitation to Research in Practical Theology* (Routledge, 2018). Her most recent work considers public theology as a form of Christian apologetics: *Between a Rock and a Hard Place: Public Theology in a Post-Secular Age* (2013) and *Apologetics without Apology: speaking of God in a world troubled by religion* (2017).

Carla A. Grosch-Miller has spent more than 20 years in parish ministry in the United States and the United Kingdom and 15 years as a staff or short-course theological educator in diverse ministerial training institutions, including the South West Ministry Training Course, the Southern Theological Education and Training Scheme and the Cambridge Theological Federation. As Senior Minister of a Chicago area United Church of Christ between 1996 and 2003, she led the church through responses to the Columbine High School shooting, the 9/11 terrorist attack and the disappearance of a teenaged member, as well as less extraordinary church family crises. She is the author of *Psalms Redux: Psalms and Prayers* (2015).

Mia Kyte Hilborn is Head of Spiritual Healthcare, Hospitaller and Chaplaincy Team Leader at Guy's and St Thomas' NHS Foundation Trust. She is also senior Brigade chaplain for the London Fire Brigade and trustee and chaplain for the Firefighters Memorial Trust. Mia has extensive experience in the field of trauma and is coordinator of a Foundational Chaplaincy Course for Chaplaincy Volunteers, Postgraduate Students and Fire, Trauma & Disaster Chaplaincy, sponsored by the NHS Foundation Trust. Mia is co-author of 'Do Oncology Outpatients Need Chaplaincy Services?' in *Health and Social Care Chaplaincy*.

Hilary Ison has been a parish priest, hospice chaplain, adviser for women in ministry and member of a bishop's senior staff team, a theological educator, and, latterly, a member of the team of Selection Secretaries overseeing the national selection panels for those offering for ordained ministry in the Church of England. Her recent training is in systems constellations, a method of exploring traumatic events and difficult personal and organisational issues in individual or group settings. Her freelance work has included individual supervision, facilitation of reflective practice groups and practical theology research projects as an associate member of the Oxford Centre for Ecclesiology and Practical Theology, Ripon College, Cuddesdon.

Ruth Layzell is Director of the Institute of Pastoral Counselling and Supervision (IPCS) and of the Sherwood Psychotherapy Training Institute and has a passion for making links between theology and psychology. She has held posts in social work (including working in adoption and fostering) and teaching (she was Lecturer in Pastoral Care and Counselling and then Director of Counselling at St John's College, Nottingham). Alongside her work as a counselling and pastoral supervision trainer with IPCS, she is a British Association of Counselling and Psychotherapy accredited counsellor in independent practice. Ruth is co-author with Sara Savage and Fraser Watts of *The Beta Course*.

Karen O'Donnell is Coordinator of the Centre for Contemporary Christianity at Sarum College. She describes herself as a feminist, ecumenical, practical theologian whose interdisciplinary research interests span theology, spirituality and pedagogy. Karen is the editor of Interdisciplinary Press's 2016 volume *Ruptured Voices: Trauma and Recovery*. Her publications include the monographs *Broken Bodies: The Eucharist, Mary, and the Body in Trauma Theology* (2018) and *Digital Theology: Constructing Theology for a Digital Age* (forthcoming 2019).

Christopher Southgate is Professor of Christian Theodicy at the University of Exeter and Director of the Tragedy and Congregations project. In the past he has been a biochemist, a bookseller, a house-husband and a lay chaplain in university and mental health settings. He trained ordinands for the South West Ministry Training Course for 16 years, serving as Principal from 2013 to 2017. His theological monographs include *Theology in a Suffering World: Glory and Longing* (2018) and *The Groaning of Creation* (2008). He is also the author of eight collections of poetry.

Megan Warner is Postdoctoral Researcher to the Tragedies and Congregations project at the University of Exeter and Visiting Fellow of King's College London's Department of Theology and Religious Studies. Her primary field of scholarship is Biblical Studies, specialising in Old Testament/Hebrew Bible. Megan is a Licensed Lay Minister and a member of the General Synod of the Church England. She is the author of SPCK's 2016 Lent Book *Abraham: A Journey through Lent* and *Re-Imagining Abraham: A Re-Assessment of the Influence of Deuteronomism in Genesis* (2018).

Kate Wiebe is an organization consultant specializing in education, coaching, and therapeutic services following crises, trauma or disaster. Founder and Director of the Institute for Collective Trauma and Growth, she includes among her practical experience pastoral care and counselling, relational psychotherapy, marriage counselling, group critical incident debriefings and serving as a volunteer National Responder for Presbyterian Disaster Assistance. She has studied relational psychoanalysis, group and organizational dynamics and community care after disasters for 20 years.

Introduction

Megan Warner, Christopher Southgate, Carla A. Grosch-Miller and Hilary Ison

Bad things happen – things that knock the wind out of us, that bring us to our knees, that shatter the world as we knew it. They can come from the unruly earth, with its wild weather, tilting tectonic plates and surging seas. Or they can come from the deeds or misdeeds of other human beings, from malevolence, greed, ignorance or negligence. Sometimes, as in the case of climate change, they come from both.

Theology has long grappled with the question of why bad things happen. If God is good and all powerful, why does God allow this? Reams have been written wrestling with the questions of theodicy, and, later on in this book, more ink will be spilled on the topic. But this book begins not with the theory of bad things happening but with an examination of the experience of bad things happening. What happens when a person is traumatised? What light may the experience of trauma shed on theology?

The relatively new field of traumatology took off when researchers began to focus, first, on the experience of returning veterans of war and, second, on the experiences of victims of sexual abuse.[1] The focus on actual lived experience – enhanced by developments in neuroscience, developmental psychopathology and interpersonal neurobiology – has led to greater understanding and more effective treatment. It is now clear that trauma is not in an external event. Rather, it is a specific and automatic collection of physiological responses to an event, which are triggered when an individual's or community's adaptive capacity is overwhelmed. In individuals, neurological responses of flight, fight or freeze (immobilisation) are triggered in a whole-body response that aims to preserve human life in the face of threat. In communities, systems may become more dysfunctional and conflictual. One of the powerful effects of trauma, in individuals and communities, is that connections are broken and assumptions about how the world is supposed to be are shattered. For Christians, this can include assumptions about who and how God is in the world. One of the tasks in trauma recovery (or

1 Bessel van der Kolk, *The Body Keeps the Score: Mind, Brain and Body in the Transformation of Trauma* (London: Penguin, 2014).

remaking) is to piece together from the shattered fragments a coherent view of God and the world.

This was brought home to the project team in the most vivid way when, in the summer of 2017, a series of high-profile tragedies struck the United Kingdom. A terrorist bombing in the Manchester Arena, targeting a concert attended by young teenage girls, was followed in swift succession by terrorist attacks on the Westminster and London Bridges and Borough Market, an attack on the London Tube system and an unimaginably horrific fire in London's Grenfell Tower.

The interest of the editors of this volume was focused on the profound impact that these disasters had on nearby churches. In some cases, churches lost congregation members and found themselves mourning the loss of their own, as well as supporting survivors of the disasters and family and friends of those killed. In other cases, even though churches had relatively few direct links with survivors and the bereaved, they nevertheless found their day-to-day activities being completely overturned and overwhelmed as a result of proximity to the disaster, becoming gathering places for survivors and mourners, as well as collection and dissemination points for donations and information.

For most people, this impact on nearby churches came as a surprise that challenged previous assumptions about churches – what they were about and what they could offer their communities. This was true both for the churches themselves and outsiders. For the churches, the disasters brought mixed blessings. On one hand, congregations reported experiencing increased senses of well-being and value as members pitched in and helped out in ways that made significant contributions to their local communities and even to the nation as a whole. On the other, a number of congregations reported feelings of absolute overwhelm and urgent and desperate desire to be allowed to return to 'business as usual'. For those outside the churches, the roles taken by clergy and congregations sometimes came as complete revelations. Churches were revealed to be organisations deeply rooted in their communities, often with strong ties to synagogues, mosques and other places of worship, bringing with them armies of swiftly mobilisable volunteers and accessible gathering places with facilities for the production of meals and endless cups of tea and coffee. In the case of the Grenfell Tower fire, again, the differences between what local churches and local government were able to offer the community were placed in sharp relief, as anger with local authorities grew, while the churches became places of refuge and neutrality for conversation between angry locals and besieged council representatives.

While these were the kinds of roles played by local churches, larger churches and cathedrals made their own distinctive contributions. The 'National Memorial Service' held at St Paul's Cathedral six months after the Grenfell Tower fire, for example, played a vital role in recovery for the nation as a whole as well as locally. The same is true of the 'Services of Hope' conducted at Southwark Cathedral following the London Bridge attack. We also saw an increasing profile of 'reclaiming liturgies' conducted by clergy in public areas impacted by disaster, such as those held in the Maltings, Salisbury, following the March 2018 nerve agent attack, and on London Bridge and around Borough Market following the attacks there. These observances of blessing and 'reclaiming' seemed to speak to local people who might not ordinarily attend a church but for whom a ritualised response to the shattering of the peacefulness and order of their places of business and leisure contributed to healing and a return to normality.

The lasting impact of these church responses on both individual congregations and churches in the United Kingdom as a whole may prove to be significant. Already some changes are apparent. For example, clergy are now, for the first time, being admitted inside disaster cordons as police begin to appreciate the gifts of pastoral care and local knowledge that ministers can bring to a trauma scenario. Similarly, while churches have for a long time been included in the disaster response plans of local authorities, they are now being placed at the very centre of such plans, and their participation is being sought at the beginning of planning, instead of being something of an afterthought as has often been the case in the past. Time will tell whether disaster response will, in an increasingly unpredictable and disaster-prone future, become a central focus of the role of churches in their communities and the nation or whether the expectations placed on churches may perhaps become too great for them to bear.

The Tragedy and Congregations project

The research project that gave rise to this volume started before the string of disasters that rocked the United Kingdom in the summer of 2017. The Tragedy and Congregations project was established under the leadership of Christopher Southgate in late 2016. It was funded by the Templeton World Charities Foundation, Inc., and based at the University of Exeter, where Southgate is Professor of Christian Theodicy. The Revd Hilary Ison and the Revd Canon Dr Carla A. Grosch-Miller are also foundation members of the project, having worked with Southgate several years before on the South West Ministry Training Course. Dr Megan Warner was appointed once the project had got underway, as its postdoctoral researcher. While this volume is at the centre of the project's output, the project team has also undertaken extended travel and teaching projects, visiting theological education institutions, dioceses and other regional church centres to teach between one- and five-day programmes, as well as interviewing ministers and lay members of congregations that have experienced trauma. The project maintains a website (www.tragedyandcongregations.org.uk) that offers information about the project and project team and includes helpful background information, news and links and an extensive bibliography.

The focus of the project has been on understanding the physiology of trauma response and applying that knowledge to the experience of Christian congregations in the United Kingdom, with the goal of resourcing ministers to lead their congregations through experiences of disaster and trauma response. Work of this type had been done in the United States in the wake of events such as the Columbine and Virginia Tech shootings and the Boston Marathon attack, but had not previously been undertaken in the United Kingdom. The team has benefitted particularly from the work of Kate Wiebe and her team at the Institute for Collective Trauma and Growth in California, and we are extremely grateful for her contribution to the project and for her essay in this volume. Even before the string of disasters in the summer of 2017, the team was persuaded that taking on this work, with its particular focus on the UK experience, would be important, but living through that period brought home to us in the most sobering way that this work was not only necessary but urgent.

The founding members of the project team were clear from the inception of the project that it should take as its focus not only major public disasters of this kind but also more prosaic, yet still traumatic, events that rock congregations from within – suicides, murders and other shock deaths, financial embezzlement, sexual and other forms of abuse, destruction of church property by fire or floods and the apparently lesser institutional traumas arising from the arrivals and departures of ministers, elders and other authority figures – that can give rise to trauma within congregations and that tend to fester and grow when not addressed and healed. This kind of trauma experience can be every bit as damaging as that occasioned by dramatic external events, and often even more so as the aftermath is complicated by questions of fault, blame and shattered identity that exacerbate the relational ruptures that are the inevitable product of trauma.

The team's best intentions notwithstanding, we have not managed, in this volume at least, to achieve our goal of finding a balance between showcasing the impact of major, external disasters *on* congregations and the effects of perhaps smaller, internal disasters *within* congregations. It will be apparent to readers that the bigger, public tragedies get more airtime in these pages and probably also in our teaching. We have been reflecting on why this might be. Possibly it is simply the case that major disasters are easier to spot – we know whom to contact in response to a major disaster, while equally traumatic, but localised, events go on under the radar in individual congregations, where they can be kept, largely, hidden from public view.

But it is possible, too, that there are other, slightly less satisfactory reasons for the imbalance. Does attraction of the team, and those we talked with, to the exploration of congregational responses to major public disasters reflect a residual 'hero complex' in Christians that wants to be able to proclaim to the world that the Christian churches, far from being irrelevant and impotent as is so often assumed, are able to offer to the secular world exactly what it needs at the moments of its greatest vulnerability? Might we perhaps see public disaster response as a kind of 'fresh expression' of church – a way of demonstrating our continuing relevance to the world and so building our brand? Perhaps we just want to be 'good Christians' who 'do stuff' for others.

Possibly, the truth is even less palatable than this. Perhaps focusing on what the church can do for others allows us to avoid facing fully some uncomfortable truths around the fact that members of Christian congregations are every bit as capable of generating traumatic events and situations as our non-churched sisters and brothers. A focus on the trauma of others may allow us to shy away from the thornier questions about who we are and how we relate as Christians, and how we understand God to be at work in a world in which disaster and suffering seem to be doled out far too often and without regard to any apparently meaningful or defensible plan.

Whatever the reasons, there are more stories told in this volume of large, public traumas, than of internal, congregational disasters. Amongst the public traumas, the series of attacks and the Grenfell Tower fire of 2017, and church responses to them, are prominent, and we are especially grateful to clergy and ministers who have graciously allowed us to have access to, and in many cases to publish, the liturgies they prepared in response to them. That does not mean that stories of intra-congregational traumas are missing from these pages, but it does mean that those that have been shared with us can tend to do heavy duty in the essays collected here. One story deserves special mention because it is highlighted in a number of these essays. In Chapter 2, Carla A. Grosch-Miller tells the story of a parish that experienced the suicide of the fourteen-year-old daughter of faithful and much-loved congregation members. The girl herself had been an involved member of the congregation all her life and, at the time of her death, sang in the church choir. This story resurfaces in subsequent essays in the volume not only because it is one of the stories of internal trauma collected by the project team, but also because it offers an unusually telling illustration of many of the themes of the book: the needs of immediate response and pastoral care; the sharp challenges that can be faced by liturgists in the wake of disaster (with little opportunity for reflection or polishing); the acute dilemmas around theology and identity that can be thrown up by particular disasters, both for ministers and congregations; and the challenges *and* opportunities that can be presented for post-traumatic remaking. We are immensely grateful to the team rector of the parish in which this disaster happened for sharing with us so much of the congregation's experience and his own.

This volume

The team has invited contributions to this volume from a wide range of scholars and practitioners in the field and is delighted that the contributors represent such a broad, and deep, range of specialisms and expertise. We are proud that the present volume is genuinely ecumenical in its outlook, representing the experiences of theologically conservative and liberal, established and non-conformist, majority and minority church traditions, and we are grateful to those who have shared their particular expertise in these matters from a wide range of perspectives.

This collection of essays is designed to be accessible, and of value, to both academic audiences and those working at the sharp end of disaster and trauma response in UK churches, chaplaincy and community settings. The essays collected here are based on a combination of the most recent research, both from the UK context and internationally, and the personal experiences of the participants. Readers will discern a variety of voices in these collected essays. Some are of a more academic nature, while others are more reflective of personal experience or simply speak in a manner that both ministers and those without formal theological training will find easily accessible and essentially practical in outlook. Such variety might be thought to be a limitation in a collection of essays, but it can just as easily be seen as a strength, and any reader sufficiently interested to pick up this book will be sure to find in it something that speaks particularly to their own concerns. Readers will find some limited degree of repetition of information across the chapters. Again, what might be considered a flaw is also, in fact, a strength, as a particular writer with a particular voice may be able to convey meaning to certain readers in a way that other writers are not. Together, these essays, in all their variety, present a rounded picture about what is desirable (and what is best avoided) in church responses to experiences of disaster, both within and without.

The book is organised into six sections, each of which opens with a brief introduction to the included essays and their relationship with one another.

Part I presents two essays that offer an introduction to theological reflection on the experience of trauma. Elaine Graham opens the volume with an exploration of a range of approaches to theological reflection. Carla A. Grosch-Miller's essay focuses on a single model of theological reflection in some detail. Her essay also introduces the story of the teenage suicide mentioned above, as a case study of an 'internal' congregational trauma that has been especially challenging and informative for the team and to which subsequent essays also refer.

In Part II, Kate Wiebe and Hilary Ison draw our attention to the physiological aspects of trauma experience. They present a wealth of recent trauma theory and explore the ways in which trauma is 'stored' in the body and how, as a result, we need to consider the body and its processes when thinking about the addressing and healing of trauma. Kate Wiebe, to whom we have already referred earlier, brings to her essay her extensive US experience and a deep engagement with trauma literature. Hilary Ison, like Grosch-Miller, presents a case study of an internal congregational trauma in her essay, in this case to illustrate how a single traumatic event may affect witnesses in different ways, and how the impact of previous, unresolved trauma may be 'held' in the body and may have unexpected consequences for the response of body and psyche to new traumatic events.

Part III includes five essays that approach the challenges that disasters throw up for theology from a variety of viewpoints. Megan Warner opens

Part III with an essay that considers the relationship between the Bible and traumatic experience and the theological, practical and pastoral implications of reading biblical text through the interpretive lens of trauma. Roger P. Abbott follows with an essay that presents an evangelical response to disasters and the challenges they pose for thinking about God's role in a violent and dangerous world. His essay focuses particularly on the theme of providence. Christopher Southgate picks up the baton from Abbott and continues to press difficult questions of theodicy, offering a systematic approach to responding to different categories of disaster experience, and drawing on reflections arising from the Holocaust. Southgate is responsible for the next essay as well, which picks up on the theme of 'story', already highlighted by Grosch-Miller and Warner. Southgate presents and contextualises earlier work focusing on the use of narrative approaches to working with congregations, bringing this body of work into conversation with the literature on the collective experience of trauma in Christian congregations. Deanne Gardner, bringing this section to a close, and building on both her academic expertise and personal experience, offers a window into the practical theology of black-led congregations in the United Kingdom, particularly with reference to disaster response.

The first essay in Part IV, which considers liturgical responses to trauma, is the work of the team as a whole, led on this occasion by Grosch-Miller, and is based on a series of interviews conducted by team members with ministers who have conducted liturgies in the wake of major traumas, including each of the disasters of the summer of 2017, mentioned earlier. It links closely with the liturgical materials collected in the Appendices to this volume. It is followed by an essay by Megan Warner that focuses on the oft-overlooked tradition of lament, with particular reference to the lament psalms of the Old Testament. Warner's essay considers not only lament as tradition but also explores practical considerations for working with lament psalms with individuals and communities that have experienced trauma. Finally, Karen O'Donnell addresses the gifts and the challenges – theological, practical and pastoral – of Eucharistic liturgies in contexts marked by trauma.

Part V, which focuses on specific pastoral issues and challenges, opens with two essays by Mia Kyte Hilborn. In the first, Hilborn explores the ethics of trauma response, and in the second, she offers an extended exploration of the particular challenges of pastoral response to trauma in chaplaincy contexts. This latter essay includes a discussion of pastoral trauma response with young children. Ruth Layzell's essay in Part V draws together many of the themes, especially pastoral themes, that are touched on in other essays, in the particular context of ministry with traumatised congregations. The final essay in this section is by Carla A. Grosch-Miller. From her research and experience of working with church hierarchies on the handling of ministerial sexual abuse, she addresses the distinctive features and challenges of responding to congregational trauma following sexual abuse.

The final section of the book, Part VI, contains an extended transcript of an interview with Sarah Horsman, conducted by Christopher Southgate. Horsman is Warden of Sheldon, a Devon retreat centre run by the Society of Mary and Martha. Sheldon has a particular vocation to support the health and well-being of clergy and ministers, and Southgate asks Horsman to share her experience and wisdom, accumulated both as a result of her medical background and many years work at Sheldon, on the subject of clergy self-care in the context of trauma.

Acknowledgements

This volume could not have come about without the dedicated work and generous support of many people. We wish to acknowledge the very generous financial backing of the Templeton World Charities Foundation, Inc. The views expressed here are those of the contributors, not the Foundation itself. We are grateful also to the University of Exeter's Department of Theology and Religion for being a 'home' for the project. The team extends its heartfelt thanks to each of the contributors of essays to this volume, some of whom delivered their promised contributions against backgrounds of intense personal difficulty and challenge.

Those who work in the field of trauma report with remarkable regularity that their personal lives, as well as their professional interests, come to bear the marks of trauma. The experiences of both team members and guest authors during the gestation period of this volume, regrettably, bear out this testimony, and the team considers it a tribute to all involved, and a mark of grace, that the volume exists in its current form.

We are additionally grateful to those who contributed to the volume behind the scenes, as interviewees, as consultants and as members of the project's advisory panel. In that regard, we would like to acknowledge, in particular, the contributions of Lynn Stoney and Professor Ruard Ganzevoort, who gave time as consultants to aspects of the project. We are indebted, also, to those who have given the necessary copyright permissions, allowing us to append the extensive collection of liturgical resources.

Two final words of thanks. First, to the Right Revd James Jones, KBE, former Bishop of Liverpool, who has written the fine Foreword to the volume. Probably no living senior church figure in the United Kingdom has worked more closely, or extensively, with the consequences of collective trauma for the church and society. Bishop Jones made his name in the field of trauma support as chair of the Hillsborough Independent Panel, and his services are now keenly sought after in the field of collective trauma. We are honoured that he has agreed to provide us with what we are calling a 'Foreword' to the volume but which is, in truth, a valuable contribution in its own right. Second, we wish to express our gratitude to the staff of Routledge who have been so supportive of this volume and who have helped us to hasten its publication. We hope that it will be a repository of knowledge and guidance that resources, richly, those who find themselves ministering in the face of trauma.

Shalom and Godspeed
The Project Team
Megan Warner, Christopher Southgate, Carla A. Grosch-Miller and Hilary Ison
London
Ash Wednesday, 6 March 2019

Part I

Trauma

The presenting issue

Introduction to Part I

Just as traumatologists have been able to refine their response to trauma by focusing on the lived experience of it, so too a focus on the lived experience of trauma aids theologians in their task of speaking of God. The theological discipline particularly well suited to working with human experience is Practical Theology, which also has had a resurgence and enrichment in recent decades. With expanding methods and understandings, Practical Theology provides tools for examining lived experience for the clues and glimmers it offers about the nature of God and human life and for discerning how Christians and Christian communities may best respond.

In the first chapter, practical theologian Elaine Graham turns a wide-angle lens to the question of how theological reflection on the experience of trauma has impacted upon understandings of God and the Christian vocation. One of the authors of *Theological Reflection: Methods*,[1] Graham considers the aim of theological reflection as nurturing practical wisdom for the church. Drawing on Shelly Rambo's groundbreaking work on the theology of trauma, she explores essays in *Post-Traumatic Public Theology* (2016)[2] and Alan Everett's reflection on the Grenfell Tower fire in London,[3] in order to ground a discussion of how different methods or modes of theological reflection on the experience of trauma may renew, expand or challenge theological and secular understandings. Constructive narrative theology is shown to fund the rereading and reclaiming of Scripture. Canonical narrative theology, drawing on the suffering of Jesus, resources healing for veterans and challenges a social narrative that has silenced the lived experience of war. Reflection on the experience of marginalised people emphasises the importance of right action over right belief. And the incarnational ministry

1 Elaine Graham, Heather Walton and Frances Ward, *Theological Reflection: Methods* (London: SCM, 2005).

2 Stephanie N. Arel and Shelly Rambo, eds., *Post-Traumatic Public Theology* (London: Palgrave Macmillan, 2016).

3 Alan Everett, *After the Fire: Finding Words for Grenfell* (London: Canterbury, 2018).

of local churches is held up to be where God takes place. In Graham's assessment, theology is in dialogue with science, art and communal and personal experience to enable the nurturing of faithful personal and communal discipleship and engagement with the wider world.

In Chapter 2, Carla A. Grosch-Miller fixes a narrower gaze on what happens when a traumatising experience shatters a particular and potentially foundational theological understanding. Working with a case study of how the suicide of a young teenager rocked a church and its priest, she explores the power of the stories on which we build our lives and the urgency of experience as a driver for reframing those stories. Grosch-Miller proposes a model of the pastoral cycle which takes seriously lived experience and embodiment in critical-liminal conversation with theological and other sources and which can chart the remaking of tradition. Like Graham, she finds Rambo's articulation of the 'middle' space (between Good Friday and Easter Sunday) – which holds both death and hope of God's overcoming of death through enduring love – a particularly fruitful concept.

1 After the fire, the voice of God

Speaking of God after tragedy and trauma

Elaine Graham

'How can we find the language to express our grief at the loss of so many people in unimaginably terrifying circumstances?'[1] So writes Alan Everett in the aftermath of the fire that engulfed Grenfell Tower in London in June 2017. His reflection on the trauma unleashed by those terrible events tries to find meaning out of what happened. One grain of consolation was the response of faith communities and the reserves of practical help and volunteers they were able to muster in the vital hours and days after the tragedy. But Everett is also struggling to make sense of what happened theologically: how to find the language to articulate the depths of human emotion; how to speak of God. Where was God in these events?

As Jeffrey Alexander argues,[2] injury and suffering are not just events that happen. Rather, trauma that is experienced by a community is a product of the cultural imagination insofar as events emerge from, and help shape, collective identities and actions. Responses to social suffering are certainly material, but they also involve cultural processes of meaning-making. How are narratives about suffering, its causes and effects, constructed and mediated? We must clearly address the practical and political implications of collective suffering and trauma, but also attend to their discursive and symbolic dimensions: questions of meaning, attribution, purpose and narrative. So theological engagement is also necessary in order to consider how understandings of the will of God, the suffering of Christ and the meaning of redemptive hope function within our cultural imaginations.

In this chapter, I want to bring some ideas about what it means to 'reflect theologically' together with some recent writings on tragedy and trauma. I argue that theological reflection has always been part of Christian tradition and has always emerged in response to three key practical tasks: the formation of Christian character, building and maintaining the community of faith and communicating the faith to the wider world.[3] I want to demonstrate

1 Alan Everett, *After the Fire: Finding Words for Grenfell* (London: Canterbury, 2018), 117.

2 Jeffrey C. Alexander, *Trauma: A Social Theory* (Cambridge: Polity Press, 2012).

3 See, further, Elaine Graham, Heather Walton and Frances Ward, *Theological Reflection: Methods* (2nd ed.; London: SCM, 2019), 11–12.

how these imperatives make use of different elements of the Christian tradition – notably Scripture, tradition, cultural information and experience, both individual and corporate – to generate ways of speaking that are capable of inspiring and nurturing a 'practical wisdom' for the Church.

Methodology in theological reflection

Theological reflection has been the term of reference for the practical end of the theological spectrum for more than 30 years. There is no single method in theology today, and a plurality of approaches is generally accepted and expected. Most theologians and ministers, however, understand that theological reflection deals with the connection between theological sources and the issues, experiences, trends and possibilities of contemporary life. In *Theological Reflection: Methods*,[4] together with my co-authors, Heather Walton and Frances Ward, I argued that theological reflection has always been about resolving practical dilemmas arising from everyday life. Different methods of theological reflection, then, are not abstract constructs imposed on experience but, rather, ways in which Christians have come to formulate their ideas and understandings of God in and through their particular contexts and concerns. Theological reflection 'enables people of faith to give an account of the values and traditions that underpin their choices and convictions and deepens their understanding'.[5]

We based our exploration of theological method on the assumption that practical theology is not simply a matter of examining practice through the lens of theology. Rather, it is a work of constructive theology which is not confined to the academy but is at the heart of a lifelong learning that characterizes faithful discipleship:

> At the heart of theological reflection . . . are questions about the relationship of theory and practice, and how to connect theological discourse about the nature of God to the exercise of faith. This is an endeavour shared by laity and clergy. Christian practice is not simply about the duties of congregational ministry but the entire life and witness of the Church. It is predominantly a critical interrogative enquiry into the process of relating the resources of faith to the issues of life. The exercise of theological reflection is thus one 'in which pastoral experience serves as a context for critical development of basic theological understanding'.[6]

Fundamentally, theological reflection arises from practical discipleship. It aims to articulate the nature of God in order that people might lead godly lives. In particular, it serves the following main purposes: facilitating Christian

4 Graham et al., *Theological Reflection*.
5 Graham et al., *Theological Reflection*, 6.
6 Graham et al., *Theological Reflection*, 6, citing Burck and Hunter, 1990, p. 867.

nurture, describing the normative ethos and contours of the faithful community and engaging in dialogue and apologetics with the wider world and those who hold different worldviews. These three tasks constitute theology as a form of 'practical wisdom' within which faithful discipleship is shaped. Christians have turned to the sources of their faith, such as Scripture, experience, church practice and cultural information, in order to articulate the normative horizons by which authentic living can be guided.[7]

In what follows I consider what this understanding of reflecting theologically on practice might mean for work that responds to tragic or traumatic events and, in particular, what can be learned about the key tasks of doing theology as a practical undertaking. I refer extensively to the collection of essays published in 2016 titled *Post-Traumatic Public Theology*,[8] which was, in part, inspired by responses to the bombing of participants and spectators at the Boston Marathon in 2013. As with Alan Everett's reflections on Grenfell Tower, the core problematic is this: how to speak of God in ways that can both make sense of the initial impact of tragic events and inform a continuing ministry of support and care.

Narrative: nurture, narrative and identity

It is not surprising that narrative features strongly in theological treatments of tragedy that explore means of effecting healing in the wake of suffering and trauma. Here, the emphasis is on a generic human capacity to tell and live by stories. It has clear connections to traditions of cultural anthropology which emphasize the 'storied' nature of culture. Through narrative we construct meaning, and the stories we live by are redolent of spiritual, religious and moral worlds.[9] Some may interact with the sacred narratives of the Bible. Those writing from therapeutic and spiritual direction contexts also demonstrate that narrative is a prime bearer of meaning and is fundamental to the formation of subjectivity. Narrative approaches also function within theological reflection as means of bringing to speech hitherto

7 In *Theological Reflection: Methods*, we set out seven different types or methods of theological reflection according to the differential emphasis placed on the key resources of scripture, reason, culture and experience. The selection consists of (1) 'Theology by Heart: The Living Human Document' (records of personal experience), (2) 'Speaking in Parables: Constructive Narrative Theology' (parabolic and other metaphoric narrative), (3) 'Telling God's Story: Canonical Narrative Theology' (the scriptural witness), (4) 'Writing the Body of Christ: Corporate Theological Reflection' (the credal and ritual expressions of the church's life), (5) 'Speaking of God in Public: Correlation' (the relation of theological thinking to culture and non-theological forms of discourse), (6) 'Theology in Action: Praxis' (performance-based knowledge such as liberation theology) and (7) 'Theology in the Vernacular: Contextual Theologies' (the particular form of the gospel's expression in any specific place and time).

8 Stephanie N. Arel and Shelly Rambo, eds., *Post-Traumatic Public Theology* (London: Palgrave MacMillan, 2016).

9 R. Ruard Ganzevoort, 'Scars and Stigmata: Trauma, Identity and Theology', *Practical Theology* (2008): 19–31.

marginalized voices. In that respect, we can see how the specific and concrete nature of lived experience as mediated through narrative serves to challenge the abstractions and absolutes of more generic forms of theorizing and representation.

Some of the essays in *Post-Traumatic Public Theology* address these issues. Drawing both on contemporary narratives and biblical literature, Shelly Rambo begins to construct a form of engagement with Scripture that can adequately address the complexity of trauma.[10] She uses Rebecca Chopp's work on poetics to propose a root-and-branch revision of doctrines of the Resurrection and our interpretations of the biblical narratives. Mindful of the insights gained from dialogue with trauma theory and therapeutic practices, she argues, when approached from different perspectives and viewed through new hermeneutical lenses, sacred texts can yield up hitherto hidden wisdom.

Thus, theologians can turn to the resources of Scripture and tradition in search of new perspectives. Focusing on the Johannine accounts of Jesus's post-resurrection appearances to the disciples (Jn 20:24–8), Rambo stresses the ambivalence and persistence of post-traumatic experience. As Christ shows his wounds to his disciples, he demonstrates the interconnection between suffering and hope, death and life. The disciples are vividly reminded of the realities of the Cross, and yet in the showing of wounds, they are bound together into a community that can testify to the possibility of wounded life. This is the 'middle' space between death and resurrection, where suffering and defeat cast a deep shadow and yet where life and hope for the future are not extinguished. Just as the Johannine account bears witness to a world in which life and death are intermingled, its legacy is to challenge the Church today to find language in which to speak about the enduring remainders of suffering in those who live on:

> [The disciples] are on lockdown in the aftermath of his death. It is unclear how long they have been there, but he appears in their midst, as if out of nowhere. He offers no explanation for the display of the wounds. Some say it was to confirm his identity, to prove he was the one he claimed to be. But the wounds bring back memories. They remind them of what they wanted to forget. The events in the Upper Room tell a story about wounds that surface, testifying to wounds that have never passed away'. Histories of suffering return in this space, both perilous and promissory. His body tells truths about the past, but it also signals a future. It speaks something more, not beyond history but across it. The past is alive, but they hold its difficult truths in

10 Shelly Rambo, 'Introduction', in *Post-Traumatic Public Theology*, 1–21. See also Shelly Rambo, *Spirit and Trauma* (Louisville, KY: WJK, 2010) and *Resurrecting Wounds: Living in the Aftermath of Trauma* (Waco, TX: Baylor University Press, 2017).

tension. He sends them out, with life-giving breath. Stepping out, a new collective life takes shape.[11]

In *Theological Reflection: Methods* we identified several approaches which emphasized the importance of narrative for Christian identity and discipleship. Rambo's disruptive reading of biblical literature corresponds with what we term 'constructive' narrative theology and, in particular, the growing interest within theological studies in the discipline of 'theopoetics'.[12] Using literary theory and especially readings informed by post-structuralism and deconstruction, Rambo reads against the grain of dominant interpretations, especially within canonical biblical texts that appear to justify passivity or resignation in the face of violence. Rambo's method highlights the extent to which engagement with sacred texts opens ambiguity and tensions in both human and divine accounts that cannot be easily resolved through narrative closure. This opens new possibilities for re-reading and reclaiming Scripture.

Rambo uses the metaphor of 'haunting' to convey the sense of an experience that lives on in the margins of consciousness and public discourse – that which is 'present but not visible' – beckoning to dimensions of reality that are otherwise difficult to account for.[13] Her reading of the post-resurrection appearances of the risen Christ to the disciples in the Gospel of John talks about abiding and haunting: an imperative to live on in the shadow of trauma, empowered by the enigmatic and haunting presence of Jesus in the form of the Spirit. 'What is handed over is the haunted [we might also say haunt*ing*] figure of love, seeking readers, seeking followers, seeking a name, seeking forms of life that are not necessarily triumphant but nonetheless sustaining.'[14] This represents an invocational presence.

Rambo's reading of tradition also seeks theological alternatives to atonement theories that emphasize the substitutionary sacrifice of Christ and in the process glorify redemptive suffering, and to Resurrection theologies which stress the victory of Easter Day over Good Friday without adequately resting in the reality of Holy Saturday.[15] The 'open wound'[16] and 'remainders' of trauma in the shape of physical, psychological and psychosomatic ailments represent the reality of lived experience for most people and the 'precarious middle' must be protected as the place from which theological work must begin.[17]

11 Rambo, *Resurrecting Wounds*, 71.

12 See, for example, L. Callid Keefe-Perry, *Way to Water: A Theopoetics Primer* (Eugene, OR: Cascade, 2014).

13 Shelly Rambo, 'Haunted (by the) Gospel: Theology, Trauma and Literary Theory in the Twenty-first Century', *PMLA* 125, no. 4 (2010): 936–941, 939.

14 Rambo, 'Haunted', 940.

15 Rambo, *Spirit and Trauma*, 137.

16 Rambo, *Spirit and Trauma*, 6.

17 Rambo, *Spirit and Trauma*, 126.

Narrative: canonical narrative theology

An alternative way of engaging with Scripture in theological reflection is termed 'canonical' narrative theology. This is rooted in the belief that the life and death of Christ normatively grounds Christian identity and formation. Scripture shapes patterns of discipleship. 'The Story' of God is definitive in determining 'our stories' of individual and corporate discipleship.

In considering recovery from the traumas of active military service, Willie James Jennings draws close analogies between the stories of veterans of armed combat and the sacrificial sufferings of Christ.[18] What does it mean to remember, especially if national or public memorial is out of step with individuals' complex emotions and memories? Abstract ideals such as democracy, sacrifice or freedom serve as templates for dominant discourses but rarely reflect lived experience. This leads to massive contradictions between public and private. 'In this regard, veterans are often invited into a kind of remembering that renders them lifeless monuments who should be seen but never heard, even when they speak.'[19] Those who fight in and survive armed conflict have to come to terms with their own complicity in violence and the guilt of their survival. This complicates the binaries of hero/villain, guilt/innocence and good/evil. The theological task here, then, is to unmask the dominant cultural ideologies that fall far short of the profundity of sacrificial suffering for which only the death and Resurrection of Christ provide the definitive narrative.

For Jennings, the interaction between God's word and human story serves as a powerful hermeneutical event. One strategy is to learn from Karl Barth's theological method in the face of Nazism.[20] The authority of the Nazi state in the 1930s was regarded as absolute; Barth's response was to deny its legitimacy – not least the discursive narrative of the God-given destiny of the German people – by positing an alternative, divine power. Barth's description of Christian identity is rooted in the foundational stories of the Bible; only the revelation of the Word of God through Scripture can expose the hubristic nature of human discourse and its tendency to fuel dangerous idolatries.

This revelation rests in the person and work of Jesus, the innocent who has been put to death but who offers forgiveness and reconciliation from a body marked by suffering and violence. 'In Jesus, we learn that God remembers . . . God remembers what others have forgotten.'[21] Jesus heals our wounded humanity by inviting us 'into the compassion that constitutes

18 Willie James Jennings, 'War Bodies: Remembering Bodies in a Time of War', in *Post-Traumatic Public Theology*, 23–35.

19 Jennings, 'War Bodies', 26.

20 See Karl Barth, *The Word of God and the Word of Man*, trans. D. Horton (Boston, MA: Pilgrim, 1929); David F. Ford, *Barth and God's Story: Biblical Narrative and the Theological Method of Karl Barth in the Church* (Frankfurt: Peter Lang, 1981).

21 Jennings, 'War Bodies', 31–32.

God's knowing and remembering'[22] – his Resurrection is an abiding presence, an ever-present memory. The believer's encounter with the wounded body of the risen Christ, rather than being a site of repetitious trauma, becomes an occasion of grace:

> Pastoral intervention that intends to address moral injury needs a theological vision that draws veterans into God's own memory work. For Christians, we serve a God who remembers and invites us to enter the divine reality of remembering in ways that remind us not only of who we are but also who God has been for us and will be for us.[23]

There is a question here between constructive and canonical approaches about whether narrative reveals or constructs meaning, but nevertheless, the significance of narrative in relation to the theological task of shaping identity rests on the power of stories not just to convey meaning but also as ways of engaging with the sources and resources of sacred texts and eliciting new and potentially liberatory meanings, as well as being a crucial medium through which identity – personal and corporate – is articulated *in imitatio Christi*.

Writing the body of Christ

Theological reflection that attends to the formation of the community of faith describes this process as a corporate activity that often uses metaphor and ritual to construct a sense of shared identity. Faithful theological thought is an activity of the community, not the isolated individual. Paul's letter to the church in Corinth provides a clear biblical example of corporate theological reflection using the metaphor of the community as the body of Christ.

The notion of the Christian community as a body is therefore well established, but it may be helpful to revisit that idea in relation to a multiplicity of meanings: body or community in its material, physical and virtual manifestations. It is to the latter, and to the life-enhancing effects of the corporate ministry of an online version of church, that Deanna Thompson turns her attention. She writes of the support offered following her diagnosis of cancer, identifying such life-changing illness as a form of trauma and its long-term effects as a type of post-traumatic stress disorder.[24]

The fact that the apostle Paul conducted much of his ministry with the earliest churches via a virtual, epistolatory conversation reminds us of the dispersed nature of the Body of Christ and the potential of ties that

22 Jennings, 'War Bodies', 32.

23 Jennings, 'War Bodies', 26.

24 Deanna A. Thompson, 'The Virtual Body of Christ and the Embrace of those Traumatized by Cancer', in *Post-Traumatic Public Theology*, 155–172.

transcend physical proximity for talking meaningfully about Christian community. Digital technologies, such as social media, return us to a contemporary virtual version of the Church. Online communities become vital arenas for sharing and articulating experience and meaning-making, as well as giving and receiving moral support.

Writing about her own experience of the online network known as CaringBridge, Deanna Thompson remarks, 'What I'm talking about is a breathtakingly broad embodiment of Christ's hands and feet ministering to me and my family during our walk through the valley of the shadow of cancer.'[25] The 'virtual incarnation of Christ's body via digital technology' becomes not only the medium for support but also a space for theological reflection and practices of solidarity. The open-ended nature of this network has also enabled those persons to participate in forms of online Christian activity who would not have normally done so offline, something which, for Thompson, 'means reconsidering the parameters of the body of Christ [which] expands – even disrupts – conventional Christian notions of boundaries of the church universal'.[26]

Once more, this method begins and ends in practice. The practices of curating and participating in a virtual network of mutual aid reshape ecclesiology (new ways of thinking about, and being, church). In some respects, we may experience social media, new technologies and virtual cultures as disembodied, even alienating, and yet, paradoxically, as Thompson demonstrates, they also enable new understandings of what it means to be incorporated into the Body of Christ.

Liberating praxis and the life of the Church

An emphasis on the practical nature of theology is strongest in modes of reflection which maintain that the primary concern of theological reflection – specifically practical theological reflection – is right action (*orthopraxis*) over right belief (*orthodoxy*). From this perspective, no theological claim, no matter how philosophically acute, can reflect God's work in the world if it does not contribute to liberation and justice. 'The starting point of this method of theological reflection has . . . never been abstract speculation on timeless truths.'[27] Rather, theology begins with concrete experience and asks questions about transformative values that will help people resist oppression. This theological method is relevant in pastoral and clinical work with those who are marginalized because of gender, race, social class, sexual orientation, or disabilities.

25 Thompson, 'Virtual Body', 161.
26 Thompson, 'Virtual Body', 164.
27 Graham, Walton and Ward, *Theological Reflection*, 186.

Writing about racism as a cultural trauma, Dan Hauge reflects much of this sensibility.[28] First, this approach is premised on a commitment to view the world 'from the underside of history' and to privilege the voices and perspectives of those least advantaged. The most urgent task is thus to affirm the humanity of people of colour and other oppressed cultures in the face of dehumanizing socio-political-economic structures, narratives and representations. The theological task is one of restoring or asserting the irreducible stamp of the imago Dei. The aim of praxis-oriented practical theology is not to preach right belief but, in the words of Gustavo Gutiérrez, 'Modern theology tries to answer the challenge of the "non-believer"; but in contrast, liberation theology listens to the challenging questions of the "non-person".'[29]

The everyday trauma of racism cannot be framed either as the personal aberrations of malicious individuals or a historical set of policies now discredited. It is an everyday experience, embedded in social structures and institutions, manifested in small but insidious instances of 'microaggression' towards people of colour.[30] Specific acts or events may engender primary trauma, but these things exist within a wider context of discrimination, danger and abuse at the hands of others. A failure to apprehend this simply compounds the trauma.

Black theologies call for wholeness and liberation, whereas white theologies sanction a culture of oppression and racism, not least in the way they exclude others from their conceptual frameworks. As conceived within such a framework of privilege, white theologies are unable to speak of God's preferential option for the poor. As a result, oppressors can say nothing meaningful about the experience of the oppressed or God's liberation. Healing and reconciliation are impossible until the root causes of the problem – including and especially the hegemony of 'whiteness'[31] are addressed.

This amounts to a theology of liberation that simultaneously demands the emancipation of marginalized communities from structural and institutional discrimination and the liberation of oppressors from their own privilege and predominance. Similarly, Shelly Rambo issues a call to white Christians to acknowledge the wounds of racism; theology cannot speak so long as they are in denial:

> By placing black-lynched bodies as the object of gaze for the witnesses at the foot of the cross, [James] Cone insisted that Christian witness is intricately tied to the suffering of black peoples. In turn if the good news

28 Dan Hauge, 'The Trauma of Racism and the Distorted White Imagination', in *Post-Traumatic Public Theology*, 89–114.

29 Gustavo Gutiérrez, *The Power of the Poor in History* (Maryknoll, NY: Orbis, 1983), 57.

30 Dan Hauge, 'Trauma of Racism', 95.

31 Tom Beaudoin and Katherine Turpin, 'White Practical Theology', in *Opening the Field of Practical Theology*, eds. K.A. Cahalan and G.S. Mikoski (New York: Rowman & Littlefield, 2014), 251–69.

> of resurrection is to be proclaimed by Christians the witnesses positioned at the site of wounds returning must think in terms of the ongoingness of crosses. . . . Thus resurrection involves the return of the wounds that white America does not want to see. Wound-work then has to take place according to a different register, targeting the affections.[32]

This is not to claim false parallelism, however, since the prescription for change must come through authentic listening to the voice of the oppressed and by actions that release their agency, not through the goodwill of the oppressor.

For this mode of theological reflection, the task of *Christian formation and nurture* is one of empowerment and liberation and transforming those on the margins from objects of others' abuse into subjects in control of their own destiny. The task of *building up the community of faith* involves taking a stand for human dignity and reconciliation in solidarity with those of all faiths and none who are similarly called to resist inequality, oppression and violence.

Where God takes place: Church as incarnation and sacrament of the local

A further method of theological reflection for Graham, Walton and Ward focuses on the significance of local place and space. This method pays attention to the theologies that can be constructed from everyday language, the various ways in which people speak of and practise their beliefs, and popular culture. It stresses the incarnational nature of discipleship and church life and reminds us that all theologies are embedded in social, historical, geographical and political contexts. In this light, all theology is contextualized and local. Theological discourse, therefore, will be multiple and multi-voiced; it will be articulated 'in the vernacular'.

Here, for our best example, we return to Alan Everett's meditations on the role of the church in addressing the tragic events of Grenfell Tower. His is a strongly incarnational theology in which the oddities of the Church of England parish system, with its commitment to minister to an entire geographical community, provides the foundations for a strongly local and sustainable form of social capital. Faith communities offer advantages of localism, trust and place of refuge, symbolized by the open door.[33] This enables the ministry of enduring presence to be maintained long after the emergency vehicles and media cameras have left the scene. It speaks of God in creation, in human form and indwelling and inspiring human collectives:

> There is no place that is Godless. When we arrive in a new place, we find that God is there before us; it is God's place before it is ours . . .

32 Rambo, *Resurrecting Wounds*, 92.

33 Everett, *After the Fire*, 48.

> Second, Christ is among us, having in some way renewed and restored the image of God. . . . Third, the Holy Spirit offers us reassurance and comfort, while helping us to break free from the prisons in which we find ourselves: of narrowness, prejudice, judgementalism and rigidity. The Holy Spirit gives us the energy to change, the courage to reach out to others, and the wisdom to discern the way forward.[34]

This roots a theological response firmly in a sense of place and in the 'vernacular', or ordinariness, of quotidian existence and an affirmation of the essential sacredness of creation. God is not imported but revealed in any given local context. From the fundamental principle of the Incarnation, Everett reflects on themes of solidarity in suffering as exemplified in the Crucifixion and Resurrection of Jesus. It connects with the post-traumatic context of Grenfell, enabling an identification with the events of Good Friday and the violence it represented, as well as the hope of God's overcoming of death through enduring love. Like Shelly Rambo, however, Everett refuses both the narrative of substitutionary atonement and the easy victory of resurrection. Instead, the Cross can be used as an aid to take us to that 'middle' place:

> The cross creates a space where we can place our needs, our anxieties and our grief. It has the capacity to open up a deep, hidden place within us, a place that in the usual course of events we may find difficult to access. Entering into this hidden, sometimes dark space is potentially therapeutic, providing we can be certain that we are being safely held.[35]

Grenfell revealed how, in the aftermath of tragedy, the church was highly effective in translating its reserves of 'social capital' into bonds of solidarity and neighbourliness.[36] Strategies for mission as personal evangelism need, therefore, to be complemented by ministries of presence, service and prophecy in order for parish churches to remain 'hard-wired' into their communities:

> The Grenfell disaster has shown us that worshipping communities have a significant capacity to elicit trust, to build bridges, to assist in conversation and mediation, and to become safe spaces for healing and advocacy. However, in order to serve in a crisis, they need to be in a state of readiness, with a record of authentic prior commitment.[37]

34 Everett, *After the Fire*, 68.
35 Everett, *After the Fire*, 80–81.
36 See Robert Putnam, *Bowling Alone: The Collapse and Retrieval of American Community* (New York: Simon and Schuster, 2000).
37 Everett, *After the Fire*, 126.

Yet it is clear that Everett speaks out of an enduring tradition of theology and practice that is rooted in the Incarnation and the Eucharist, which sees the world as a constant and unfolding sign and sacrament of the presence of God in all things. 'The incarnation and the sacraments are part of a continuum, in which the physical world is part of a sacred network: apparent in water, oil, light, the sign of the cross and human touch.'[38]

Speaking of God in Public: Correlation

The method identified as 'Speaking of God in Public: Correlation' brings theological and religious perspectives into dialogue with scientific, artistic, and socio-economic perspectives in order to construct new religious and theological propositions.[39] Starting with the correlative method as a model for understanding how theological language influences and is influenced by the language of others' worldviews, this approach also describes the ways in which Christian thought and practice are mediated into in public contexts broader than explicitly Christian communities. Since major public tragedies are framed within the discourse of trauma, how then does this method of theological reflection manifest itself?

Traditionally, the correlative model regards itself not only as a theological commentary on public issues – a form of Christian social ethics – but a form of theological practice that emphasizes the need to conduct itself in public: open to the critical and constructive perspectives of worldviews beyond the purely ecclesial. This dialogical method is also apparent in some contributions to *Post-Traumatic Public Theology*, as its title suggests. It is important to gauge how theologies of trauma play out in the public realm when subject to this kind of scrutiny.

As Phillis Shepherd argues, to begin from theological categories in isolation is to be fatally self-referential and will have nothing to say to the world beyond the boundaries of its own discourse:

> Historically, theology has often taken its categories or doctrines as the lens from which reflection embarks. The efficacy and result of this theological reflection is in the service of rationality over experience and thinking about theology, rather than those who should be the epistemological basis of theological reflection. If our theology is not *of* those who live with trauma and, I might add, subject to their reflection, it is dangerous talk *about* theology, and its danger lies in its power in theological discourse and theological practices to produce trauma.[40]

38 Everett, *After the Fire*, 71.

39 Graham, Walton and Ward, *Theological Reflection*, 151–184.

40 Phillis Shepherd, quoted in 'Afterword', in *Post-Traumatic Public Theology*, 291–300, 292.

Conducting a dialogue between trauma studies, theology and jurisprudence in the context of examining practices of restorative justice, Stephanie Arel notes the tension between rehabilitation and punishment, especially in light of the deep challenge of listening to perpetrators' stories, which call forth many questions of complicity, guilt and forgiveness.[41]

She advocates the theological learning that can take place through listening to different parties, attending to conflicting narratives from different protagonists, processing physiological, cognitive and affective responses to stories of trauma or abuse and negotiating between different disciplinary frameworks – legal, psychological, theological, sociological – that inform different models of criminal justice. Theologically, 'we find ourselves moving back and forth between the ideas that shape and order our understanding of God and the world we inhabit and the raw data of life as it is lived. In the best case, each informs the other in a process of continual enrichment.'[42] Similarly, theology must be open to interdisciplinary scrutiny and make itself vulnerable to critique at points where it has colluded with or perpetuated cycles of violence or victimhood. This will also involve listening to many dimensions and levels of the experience, including the affective.

Another strategy of cross-disciplinary listening to the voices of the wider public domain is to consider how popular culture beyond that of the church understands the dynamics of trauma and tragedy. Bryan Stone adopts a correlative approach by interrogating reality TV as a site of meaning-making – a parallel cultural milieu to that of theology but potentially one that serves to construct and mediate notions of surrogate religion and sacred space.[43]

Reality TV often serves as a showcase for personal narratives of trauma, tragedy and pain for the sake of entertainment. It transforms the everyday and ordinary into objects of public spectacle. Trauma has become a major cultural trope, informing many genres of documentary and confessional talk shows as well as reality TV, 'permeated with narratives of victimization, survival, trauma, and recovery'.[44] This is positive insofar as it gives voice and visibility to those experiencing various kinds of injury, abuse, injustice or tragedy, but to what extent has it been manipulated and co-opted by the very media responsible for its coverage? Does reality TV in some ways become a surrogate religion as a site of confession, testimony and reparation?

Reality TV enables us to witness such experiences and identify with them, but its idealized and sensationalized format precludes any authentic engagement. In addition, such public scrutiny can induce longer-term effects on participants. In the interests of entertainment, the 'remainder' of trauma of which Shelly Rambo speaks is suppressed. Experiences of suffering are

41 Stephanie N. Arel, 'Examining Restorative Justice: Theology, Traumatic Narratives, and Affective Responsibility', in *Post-Traumatic Public Theology*, 173–191.

42 Everett, *After the Fire*, 105.

43 Bryan Stone, 'Trauma, Reality, and Eucharist', in *Post-Traumatic Public Theology*, 37–62.

44 Stone, 'Trauma, Reality, and Eucharist', 44.

removed from wider socio-economic contexts; complex moral questions of causation, blame and reconciliation are glossed; and lives and bodies in pain are effectively (re)victimized and commodified for public consumption. Narratives of redemption have been collapsed into forms of cheap grace by televised therapy-as-makeover.[45]

This 'testimony to the middle'[46] beyond the simplistic renditions of atonement or triumph offers resources for an alternative theological engagement with popular cultural representations of tragedy and trauma. Once again, an emphasis on the practices of faith rather than propositional belief play a major part in this method of theological reflection. The theology that emerges out of such reflection is less cognitive than performative, as practices build discursive and material worlds which enable a community to narrate and embody its reality differently. Rambo and Stone both suggest that rituals such as the Eucharist enable the church to inhabit the middle in ways that acknowledge the wounds of suffering, yet through participating in the life of the risen Christ, they express a corporate identity that embodies hope in solidarity and healing. In this respect, theology works on both sides of the Cross; as Shelly Rambo might say, the vocation of theology is one of working between 'the *as is* and the *otherwise*',[47] or the transfiguration and transformation of this world into the next. As a work of *anamnesis*, the very heart of the Eucharist is remembering – and re-membering. As the community shares the bread and wine, they invoke the advent of the Holy Spirit to make them one in Christ who lives on in the church's acts of justice, solidarity and transformation:

> Gathered around the table as a people who all possess our own scars and wounds, the Eucharist is a meal in which the real is both revealed and performed as we give witness to suffering without pretending that it is redemptive, on one hand, or that it can be neatly erased, on the other.[48]

Conclusion: the practical task of theological reflection

Theology is practical through and through. It begins with the immediate tasks of nurturing the believer, forming the community of faith and negotiating the boundaries between 'Church' and 'world'. Yet the aim is also to express, in deed and word, the means by which Christians, individually and collectively, can experience the grace, love and forgiveness of God – realities that are themselves mediated incarnationally through practices of faith. It is one of naming and challenging dominant discourses and representations and of facilitating counter-movements of compassion and change.

45 Stone, 'Trauma, Reality, and Eucharist', 48–49.
46 Rambo, *Spirit and Trauma*, 151.
47 Rambo, 'Introduction', 3.
48 Stone, 'Trauma, Reality, and Eucharist', 57.

All the theological reflections on trauma and tragedy I have considered have therapeutic, political, constructive and prophetic dimensions, but essentially they are all practical from beginning to end, 'deemphasizing beliefs as cognitive assertions and, instead, concentrating on the development of ways of being that are cultivated over time'.[49] The emphasis is on the practices of faith – textual, sacramental, pastoral and public – that enable living well and promoting healing and virtue. They concern questions of how to negotiate elements of tradition and practice as theological resources and how new practices of reading, telling, blessing and caring might embody a new way of speaking of God in the light of tragedy.

Select references

Arel, Stephanie N. and Shelly Rambo, eds. *Post-Traumatic Public Theology*. London: Palgrave MacMillan, 2016.

Everett, Alan. *After the Fire: Finding Words for Grenfell*. London: Canterbury, 2018.

Graham, Elaine, Heather Walton and Frances Ward. *Theological Reflection: Methods*, 2nd ed. London: SCM, 2019.

Rambo, Shelly. *Spirit and Trauma*. Louisville, KY: WJK, 2010.

Rambo, Shelly. *Resurrecting Wounds: Living in the Aftermath of Trauma*. Waco: Baylor University Press, 2017.

49 Rambo, 'Introduction', 13.

2 Practical theology and trauma

The urgency of experience, the power of story

Carla A. Grosch-Miller

In September 2015, the parents of a 14-year-old girl returned home from a church film night to find that she was not home. Her father and brother went looking for her in a place near a park and river where they knew she and her friends liked to gather. Her brother found her dead, hanging from an electricity pylon.

The family were active members of a broadly evangelical, thriving church in an affluent suburb of a large city. Facing into the horrific trauma, the minister and church did all the right things to attend to the needs of the family and the larger community. They cared for the family, gathered the community, made space for young people to grieve, provided lots of pastoral care, arranged work on suicide at the high school and hosted a big public funeral.

Three months later at the Coroner's Court hearing, a bombshell dropped: an examination of the girl's phone and search history had revealed the question, *Can I be gay and Christian?* She had been depressed and unable to believe that God loved her. Only her friends and fellow choir members knew she was gay. This teenage girl appeared to have killed herself because she did not think that being gay was acceptable to God or to her church.

The teenager's tragic death is not an isolated event. The Oasis Foundation published a report in 2017, titled *In the Name of Love: The Church, Exclusion and LGB Mental Health Issues*,[1] that highlights the negative impact on lesbian, gay and bisexual people of church teaching on homosexuality, which includes a significantly higher risk of suicide for young people.[2] This

1 Steve Chalke, Ian Sansbury and Gareth Streeter, *In the Name of Love: The Church, Exclusion and LGB Mental Health Issues* (London: The Oasis Foundation, 2017).

2 The report cites a survey of 7,000 lesbian, gay, bisexual and transgendered (LGBT) youth in the United Kingdom, of which 44% had thought about suicide as compared to 26% of the heterosexual, non-transgendered respondents. That young people who identify as homosexual or bisexual have a higher risk of suicide ideation, attempt and completion has been documented in a number of studies. A meta-analysis of American studies (Michael P. Marshal et al., 'Suicidality and Depression Disparities Between Sexual Minority and Heterosexual Youth: A Meta-Analytic Review', *Journal of Adolescent Health* 49 [2011]: 121) concluded: 'This study provides strong evidence that sexual minority youth experience significantly higher levels of suicidality and depression symptoms than heterosexual youth. The robust

phenomenon raises the questions: How does the church consider experience vis-à-vis Scripture and tradition as it seeks to make sense of such tragedies? What gets in the way? What may help?

Practical Theology is the discipline that takes human experience seriously in the search for a faithful, real-life response. After a discussion of how theology has apprehended experience, and in the light of the methodologies outlined by Elaine Graham in the previous chapter, this chapter proposes a method of theological reflection that seeks to describe the embodied experience of sense-making in the aftermath of trauma and to chart a way forward that enables human experience to influence the development of tradition.

Experience as a source for theology

The Church has long operated under the assumption that the truth of all things in God has been revealed once and for all and captured in the stories and symbols that make up the Christian faith. Theologian Edward Farley describes this as the 'house of authority' paradigm.[3] Scripture is considered the primary source of theology, supplemented by tradition and reason (which, in turn, interpret Scripture).[4] Experience as a source of revelation about God has been regarded as slippery and particularly problematic.[5]

Yet experience, in fact, has been the silent partner to Scripture and to tradition. The Bible, first and foremost, was written to testify to people's experience of God in the world; the witness of Scripture is that God is revealed through human experience in the body.[6] Tradition, too, bears the fingerprints of experience, developing over time through argument and innovation.[7] Scripture and tradition are 'codified collective experience'.[8]

---

pattern of results, particularly regarding suicidality, highlights the severity and pervasiveness of disparities between sexual minority and heterosexual youth . . . on average 28% of sexual minority youth reported a history of suicidality as compared with 12% of heterosexual youth.'

3 Edward Farley, *The Fragility of Knowledge: Theological Education in the Church and the University* (Philadelphia, PA: Fortess, 1988), 125. Farley further observes (128–129) that the 'house of authority' paradigm is inadequate to wrestle with the growing acknowledgement of the historicity of all knowledge.

4 Adrian Thatcher, 'Introduction', in *The Oxford Handbook of Theology, Sexuality, and Gender*, ed. Adrian Thatcher (Oxford: Oxford University Press, 2015), 8–9.

5 Ellen T. Charry, 'Experience', in *The Oxford Handbook of Systematic Theology*, ed. John Webster, Kathryn Tanner and Iain Torrance (Oxford: Oxford University Press, 2007), 413–418.

6 Luke Timothy Johnson, *The Revelatory Body: Theology as Inductive Art* (Grand Rapids, MI/Cambridge, UK: William B. Eerdmans, 2015), 2–3, 7.

7 Alasdair MacIntyre, *After Virtue* (3rd Ed.; London: Duckworth, 2007), 222; Donald Winnicott, *Playing and Reality* (London/New York: Routledge, 2005), 134; Thatcher, 'Introduction', 10.

8 Rosemary Radford Ruether, 'Feminist Theology: Methodology, Sources and Norms', in *Theological Reflection: Sources*, ed. Elaine Graham, Heather Walton and Frances Ward (London: SCM, 2007), 295.

The collective experience behind the house of authority has been the specific experience of heterosexual males.[9] The patriarchal cultures of the ancient near east left more than their fingerprints on the sacred texts; they significantly shaped them. Theology thus has had an inherent ignorance of the experience of God in the lives of the invisible and the underclass. This was true until the last fifty years, which have seen an explosion of theological scholarship exploring the embodied, revelatory experience of people of colour, women, and lesbian, gay, bisexual and transgender people.[10]

Exploring experience for glimpses of God is challenging. How does one know that an experience is of God? Does the subjectivity of human experience obfuscate the divine? How is experience reliably to be interpreted? Scripture and tradition also come with challenges of interpretation, but the interpretation of experience is more baldly problematic: experience is highly personal, seen through a lens formed by past experiences and dialogical with one's interpretation of Scripture and tradition.

Yet Scripture itself assists in the interpretation and validation of experience. The Gospel of Luke reports that when the followers of John the Baptist asked Jesus 'Are you the one to come?', he replied, 'Go and tell John what you have seen and heard: the blind receive their sight, the lame walk, the lepers are cleansed, the deaf hear, the dead are raised, the poor have good news brought to them' (Lk 7:18–20). Likewise, the Johannine community criticised people for not recognising Jesus despite seeing the works that he did in God's name (Jn 10:22–39). The faithful, too, are instructed to recognise the works of God by the fruits of the Spirit – attributes that will be obvious in the follower's life (Gal 5:16–26). One can discern whether an experience reveals God by looking at the fruits of the experience – did it beget the flourishing of life, love and justice? Did it call forth action that would enable such flourishing? Rowan Williams conceives of revelation as God establishing Godself among us as 'the loving and nurturing advent of *newness* in human life – grace, forgiveness, empowerment to be agents of forgiveness and liberation'.[11] These things are manifest in human experience and recognisable.

Given the importance of experience to the whole theological endeavour and the limitations of a primary source that comes out of ancient cultures, theology is best understood as an inductive art,[12] or as historically situated reflection and interpretation,[13] the purpose of which is to discern how to

9 Ruether, 'Feminist Theology', 295.

10 See, for example, James H. Cone, *A Black Theology of Liberation* (Maryknoll, NY: Orbis, 1970); Mary McClintock Fulkerson and Sheila Briggs, eds., *The Oxford Handbook of Feminist Theology* (Oxford: Oxford University Press, 2012); Marcella Althaus-Reid, ed., *Liberation Theology and Sexuality* (Aldershot/Burlington, VT: Ashgate, 2006).

11 Rowan Williams, 'Trinity and Revelation', in *Theological Reflection: Sources*, 30 (emphasis in original).

12 Johnson, *Revelatory Body*, 7.

13 Farley, *Fragility of Knowledge*, 128, 133–162.

respond faithfully to God's presence in the world. It is this task of discernment that practical theological reflection can assist.

Theological reflection after trauma

Returning to the teenager's suicide, how were individuals and the church to make sense of the death of a child that apparently resulted from Scripture? Was it a matter of the wages of sin being death – a tragic sacrifice that maintains the coherence of a literalist interpretative schema? Or would her death necessarily spark a deeper inquiry into the church's understanding of how to read Scripture?

For the girl's minister, it was the beginning of a searching inquiry. A child had died 'on my watch'.[14] While the minister and his colleague did not hold homophobic views, they had not raised the issue with the congregation, it being is a divisive issue in the evangelical world to which the congregation belongs. When the coroner revealed the apparent underlying cause of the girl's death at the hearing, the newspaper evening news ran the story in a way that painted the church as being in some degree responsible. The story went viral. In response, the ministers of the church published a statement saying that they wished the girl had told them that she was struggling because she would have been met with a lot of warmth and acceptance, but that they nevertheless realised that the gap had been too big for her to cross. They committed to doing a root-and-branch inquiry of how the church looked at sexuality.

The next month the governing body of the church unanimously passed a statement of inclusion that articulated the church's new public stance. The statement was met by parishioners with cheering, indifference or (among a small minority) aggressive resistance. In the aftermath of that decision, both the minister and the congregation undertook a process of reflection and education which included listening evenings facilitated by an outside theological educator. The minister – realising that while he was not confused about how to respond pastorally to gay people, he was confused as to how to reinterpret God in the light of what had happened – saw a Jesuit psychotherapist for over a year. He describes his journey as an enormous process of dismantling how he read Scripture and understood faith and rebuilding – a process that continues.

When a traumatising event happens, the embodied experience is powerful and unavoidable. In the chapter by Hilary Ison that follows, the impact of trauma on the human body is described in some detail. Put briefly, traumatising experiences trigger the limbic system, flooding the body with stress hormones and cutting off the cerebral cortex. The body is enabled to react quickly, aiming to preserve life. Cognition and reflection are temporarily inhibited. Normally full function is restored in four to six weeks.

14 Personal communication, March 21, 2018.

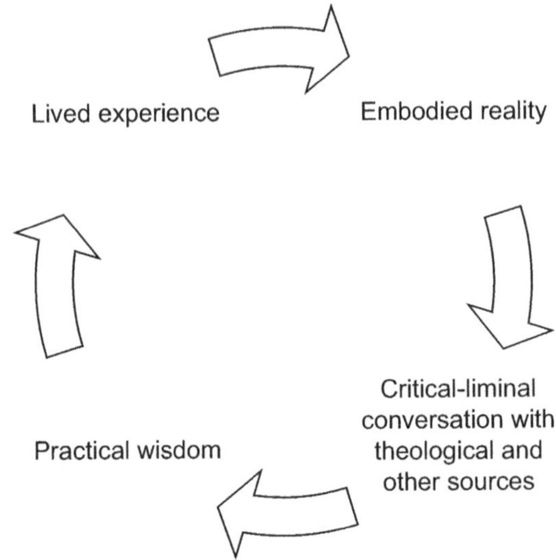

Figure 2.1 Theological reflection after trauma

But individuals in a congregation will have different reactions and different rates of recovery, depending on their physiology and past experience. The church's capacity to make sense of an experience of trauma that has shattered its framework of meaning will typically take much longer. Kraus *et al* observe that a traumatic event is the start of a journey that can take years.[15]

The process the minister and some of the congregation undertook to make sense of the girl's suicide can be mapped as shown in Figure 2.1.

This version of the pastoral cycle,[16] like all others, oversimplifies the process of sense-making and discernment. While reflection begins with lived experience and is shaped by embodied reality, the process is not linear, nor is it entirely conscious. Individuals pick up the pieces and reshape their framework of meaning in diverse ways; there are setbacks and new challenges that arise.

The critical-liminal conversation part of the cycle attempts to describe the process of bringing together experience with the other sources of theology (Scripture, tradition, reason) and with other knowledge (e.g., social and physical sciences) to make sense of an event. The conversation is critical in that critical thinking is employed: in the case of the girl's suicide, there are

15 Laurie Kraus, David Holyan and Bruce Wismer, *Recovering From Un-Natural Disasters* (Louisville, KY: Westminster John Knox, 2017), xiv.

16 The pastoral cycle is a tool of theological reflection that derives from David Kolb's theory of adult learning. See, for example, Judith Thompson with Stephen Pattison and Ross Thompson, *Theological Reflection* (London: SCM, 2008), 21, 51–60.

a number of respects in which Scripture may be re-examined critically. For example, one might choose to take into account its historical context and, in particular, the role of sexuality in a time when maximum procreation was necessary for survival of the clan. Similarly, one might explore new insights from the science of human sexuality or insights from the social sciences that illuminate the phenomenon of youth suicide. The conversation is also liminal. The word *liminal* derives from the Latin *limen*, meaning 'threshold'.[17] Liminal spaces and processes enable people to move from one way of being to another. They are places of wrestling and places of grace, working in deep ways (conscious and unconscious) and holding emotion, competing claims, cognition and imagination. One does not so much marshal facts in liminal space as encounter the inexplicable. These spaces and processes enable the integration of an experience into a person's life story. Ritual, art, prayer, poetry and play are liminal activities.

As meaning is made and experience is integrated, an individual or community crafts a practical wisdom that will enable them to make sense of what has happened and to move into the future with new insights and behaviours that enable the flourishing of human life. That wisdom is taken into daily life and life together and tried and tested by further lived experience.

The girl's minister characterises the journey the church has been on as both painful and ultimately liberating for the congregation. Some people left the church, but more joined as people who were looking for an inclusive church found a welcome there.

> A lot of the things that have changed in our church are difficult to define. It's the tone of the conversation with ourselves that has changed. Bring all of yourself; it's all absolutely fine. . . . Suddenly we aren't in a holiness competition and it's just amazing. . . . We're all being a bit more honest about ourselves.[18]

He reflected further that when another crisis arose, the church took it in its stride and handled it with equanimity. The framework was not shattered. Yet he is aware that he himself is still a work in process, occasionally falling into old ways of understanding Scripture as he reaches for a word to speak to the people. He is slowly trying to 'work out how to tell the good news and build good things in a way that is not naïve and is honest', merging probing analysis and telling a good story.[19] The worship services reflect the change more than preaching: in the Services of the Word, there is always an anointing of oil and anyone can come for it for any reason. 'Whatever you

17 Victor Turner, *The Ritual Process: Structure and Anti-Structure* (New Brunswick/London: Aldine Transaction, 2008), 94.

18 Personal communication.

19 Personal communication.

are wrestling with, it's your thing; we'll bless what that is about without knowing it. We don't have a barrel full of answers.'[20]

The story of who we are

What has been happening in the teenager's minister and congregation as they integrate the experience of her suicide is that they have been reframing the story of who they are and how God relates to the human family.

Humans are story-makers and storytellers. Neuroscientist Antonio Damasio believes that storytelling is 'probably a brain obsession . . . [that precedes] language, since it is, in fact, a condition for language, and it is based not just in the cerebral cortex but elsewhere in the brain'.[21] He theorises that the self is made up of the nonconscious neural signalling of an individual organism which begets a nonverbal 'proto-self', which permits 'core self' (transient, conscious and noninterpretive) and 'core consciousness', enabling an 'autobiographical self' derived from the core self and autobiographical memory.[22] He concludes:

> The idea each of us constructs of ourself, the image we gradually build of who we are physically and mentally, of where we fit socially, is based on autobiographical memory over years of experience and is constantly subject to remodeling. I believe that much of the building occurs non-consciously and that so does the remodeling. Those conscious and unconscious processes, in whatever proportion, are influenced by all sorts of factors: innate and acquired personality traits, intelligence, knowledge, social and cultural environment.[23]
>
> The core *you* is only born as the story is told, *within the story itself*.[24]

The story of self is what gives an individual identity. Events are interpreted, synthesised and plotted to give a life an intelligible shape.[25] The plot not only allows the integration of experience into one's life story but also gives the story direction: there is an end towards which the story moves.[26] It is this end, according to virtue ethicist Alisdair MacIntyre, that enables moral unity and action.[27]

20 Personal communication.

21 Antonio Damasio, *The Feeling of What Happens: Body, Emotion and the Making of Consciousness* (London: Vintage, 2000), 189.

22 Damasio, *The Feeling*, 199.

23 Damasio, *The Feeling*, 224.

24 Damasio, *The Feeling*, 191 (emphasis in original).

25 Paul Ricœur, 'Life: A Story in Search of a Narrator', in *A Ricœur Reader: Reflection and Imagination*, ed. Mario J. Valdés (Toronto/Buffalo, NY: University of Toronto, 1991), 426.

26 Ricœur, 'Life', 427.

27 MacIntyre, *After Virtue*, 218–219.

The story an individual tells of his or her life – his or her identity – is not a solo project; it is intertwined with the story of the communities to which the individual belongs. The narrating *I* is formed by the stories of other *I*'s, including what Ricœur calls the 'imaginary nucleus' of the culture[28] and what MacIntyre terms 'the story of those communities from which I derive my identity'.[29] Stephen Crites, a pioneer in thinking about experience as narrative, observes that 'the *way* we remember, anticipate, and even directly perceive, is largely social'.[30] Ruard Ganzevoort, working with narrative approaches to practical theology, emphasises the importance of the audience: for whom we tell the story is also an important shaper of the story in ways that cannot be overestimated.[31] Our personal stories, unique as they may be, are intimately and powerfully shaped by other stories.

By understanding this, the shock to the system of the news of the reasons for the suicide can be seen for what it was: a shattering of the congregation's frame of reference about God, church and human sexuality that held faith and life together in a particular schema. Crites might have called this kind of frame of reference a 'sacred story', as it gives structure to individuals' sense of self and world and forms consciousness itself.[32] He writes that sacred stories are subject to change, although not by conscious reflection – sacred stories do not 'transpire within a conscious world'; people 'awaken to a sacred story'.[33] Yet sometimes parts of a sacred story must be unlearned for an individual to grasp a reformed sacred story.

The minister's testimony to his long and painful process of dismantling and rebuilding speaks to this and to the power of frames of reference or sacred stories. The process is not a simple logical adjustment to new information. Rather, a framework that has been shattered, one that holds what it means to be a sexual human being before God, needs to be painstakingly reassembled with perhaps fewer or differently shaped pieces. In the present case, the frames of reference under examination are about two of the most intimate, deeply held parts of being human: sex and God. Sexuality is

28 Paul Ricœur, 'Myth as the Bearer of Possible Worlds', in *A Ricœur Reader*, 482–483.

29 MacIntyre, *After Virtue*, 221.

30 Stephen Crites, 'The Narrative Quality of Experience', *Journal of the American Academy of Religion* 39, no. 3 (1971): 304 (emphasis in original).

31 R. Ruard Ganzevoort, 'Narrative Approaches', in *The Wiley-Blackwell Companion to Practical Theology*, ed. Bonnie J. Miller-McLemore (Oxford: Blackwell, 2012), 216–217; 'Religious Coping Reconsidered, Part Two: A Narrative Reformulation', *Journal of Psychology and Theology* 26, no. 3 (1998): 278. The audience forces the author to tell a story that is 'legitimate and plausible' (Ganzevoort, 'Coping, Part Two', 278). See also M. Carolyn Clark, 'Narrative Learning: Its Contours and Its Possibilities', *New Directions for Adult and Continuing Education*, no. 126 (2010): 3–4, who asserts that the audience shapes the structure and determines the purpose of the narrative.

32 Crites, 'Narrative', 295. According to Crites, sacred stories are mythopoeic and not necessarily about gods. Rather they 'orient the life of people through time, their life-time, their individual and corporate experience . . . to the great powers that establish the reality of their world'.

33 Crites, 'Narrative', 296.

implicated in basic human needs for relationship, touch and acceptance and is intertwined with our embodied experience; for people of faith, relation to God is an ultimate matter framing a personal worldview. It is no surprise that these frameworks are particularly resilient.

Ganzevoort, who proposes a narrative reformulation of religious coping theory, also observes the power and resilience of frames of reference (which he calls assumptive worlds, after Ronnie Janoff-Bulman).[34] In the face of a new event, the individual will try to interpret the event consistently with their personal narrative, denying or dismissing elements of the event if necessary. If that is not possible, an existential crisis will occur.[35] The resolution of that crisis, as the physiological effects of trauma subside and full brain function is again possible, happens with the reframing of the story into one that can provide coherence and meaning to one's experience.

The proposed model of theological reflection after trauma is an attempt to articulate the reframing process, a process which is ultimately mysterious and contains both conscious and unconscious workings. The key leadership task is to resource that process whilst knowing that it cannot be controlled. Congregations are collections of individuals, each of whom will be doing their own reframing work in the only way they can, which will differ from person to person. Resourcing congregational reframing includes acknowledging the pain and struggle of the event and its tear in the fabric of communal life, doing one's own personal work of reframing, making space for conversation, providing information, employing symbolic and ritual action to assist transitions and fostering an environment that helps individuals to accept that people are not all the same and will react and work through issues in their own way. As a congregation works through a trauma towards a reframing of their understanding of life before God, not everyone will come to the same conclusions. Some may have to leave. The greatest gift a leader can give the leavers is a gracious acceptance of their need to leave, acknowledging the pain of their decision for all.

Understanding the process of reframing

The process of reframing may be looked at more closely through the lens of transformative learning theory. Developed in the last quarter of the 20th century, transformative learning theory sought to explain the process of

34 Ronnie Janoff-Bulman, *Shattered Assumptions: Towards a New Psychology of Trauma* (New York: Free Press, 1992). Ganzevoort articulates (R. Ruard Ganzevoort, 'Scars and Stigmata: Trauma, Identity and Theology', *Practical Theology* 1, no. 1 [2008]: 26; conversation with Congregational Tragedy Project, 12 November 2018) Janoff-Bulman's three basic assumptions by which humans live and with which they hold together life and identity as follows: (1) that the world is a meaningful and coherent whole and not a basket of coincidences, (2) that the world is benevolent and not inclined to do harm, and (3) that I am a person worthy of care and love. He translates these into religious terms as follows: (1) the sovereignty of God, (2) the trustworthiness of God and (3) the love of God.

35 Ganzevoort, 'Coping, Part Two', 286.

learning that significantly changes a person's attitudes and actions from the inside out. Founder Jack Mezirow originally studied adult women who re-entered higher education after an extended hiatus.[36] He posited that individuals acquire habits of expectation through socialisation that assist them in making sense of the world. These meaning-making habits of expectation are the perceptual and conceptual lenses through which new experiences are interpreted. In time he called these 'frames of reference',[37] the term I have used throughout this chapter. At the start of his theorising, Mezirow envisioned the process as primarily cognitive, emphasising the role of a disorienting dilemma and critical reflection on assumptions as a part of transformative learning. As his theory developed through the work of numerous theorists and practitioners, these elements continued to be considered essential.[38] But the theory has shifted from being one that concerns a rational process to one that recognises the importance of emotion, context, intuition and relationships.[39] Some educators have made the connection between transformative learning and narrative theory, recognising that learning can be conceptualised as a narrative process and that a narrative perspective helps make sense of how transformative learning happens.[40]

In what follows, I use concepts developed in transformative learning theory to tease out the third step in the proposed theological reflection model – that mysterious, part-conscious and part-unconscious conversation that changes people's attitudes and actions from the inside out. I frame these concepts within the larger metanarrative that is at the heart of the Christian faith: death and resurrection.[41]

36 Jack Mezirow, *Education for Perspective Transformation: Women's Re-entry Programs in Community College* (New York: Center for Adult Education, Teachers College, Columbia University Press, 1978). For a review of the development of transformative learning theory, see Lisa M. Baumgartner, 'Mezirow's Theory of Transformative Learning from 1975 to Present', in *The Handbook of Transformative Learning: Theory, Research, and Practice*, ed. Edward W. Taylor, Patricia Cranton and Associates (San Francisco, CA: Jossey-Bass, 2012), 100–101.

37 Baumgartner, 'Mezirow's Theory', 109.

38 Edward W. Taylor, 'An Update of Transformative Learning Theory: A Critical Review of the Empirical Research (1999–2005)', *International Journal of Lifelong Education* 26, no. 2 (2007): 174.

39 Baumgartner, 'Mezirow's Theory', 110.

40 Clark, 'Narrative Learning', 6, 9. See, also, Ann K. Brooks and Kathleen Edwards, *Narratives of Women's Sexual Identity Development: A Collaborative Inquiry with Implications for Rewriting Transformative Learning Theory* (Stillwater, OK: New Prairie, 1997); M. Carolyn Clark, 'Transformation as Embodied Narrative', in *The Handbook of Transformative Learning*, 425–438; Kathy D. Lohr, 'Tapping Autobiographical Narratives to Illuminate Resilience: A Transformative Learning Tool for Adult Educators', *Educational Gerontology* 44, nos. 2–3 (2018): 163–170.

41 Will McWhinney and Laura Markos, 'Transformative Education: Across the Threshold', *Journal of Transformative Education* 1, no. 1 (2003): 16–37, envision transformative education as engaging the archetypal form of the path of death and rebirth that is present in many cultures around the world. Drawing on a Navajo sand painting for healing, they

Shelly Rambo, in *Spirit and Trauma*,[42] argues that Holy Saturday holds a conceptual key to the witness to trauma. In the aftermath of trauma, the line between death and life blurs. In this ambiguous and difficult middle space, Rambo finds a 'middle Spirit' that 'remains and persists where death and life defy ordinary expression; death is neither completed nor in the past, and life is neither new nor directed to the future'.[43] This Spirit 'witnesses to the depths' and 'searches for forms of life when life cannot be recognized as such', igniting the capacity to imagine beyond an ending.[44] The Spirit is a fragile breath that moves between life and death testifying to what remains – inextinguishable divine love – and powering those who abide (who receive) to give form to chaos and to imagine life.[45] The capacity to imagine is no luxury, Rambo writes, but necessary for survival and healing.[46] Post-trauma life cannot be envisioned, guaranteed or assumed; 'it must be imagined in new forms. This prior moment of imagination is the breath of witness before the breath of life'.[47] Rambo says that the Spirit's movements between life and death can be thought of twofold: attending to the losses, grief and chaos of life and sensing coming into life again, finding a way.[48] Her 'middle Spirit' is the spirit of the third step in my proposed model of theological reflection – accompanying the embodied reality of loss and death into the liminal place that encounters the depths and persists in seeking a way to live, making sense of the insensible and imagining new possibilities.

The crisis of the teenage girl's death catapulted those close to her into grief, and the later revelation of the assumed cause of her death compounded the trauma. Transformative learning theory as it has developed has noted that the pain of crisis can propel people into liminal, reflective space.[49] Her minister's shock at the coroner's revelation at the hearing, that a child 'had died on my watch', pushed him into the middle space. It is important to acknowledge at this point two things: First, working through the distress and pain caused by a traumatising event is a necessary part of the recovery process.[50] Second, the sacred stories that form our consciousness are resilient frames of reference.[51] That resilience can manifest to block or deny emotion and

---

conceive of that path as fourfold: crisis, entry into liminal space, transformative passage and reintegration into daily life.

42 Shelly Rambo, *Spirit and Trauma: A Theology of Remaining* (Louisville, KY: Westminster John Knox, 2010).

43 Rambo, *Spirit and Trauma*, 114.

44 Rambo, *Spirit and Trauma*, 115.

45 Rambo, *Spirit and Trauma*, 120.

46 Rambo, *Spirit and Trauma*, 123.

47 Rambo, *Spirit and Trauma*, 124.

48 Rambo, *Spirit and Trauma*, 160–162.

49 Kaisu Mällki, 'Rethinking Disorienting Dilemmas Within Real-Life Crises: The Role of Reflection in Negotiating Emotionally Chaotic Experiences', *Adult Education Quarterly* 62, no. 3 (2012): 219.

50 Mällki, 'Rethinking', 216.

51 Ganzevoort, 'Coping: Part Two', 286.

circumvent the possibility of engaging in critical-liminal conversation. For this and a host of other reasons, not everyone will feel the same level or kind of distress or pain in the aftermath of a tragic death.

Entering the critical-liminal process requires not only facing into pain but also a willingness to let go: of life as it was before, of cherished assumptions, of certainties and assurances. It is a symbolic death of self.[52] It is no surprise that not everyone will be willing or able to enter the process. In McWhinney and Markos's imaging of transformative learning theory as death and rebirth, passage through this liminal space may be marked by two movements. The first contains early exploratory behaviours that may include unlearning, collecting new information, exploring previously unconsidered possibilities and trying new ideas and roles on for size.[53] Playing with different perspectives is noted as potentially an important phase of meaning-making post-trauma.[54] Here, the middle Spirit holds the reality and pain of the death whilst fuelling the persistence and capacity to imagine. The second movement is more a moment: the graced *Aha!* of insight that enables the individual or group to grasp a new direction.[55] Such moments are fragile, and given the resilience of old frames of reference, it will take time for the insight to solidify. One may spend a long time in and out of critical-liminal conversation,[56] and the old ways of thinking may persist side by side with new perspectives, though less dominant.[57] Still, the middle Spirit strains towards the possibility of life anew.

A word about emotions in the middle space: not only is working through feelings necessary for recovery from trauma, but it must also be acknowledged that cognitive reasoning is not only impaired in the earliest stages, but also it is simply inadequate on its own to grapple with trauma. Sands and Tennant, studying transformative learning in the context of suicide bereavement, observed that 'no amount of cognitive processing or meta-cognitive reasoning would provide the emotional engagement necessary for healing'.[58] They note the cognitive emphasis of early transformative learning theory to be a limitation and argue that the transformation process, particularly in grief, is fundamentally extrarational and highly personal, requiring emotional engagement.[59]

52 McWhinney and Markos, 'Across the Threshold', 25.

53 McWhinney and Markos, 'Across the Threshold', 28.

54 Mällki, 'Rethinking', 220.

55 McWhinney and Markos, 'Across the Threshold', 28.

56 Mällki, 'Rethinking', 224.

57 Diana Sands and Mark Tennant, 'Transformative Learning in the Context of Suicide Bereavement', *Adult Education Quarterly* 60, no. 2 (2010): 117.

58 Sands and Tennant, 'Suicide Bereavement', 114–115.

59 Sands and Tennant, 'Suicide Bereavement', 115, 116, quoting Sue M. Scott, 'The Grieving Soul in the Transformation Process', *New Directions in Adult and Continuing Education* 74 (1997): 45–46.

Given the link between the teenager's death and Church teaching, the 'critical'/cognitive aspects of the middle way are essential. Transformative learning is a root enquiry into frames of reference that enable individuals to look critically at why they think the way they do and whether their thinking needs to be reformed. Trauma breaks open the mental horizon,[60] enabling this kind of evaluation. The resilience of frames of reference and the social nature of individual narratives underscore the importance of a community journeying together towards a new understanding. As the girl's church experienced in the aftermath of their statement of inclusion, adopting a new perspective can lead to disagreement not only within but also outside the community.[61]

Over time, the middle Spirit midwives changed perspectives and commitments that lead to a life that is wiser, aware always of a tenuous hold on life and the link between life and death.

In summary, developments in transformative learning theory alert us to the importance of certain elements of the leadership task in assisting reframing, as a congregation traverses the middle space between death and life in the company of the middle Spirit. First, facing into the traumatising event and acknowledging its pain and disorienting impact are essential. No change can happen if a disorienting event is minimised or dismissed. Lamentation and mourning open the way for the possibility of entering into the middle space where new meaning may be made. Second, while reframing is never an exclusively rational process, there is a rational component. Critical examination of the assumptions underlying a frame of reference or worldview will assist individuals who are trying to reconstruct a coherent story that includes the traumatising event. Third, making a container for strong emotion facilitates meaning-making. Elsewhere in this volume the role of ritual and liturgy in the aftermath of trauma is discussed. These kinds of liminal activities are more than cathartic; they enable the continuity of faith alongside its reformation. The church can continue to reverence the Bible through its symbolic action and structure of worship whilst providing tools for critical examination that mine the Word for reframed meaning. Providing silent spaces in liturgy or the kind of anointing that the dead girl's minister now does meets diverse people where they are and enables them to bring their pain and their need to God. Fourth, the recognition of the social construction of world view and the power of the relationships in community counsels towards community: small- and large-group events not only for worship but for emotional expression, education and re-imagining another way to understand God and human life. Alongside these elements, a leader's understanding of context will shape her or his discernment of how best to

60 R. Ruard Ganzevoort, 'Religious Coping Reconsidered, Part One: An Integrated Approach', *Journal of Psychology and Theology* 26, no. 3 (1998): 269.

61 Mällki, 'Rethinking', 223.

provide the resources needed by the congregation to reframe its story in the middle space between life and death.

The power of story: trauma remakes the tradition

The girl's minister now tells her story and the story of the church to any who want to hear it. He says to churches, 'This is Annie (not her real name), she loved kids, she played the flute, and now she's dead. Where are your Annies and what would you do?' He says it is the lived experience that gives the story the power to 'poke the hornet's nest' and provoke churches to rethink questions of sexuality.[62]

Brooks and Edwards, discussing women's sexuality narratives, write about how some stories carry more weight in the dominant discourse, while others are silent, shadowed or counter to the primary story.[63] The story of the young woman who committed suicide – a story counter to the assumed dominant discourse in her church, a story she held silently for the most part and a story that reveals the shadow side of Church teaching on sexuality – is one that has the power to remake a tradition formed and developed in patriarchal cultures.

How is tradition remade? By argument and innovation. What role may human experience play in this remaking? The literature on theological reflection is strong on working with human experience[64] but weak on how experience may function as a source of theology that remakes tradition. Thompson *et al* conclude that 'the process whereby insights drawn from theological reflection can feed back . . . into the remaking of the tradition itself' is 'largely unexplored territory'.[65] Ballard and Pritchard also note the possibility of tradition and practice needing to be changed in response to new theological understandings arising from attention to the lived experience of faith but do not theorise how that may happen.[66]

I propose a mapping of the process of human experience remaking tradition that reasserts the underlying centrality of experience in theological endeavour, as envisioned in Figure 2.2.

In this model, lived experience (Step 1) sparks an endeavour to discover ontological truth about human life (Step 2). Regarding sexuality-related enquiries, this would include an inquiry into the truth of human sexuality, its purposes and forms. Once uncovered, that truth is evaluated as a potential

62 Personal communication.

63 Brooks and Edwards, 'Women's Sexual Identity', 97.

64 Elaine Graham, Heather Walton and Frances Ward, *Theological Reflection: Methods* (London: SCM, 2005); Thompson et al., *Theological Reflection*; Paul Ballard and John Pritchard, *Practical Theology in Action: Christian Thinking in the Service of Church and Society* (London: SPCK, 1996).

65 Thompson et al., *Theological Reflection*, 200.

66 Ballard and Pritchard, *Practical Theology*, 67.

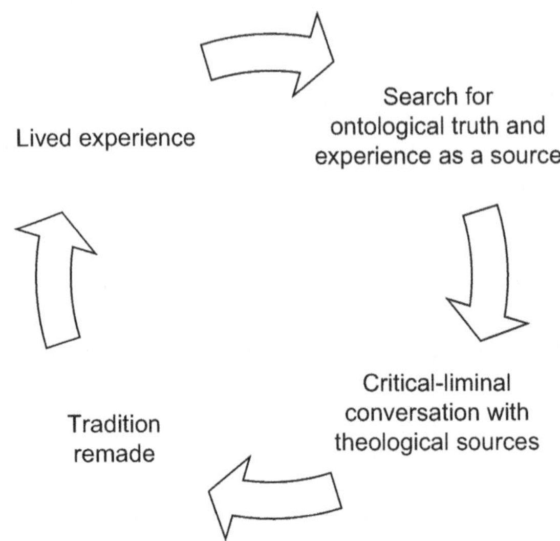

Figure 2.2 How theological reflection may remake tradition

source for understanding the divine–human relationship by considering its fruits. For example, an exploration of the role of sexuality in adolescent and adult development, and its close connection to spirituality,[67] can inform an understanding of the relationship between sexuality and human physical, emotional and spiritual flourishing.

Experience validated as a source for theology can then be invited into critical and liminal conversation with Scripture and tradition (Step 3). The conversation, like that described in theological reflection in the aftermath of trauma, is critical and creative and accompanied by the middle Spirit that leans towards life. All the theological sources are evaluated in light of the historicity of knowledge and the discerning task of theological interpretation discussed at the beginning of this chapter. An outcome of the critical-liminal conversation may be the refinement or re-imagination of the tradition so that it more fully reflects the truth of the human being in God (Step 4). Remade tradition is then validity-tested as to how it has an impact on future lived experience (Step 1).

The process is anything but linear. Understanding is formed and fomented in a more tumultuous and creative way in both the individual and the tradition as thought and feeling, insight and commitment are tried and tested. The outcome should connect real life and faith in a way that assures continuity in the tradition whilst respecting the flesh and blood, joy and pain of

67 Joan Timmerman, *Sexuality and Spiritual Growth* (New York: Crossroad, 1993).

being human as a site where God continues to reveal Godself,[68] and utilising the advances in human knowledge in other spheres.[69]

The argument for human experience remaking tradition is an argument that not only reclaims the primacy of experience in theology but also is rooted in the narrative identity and moral creativity of humankind. John Wall argues for human moral creativity as a poetic phronesis – a wisdom created out of meaning-making activity that is called forth from different others:[70] 'The "other" calls me to an imaginative self-disruption that creatively undoes, as it were, my own settled moral assumptions and calls me toward the unknown.'[71]

A teenager's tragic story disrupted the dominant narrative of her church and set her minister and church on a journey that eventually brought new life out of death, accompanied by the middle Spirit that is always witnessing in trauma to the persistent and inextinguishable love of God.

Wall sums up the opportunity and the task before humanity by turning to the first sacred story, Genesis 1 – 'To be created in the image of a Creator is one way of saying, in part, that we are perpetually responsible for fashioning new moral worlds within the multiplicity, disorder, complexity, and tragedy of human life.'[72]

Not every trauma will call for the remaking of the Christian tradition, but where that is necessary, a poetic (creative) practical theology that attends seriously to human experience, human knowledge and the movement of the middle Spirit, as well as Scripture and tradition, will find the way.

Select references

Baumgartner, Lisa M. 'Mezirow's Theory of Transformative Learning From 1975 to Present'. In *The Handbook of Transformative Learning: Theory, Research, and Practice*, ed. Edward W. Taylor, Patricia Cranton and Associates. San Francisco: Jossey-Bass, 2012, 99–115.

68 Edward Farley notes, *Good and Evil: Interpreting a Human Condition* (Minneapolis, MN: Fortress Press, 1990), 117, that 'if there is no connection between the elements in the Hebraic and Christian paradigm and the way we experience ourselves and our world, that paradigm is surely cognitively vacuous'.

69 Christian thinking that is divorced from the advances of human knowledge is deeply problematic. Surely faith is not about putting on blinders but, rather, about being able to see the world – created and loved by God – in an illuminating light. Farley argues, *Theologia: The Fragmentation and Unity of Theological Education* (Eugene, OR: Wipf & Stock, 2001), 134–135, for the importance of including in the study of theology the human, social and natural sciences.

70 John Wall, *Moral Creativity: Paul Ricœur and the Poetics of Possibility* (Oxford: Oxford University Press, 2005). Working with Paul Ricœur's theory of narrative identity and 'poetics of the will', Wall brings together two concepts that Aristotle had separated: practical wisdom (*phronesis*) and poetics (*poiesis*). Aristotle believed that phronesis is the central virtue that brings about moral action and that poiesis is simply the process of making or creating objects or literature.

71 Wall, *Moral Creativity*, 7.

72 Wall, *Moral Creativity*, 5.

Chalke, Steve, Ian Sansbury and Gareth Streeter. 'In the Name of Love: The Church, Exclusion and LGB Mental Health Issues'. London: The Oasis Foundation, 2017. https://oasis.foundation/resources/name-love-church-exclusion-and-lgb-mental-health-issues. Accessed 21 June 2018.

Crites, Stephen. 'The Narrative Quality of Experience'. *Journal of the American Academy of Religion* 39, no. 3 (1971): 291–311.

Ganzevoort, R. Ruard. 'Religious Coping Reconsidered, Part Two: A Narrative Reformulation'. *Journal of Psychology and Theology* 26, no. 3 (1998): 276–286.

Kraus, Laurie, David Holyan and Bruce Wismer. *Recovering From Un-Natural Disasters*. Louisville, KY: Westminster John Knox, 2017.

Rambo, Shelly. *Spirit and Trauma: A Theology of Remaining*. Louisville, KY: Westminster John Knox, 2010.

Part II

Trauma is in the body

Introduction to Part II

The two essays in Part II of the volume continue and intensify the focus of Part I on experience, but bring our attention to the phenomenon of the experience of trauma 'in the body'. The two consider 'body' in two distinct senses. Hilary Ison's interest is in the body of the individual. Kate Wiebe's interest is mostly in corporate bodies and the communal experience of trauma.

In Chapter 3 Hilary Ison details the brain–body trauma response and introduces the concept of the 'felt sense'. She explains the importance of the felt sense to responding in the context of social and physical environments and how working with it assists in healing individual trauma, also observing the usefulness of meditation and mindfulness in connecting brain and body to build resilience. Ison stresses the importance of the resonant, warm and caring presence of the other as the crucial ingredient in recovering from trauma. The human need for relationship, in order for people to flourish, underscores, for Ison, the theological point that we are, indeed, made for love.

Kate Wiebe considers collective trauma, which she argues is more than the sum of the trauma of wounded individuals. Identifying broken trust as a key aspect of trauma, she observes the importance of rebuilding trust to resolve health in individuals and in community. Echoing Ison's emphasis on care, Wiebe notes that responses to trauma that include personal and relational care facilitate recovery for both individuals and communities. She identifies key practices that are most likely to lead to community health and shares strategies of preparedness which may strengthen individual and collective resilience.

As in Part I, the focus in these essays on the experience of trauma, in this case bodily experience, clarifies and resources the Christian response to the bad things that can and do happen in our world. Engaging with the fullness of human experience and with biochemical and social sciences proves a fruitful means to practise theology in the face of tragedy.

3 Working with an embodied and systemic approach to trauma and tragedy

Hilary Ison

A scream – a rush of air as the body, falling from the gallery above, narrowly missed a tourist and landed on the cathedral floor. Horrified tourists, especially those who had witnessed the person climb over the high railing, looked down from the gallery, while others on the floor started to gather to see if help was needed or fled in panic. A verger and steward arrived and quickly took charge of the scene, screening off the area and attempting to administer first aid and resuscitation. Another verger dealt with the tourists and visitors, making sure that they were safely brought down from the gallery and seated in one area of the cathedral whilst those already on the ground floor were gathered and seated in another section to await the arrival of the police and emergency services. Meanwhile, drinks were brought to them and information given about what was happening. The cathedral clergy were called to assist the duty chaplain in caring for people and, together with other senior staff, took the decision to close the cathedral for the rest of the day, cancelling a major service due to take place that afternoon. While the vergers and steward involved were visibly shaken and upset by the experience, they were able to recover themselves and continue with their duties. They, together with all the staff, were given ongoing support and the offer of counselling as needed.

This was a tragedy for the person who died and the person's family and a shocking event that 'landed' in the life of the whole cathedral community as the impact of it rippled out through all its parts. Was it experienced as a 'trauma'? In this chapter, I look at how the same event within a community can leave some people traumatised while others are not and what makes the difference.

Trauma is defined as that which overwhelms our capacity to cope with our experience and which breaks connections – to ourselves, to others, to resources, to our frames of reference.[1] Sarah Peyton, an educator and writer on neuroscience, describes emotional trauma as 'the moments when what is

1 Peter A. Levine, *Waking The Tiger: Healing Trauma* (Berkeley, CA: North Atlantic, 1997), 28–29; Steve Haines, *Trauma Is Really Strange* (London: Jessica Kingsley, 2016).

happening around you is too difficult, terrifying, or painful for your brain-body to bear and it is impossible for you to integrate the experience'.[2] This chapter explores the whole-body experience of trauma and the connection between the body and the mind in the processing and integration of experience. We are very familiar with the notion of 'making sense' of things with our minds (the cognitive parts of our brain) but much less familiar and comfortable with working with the 'felt sense' – the often overlooked yet hugely important source of information that comes from our bodies, and particularly our gut, or the 'enteric brain'.[3] Simple experiential exercises in group work enable participants in trauma-related training days to begin to recognise both their felt sense in naming the sensations that alert them to what they are feeling and the impact their felt sense has on everyday social interactions and decision making.

I also look at how we can work with trauma using the felt sense. Trauma is about the overwhelm of our capacity to cope and the breaking of connections. Working with trauma requires both the inward journey of reconnecting with the experience of our bodies where the traumatic memory resides and the outward journey of reconnecting with others who can accompany us with resonant warmth and keep us grounded in a sense of safety in the present. When stress hormones are coursing round bodies in a state of high alert and arousal, nervous systems are soothed and calmed by the presence and care of another alongside us, not so much in what they say but in the visceral sense of safety conveyed by being accompanied. In the final part of the chapter I look at how findings in neurobiology show that humans are 'made for relationship' in every aspect of our being and development.

What is trauma?

Our understanding of trauma, what it is, how it impacts people and how it can be worked with, is a relatively recent phenomenon, arising over the last 40 years or so from the research of psychiatrists, such as Peter Levine[4] and Bessel van der Kolk.[5] Work with the traumatic experience of army veterans returning from theatres of war, especially in Vietnam, led to the identification and acceptance of the term *Post-Traumatic Stress Disorder* (PTSD). Likewise, the recent development of brain-imaging tools has enabled scientists to see what actually happens inside the brains of traumatised people.[6]

2 Sarah Peyton, *Your Resonant Self: Guided Meditations and Exercises to Engage Your Brain's Capacity for Healing* (New York: W. W. Norton, 2017), xxvii.

3 Peyton, *Your Resonant Self*, 162–163.

4 Peter Levine, *In an Unspoken Voice: How the Body Releases Trauma and Restores Goodness* (Berkeley, CA: North Atlantic, 2010).

5 Bessel van der Kolk, *The Body Keeps the Score: Mind, Brain and Body in the Transformation of Trauma* (London: Random House, 2014).

6 Van der Kolk, *The Body Keeps the Score*, 21.

From these developments, the understanding emerged that trauma is not, as was previously thought as late as the 1990s, an irreversible biological disease.[7] It is not just an event that took place sometime in the past, but 'it is the imprint left by that experience on mind, brain and body' and has 'ongoing consequences for how the human organism manages to survive in the present'.[8] The fundamental discovery that has changed the way trauma is understood and how it may be worked with is the realisation that if someone is traumatised, this is primarily a physiological phenomenon, an experience that resides in the body and its responses. Stress hormones and their effects need to be discharged through working with the felt sense in the body in order then to enable the experience to be integrated psychologically and cognitively.

For those people in the cathedral that day, their response to what they saw or heard would have been instinctive and felt primarily in their bodies: orienting towards a sight, a sound, a movement; sensing the atmosphere from others around them; a tightening in the chest or clenching in the gut; tensing of the muscles in face and neck and legs as their bodies primed them to fight the potential threat for themselves or others or to get away as fast as possible.[9]

These automatic and physiological responses are entirely normal. They would have happened in milliseconds, triggered by the oldest part of the brain. This part of the brain works to keep the body safe and alive whenever humans are faced with a potentially life-threatening or dangerous situation. Peter Levine writes, 'When acutely threatened, we mobilize vast energies to protect and defend ourselves. We duck, dodge, twist, stiffen and retract. Our muscles contract to fight or flee. However, if our actions are ineffective, we freeze or collapse'.[10] These are the body's coping mechanisms that have evolved in humans from very early times. 'We are wired to survive', Haines writes in his accessible introduction to trauma. '[W]e would not be here as a human species unless we had evolved ways of recovering from that lion attack, (or sudden loss of a loved one, or being abused, or being in an accident . . .)'.[11]

In an experience of trauma, the fight/flight or freeze responses are triggered when our normal capacities and resources to cope with a situation are overwhelmed. We shall see this in more detail later. If fight or flight is clearly not possible, as for those caught in the Grenfell Tower fire (London, June 2017), for example, then the body systems shut down or freeze to protect the person from experiencing the worst effects of the situation. However, trauma research shows that humans are very resilient and that in

7 Levine, *Waking the Tiger*, 37.
8 Van der Kolk, *The Body Keeps the Score*, 21.
9 Levine, *In an Unspoken Voice*, 43.
10 Levine, *In an Unspoken Voice*, 23.
11 Haines, *Trauma Is Really Strange*, 8.

communities or groups affected by a single disaster, 9 out of 10 people will naturally recover and learn and grow from the experience, many emerging stronger and wiser after being overwhelmed.[12]

For the verger in the cathedral that day, adrenaline and cortisol flooded her body in response to the scream and the horrifying sight and sound of the body as it hit the floor. Before she could even think about it, she found herself running towards the scene to see what she could do, issuing instructions to the steward, who had also arrived to cordon off the area with chairs and move others away. She had been a paramedic previously and so knew how to administer CPR. Unfortunately, the injuries were far too great, and the fallen body could not be revived. The ambulance crew arrived and took over, but the verger knew she had done what she could. Although she was shaken and upset by the event, she was able in due course to recover from it and return to normal functioning because she had been able to discharge her stress hormones in positive action; she had been able *to do* something – to have agency in the situation – even though she had been unable to save the person's life.

Trauma lies not in the event itself but in how it has an impact on us – and the degree of impact will depend on our ability to respond and on previous experiences. Another person working in a different part of the cathedral that day (who therefore did not see the falling body) felt overwhelmed on hearing about what had happened and wanted to escape, finding it very difficult over the next few days to come back into the building. If we have experienced trauma previously that has not been processed and integrated, that previous experience will have produced physiological changes in our brains and bodies. Prior trauma shapes our physiology and affects our capacity to adapt and be resilient. Prior trauma could be developmental trauma from childhood or specific traumatising events in adulthood, which may have caused the loss of meaningful things (a loved one, home, job, marriage) or injury or simply shock. These events will not hold the same meaning for everyone. As van der Kolk explains, '[b]eing traumatized means continuing to organise your life as if the trauma were still going on – unchanged and immutable – as every new encounter is contaminated by the past'.[13]

How the brain and body respond to traumatic situations

A simple, but useful, model of the brain is tripartite:[14]

1 The brain stem, situated where the spinal cord enters the base of the skull, is the oldest part of the brain. It is sometimes called the reptilian brain as it shares evolutionary aspects with ancient animal brains. It

12 Haines, *Trauma Is Really Strange*, 14.
13 Van der Kolk, *The Body Keeps the Score*, 53.
14 Van der Kolk, *The Body Keeps the Score*, 59.

is the first part of the brain to develop in babies in the womb, responsible for basic human functioning; breathing, eating, sleeping, feeling discomfort, pain and ridding the body of toxins. The brain stem and the hypothalamus that sits directly above it control the energy levels of the body and the basic housekeeping and life-sustaining functions of the body, keeping them in a relatively healthy balance known as 'homeostasis'. This is also known as the autonomic nervous system as it can override the cognitive functioning of the brain to keep the body alive. If you try to hold your breath using your thinking brain, for example, your autonomic nervous system will eventually kick in and force you to breathe.

2 The limbic system is also known as the mammalian brain because all animals that live in groups and nurture their young possess one.[15] It is the seat of emotion, feeling, pleasure, the monitoring of danger and reproductive and parental behaviour. It is the area that enables us to negotiate our complex social networks and the place where fight/flight/freeze responses are generated. The way that this part of the brain develops is very much dependent on what happens to a baby through its experiences and explorations in early life, predisposing a child towards certain perceptions of and responses to the world. If a child feels safe and loved in early experience, the brain creates pathways disposed towards play, exploration, and cooperation; if a child feels frightened, unwanted, or abused, it specialises in managing feelings of fear, abandonment and threat. The technical term for this is 'neuroplasticity'. A simple way to express this is that neurons that 'fire together, wire together'. These connections are not immutable and can be 'rewired' or modified by later experiences in life, both, for the better, by positive, resonant relationships or, for the worse, through experiences such as bullying, abuse or chronic stress.[16]

3 The cerebral cortex, sometimes called the 'neo-mammalian brain', is the most recently evolved part of the human brain, the largest part of which is the neocortex. This is involved in higher functions such as sensory perception, abstraction, spatial reasoning, conscious thought, language, planning, imagination, creativity and empathy and inhibits inappropriate behaviour.

Van der Kolk describes the first two parts of the brain, the brain stem and the limbic system, as the 'emotional brain'. This is the gateway for all the information coming in from our inner and outer worlds and is the seat of emotion and memory. Its main task is to look out for our welfare in responding to both negative and positive stimuli in our physical and social environments. The cerebral cortex, the 'rational brain', is more complicated

15 Van der Kolk, *The Body Keeps the Score*, 56.
16 Van der Kolk, *The Body Keeps the Score*, 56–57.

in structure and biochemistry and, in normal functioning, works together with the emotional brain to appraise and evaluate what has happened and how to respond.

When humans are under threat, however, this system is disrupted.

At the heart of the limbic system is the amygdala, the early warning system of the brain. This is constantly scanning the physical and social environment – as much as 100 times a second – asking, 'Am I safe?' and 'Do I matter?'[17] If the amygdala detects a potential threat it sounds the alarm within 12 milliseconds, and the hypothalamus releases a flow of chemicals to the pituitary and adrenal glands to release a flood of stress hormones, including cortisol and adrenaline, to prepare the body for action and survival (fight or flight). The connection between the limbic system and the cerebral cortex is turned off so that we can act instinctively. For example, if we see something that looks like a snake in the grass, the body is startled and jumps back. 50 to 250 milliseconds later, the prefrontal cortex comes back on-line, and we realise 'the snake' is only a coiled rope. However, if the threat is real and life-threatening, the stress responses of fight or flight escalate, and the connections with the neocortex, including the left hemisphere of the prefrontal cortex, which has functions associated with linear, rational thinking, and the ability to translate experience into words, are fragmented. We can literally become wordless.[18] If it is impossible to flee or fight and we can do nothing to escape the danger, the body's response is to switch off the escalating stress hormones. Natural opioids are secreted by the nervous system to limit the experience of pain and induce a dream-like state. The whole-body system goes into a state of helplessness and immobilisation. In effect, the person 'disappears' and enters a state of dissociation in which connections with self, others and reality are broken. As Haines writes, '[d]issociation is one of the biggest precursors to getting lost in trauma responses. The inability to feel the body and lack of connection to our internal experience often leads to pain and depression'.[19]

Whether the perceived threat is real or imagined, the body systems shift into highly energised states and if we are able to metabolise that energy successfully in fight or flight, or the threat passes and we are able to return from a state of immobilisation through metabolising the hormones (often through physically shaking) then we are left feeling relaxed and satisfied – even heroic.[20] What is also crucial in enabling the nervous system gradually to return to balance is being oriented and grounded in the present by the warm and caring presence of another or within a caring community. This is vital in generating a whole-body sense of safety so that the neocortex can strengthen its connections with the limbic system and process and integrate the experience.

17 Peyton, *Your Resonant Self*, 26.
18 Van der Kolk, *The Body Keeps the Score*, 45.
19 Haines, *Trauma Is Really Strange*, 21.
20 Levine, *Waking the Tiger*, 128, 145.

If the stress hormones cannot be discharged in effective action or resolution in the face of the traumatic event(s), then the person may become trapped in the hyperarousal state of fight/flight. The feelings of irritation–anger–rage (fight) or unease–anxiety–panic (flight) get 'stuck' in the limbic system and in the body, especially in the gut. The amygdala and the hippocampus (another limbic structure) both record memory, but the amygdala 'takes a snapshot' of the traumatic experience as it is happening in the present and records the emotions and feelings being experienced in the body and psyche.[21] In processing and integrating a painful or difficult experience, this 'implicit memory' from the amygdala is transferred to the hippocampus as a memory that is 'date-stamped' and filed away as an experience in the past. If this process is not completed, then the implicit memory stays in the amygdala so that when danger signals are detected in the future, especially those that may connect with the original traumatic experience – a sight, a sound, a smell or touch – then the amygdala goes into overdrive and the person experiences again the traumatic sensations of fear, panic and overwhelm *as though they were in the present, here and now*. When the memory of the original experience has been 'filed' in the hippocampus and made explicit, then the person has more capacity to register that something similar has triggered a state of high arousal and alert from the amygdala but that the original experience was 'then', and this is 'now', thus keeping in touch with the resources to cope and build resilience.

If a traumatic experience, either as a one-off event or as a repeated or developmental experience, has been beyond what the person can bear, rendering them helpless and unable to take any action to escape or defend themselves, then, as described earlier, the person will fall into a state of immobilisation where the only way to survive the unbearable sensations and pain in body or psyche is to dissociate and split off the experience. This is a difficult state to return from as people are often unaware of the origin of their alienation,[22] and can get stuck in an inability to feel in touch with themselves and their bodies, leading to depression, anxiety, panic attacks, addictive behaviours, rigid control of themselves and their environment and autoimmune illnesses. Traumatised individuals have vigilance about and sensitivity to threat which has a physiological basis – the symptoms have their origin in the entire body's response to the original trauma, and as van der Kolk puts it, 'the body keeps the score'.[23]

Working with the felt sense

One of the benefits of recent research in neurobiology, and the growing understanding of how trauma works in the body and brain, has been an

21 Peyton, *Your Resonant Self*, 108–112.
22 Van der Kolk, *The Body Keeps the Score*, 67.
23 Van der Kolk, *The Body Keeps the Score*, 11.

increased understanding of how healthy functioning occurs to enhance well-being and resilience in our lives and relationships. Levine speaks of learning to hear 'the unspoken voice of the body'.[24] He argues for the need for us all to acknowledge our biological commonality as instinctual beings, 'linked not only by our common vulnerability to fright but by our innate capacity to transform such experiences'.[25] The 'Felt Sense', a concept originating with the work of Eugene Gendlin in his book, *Focusing*, is not a mental experience but a physical one: a bodily awareness of a situation or person or event.[26] Levine describes how the felt sense, even when we are not consciously aware of it, is telling us through our bodily sensations where we are and how we feel at any given moment – communicating our overall experience rather than interpreting it detail by detail.[27] It is the way we experience being in 'a living body that understands the nuances of its environment by way of its responses to that environment'.[28]

We all have sensations that we experience in our bodies, especially in the gut, bowels, chest, or in our breathing, temperature changes or tingling in the skin; this experience gives us clues as to what we may be feeling at that moment which we then identify as emotions such as fear, anger, anxiety, joy, excitement and anticipation. The felt sense is how we experience the self and is 'the most basic experience of being alive'.[29] It is not always easily conveyed in language, but it is what enables us to experience a holistic sense of goodness, creativity and connection with our inner experience, with others, and with our environment, as well as alerting us to a sense of dis-ease in the face of danger or threat. We may be familiar with the term *gut instincts*, but in our Western society, we often ignore or distrust these, being more reliant on our thinking capacities, modern technologies and medicine to solve our problems and heal our bodies. As we learn to become more aware of our inner experience, to be present to ourselves and to the information coming from our sensations or 'guts', we discover the innate capacity of the body and brain to work together to promote healing and wholeness.

How does this body–brain connection work?

Between the 1930s and 1950s, the concept of psychosomatic illness was accepted as the one-way effect of mind over body. This has been the principal understanding of how the mind–body connection operates.[30] More recent

24 Levine, *In an Unspoken Voice*, 10–11.

25 Levine, *Waking the Tiger*, 35.

26 Eugene Gendlin, *Focusing: How to Gain Access to Your Body's Knowledge* (London: Random House, 2003); cited by Levine, *Waking the Tiger*, 67.

27 Levine, *Waking the Tiger*, 69.

28 Levine, *Waking the Tiger*, 69.

29 Levine, *Waking the Tiger*, 70.

30 Levine, *Unspoken Voice*, 120–121.

research shows that within our gastrointestinal wall, we have a massive network of nerves – sensory and motor neurons – which integrates our digestive and eliminatory functions. It is an intricate and complex system that functions as a diffuse brain, known as the 'enteric brain'. It also produces beneficial hormones, including 95% of the serotonin, the 'feel-good' hormone in our bodies that lets our brain know all is well when the system is in balance.[31] The two-way high road between our enteric brain and the tripartite brain in the skull is through the vagus nerve, a hefty bundle of nerves that relays information about the state of our organs and digestive system to the brain. About 80% of the fibres in the vagal nerve run up from the gut to the brain, and only 20% run down from the brain to the gut.[32] So the vast majority of information that our brain is receiving on how we are and what we are feeling, which subliminally influences our decisions and actions, is coming from our felt sense that emanates from the gut, the enteric brain.

A simple exercise, used on teaching days on trauma to demonstrate the presence and power of the felt sense, is to ask two people to stand facing each other in very close proximity. They are asked just to notice and report the sensations this provokes in their bodies. Frequently, people first report their emotions – of discomfort, embarrassment, being a threat or feeling threatened. But when asked how they *know* they are feeling this, their attention is turned to the sensations in their bodies: tension in their muscles (neck, arms, legs), tension in the stomach or chest, clenching and unclenching of the fists, averting the eyes, shallow breathing, giggling, having a strong urge to move, prickling of the skin, sweating. They are then asked to move to a position that is more comfortable for them in relation to each other and to notice what happens in their body sensations. Upon this shift in position, people often report a softening and relaxing in their muscles, a sense of well-being and calm; face muscles relax into a smile, eyes connect, and the presence of the other is experienced as supportive rather than threatening. In this exercise, people can begin to notice the power of the felt sense and the information it can give them in the experience of their nervous systems being both stimulated and calmed, within themselves and in relation to the other.

We sense threat or danger through our external sense organs (sight, hearing), and we also sense it directly through our internal sense organs (the gut and muscles), as in the exercise just described. Tension in the muscles, speeding up of the heart rate or churning in the stomach may be the first indication we have that we are sensing danger. The vagal nerve stimulates the body into action (fight or flight) through its fast lane or shuts the body systems down (immobilisation or dissociation) through switching to its slow lane. Thus, the vagal nerve is the means by which 'the body shifts the way it uses energy and how it relates to the outer world in complete dependence on

31 Levine, *Unspoken Voice*, 120–121.
32 Peyton, *Your Resonant Self*, 135.

how safe we believe the environment is'.[33] When we are relaxed and feeling safe our nervous systems enable us to explore, learn, grow and, importantly, to negotiate the complexities of social engagement, especially through sensing or 'reading' in others the tightening or relaxing of the face muscles, the focus of the eyes, and attuning to particular tones of voice.

When we are engaging well with someone, we find ourselves mirroring each other in body position, tone of voice and emotional tone. However, our capacity for mirroring also makes us vulnerable to others' negativity so that we respond to anger with mounting anger or are dragged down by another's negativity or depression.[34] Sarah Peyton describes how, 'as social animals, people get caught up in one another's cascading nervous systems'.[35] We can sense when the atmosphere in a conversation or in a meeting is warm and engaged or frosty and more hostile, and we can feel our own internal systems relax or tense up in response. However, in situations of potential danger, when the body is flooded by stress hormones, we lose connection with our thinking, rational part of the brain, and the ability to 'read' others and to engage with them at the complex level of which we would be capable when things are calm.[36] Instead, when we see or sense another's fearful, tense posture, our mirroring kicks in at a more instinctive level to tense and orient ourselves to our physical environment – 'What's the proximity of the threat; where's my line of escape?' – and in relation to others – 'Who else is with me here; who can help?' Just as with a herd of deer in the wild, the first to sense the threat of a predator will tense, with head and hears erect, and that tension and alertness will very quickly spread through the rest of the herd in readiness to respond. We rapidly and instinctively read the bodies and postures of others, even more than their faces, as recent research has demonstrated.[37] Levine calls this ability to read facial and body posture as cues to danger or fear, which bypasses the conscious mind in order to enable us to take immediate action, 'postural resonance'.[38] Through our felt sense, we resonate with the sensations and emotions of others, feeling what others feel, communicating non-verbally through postures and expressive emotions, and thus, as Levine concludes, making 'our deepest communications through empathy'.[39]

Getting in touch with the felt sense

Being able to access and trust the felt sense is key to working with trauma, but this sense is the very thing that is fragmented and defended against if

33 Peyton, *Your Resonant Self*, 135.
34 Peyton, *Your Resonant Self*, 59.
35 Peyton, *Your Resonant Self*, 137.
36 Peyton, *Your Resonant Self*, 136.
37 Levine, *Unspoken Voice*, 41–43. Levine is here borrowing from neuroscientist, Beatrice Gelder.
38 Levine, *Unspoken Voice*, 4.
39 Levine, *Unspoken Voice*, 42.

a person is traumatised. If someone has been unable to find agency and metabolise stress hormones in the face of a horrific event or events and balance has not been able to be restored, then feelings of pain, horror, rage, fear, panic and, often, shame at their response or lack of it, become trapped in the body, in the visceral senses, and are suppressed.[40] The person is stuck in a state of hypervigilance, seeking to control or avoid anything that may trigger re-experiencing the sensations and feelings. This means they can be over-reactive to life's everyday disappointments, frustrations and challenges.

Healing individual trauma, therefore, means enabling someone to get back in touch with the sensations and messages coming from their bodies through the 'felt sense', in order to discharge the unfinished business in the autonomic nervous system. Only then can the person 'make sense' of their experience. Van der Kolk observes that for the person stuck in a state of trauma, 'the rational brain is basically impotent to talk the emotional brain out of its own reality'.[41] Therefore, talking therapies that are effective in other contexts are not necessarily appropriate in the first instance in the context of trauma, as they risk the person being overwhelmed again by their sensations and feelings. Victims are likely 'to tell a story of victimization and revenge rather than being able to notice, feel, and put into words the reality of their internal experience'.[42] Healing trauma is not so much about learning to accept what happened in the past as it is about learning to acknowledge and name our visceral sensations. Helpers can then work with the traumatised by strengthening the connections between their emotional and rational brains in order to learn greater self-regulation and the ability to stay grounded in the present.[43] We all have an innate capacity for self-regulation – even if the amygdala is firing an early warning in response to possible threat or danger, so long as we are not too upset, we can learn to bring our prefrontal cortex back on-line faster and strengthen its capacity to stay connected. Neuroscientific research shows that techniques such as meditation and mindfulness increase activation of the medial prefrontal cortex and decrease activation of structures like the amygdala that trigger our emotional responses.[44] Van der Kolk describes how being able 'to hover calmly and objectively over our thoughts, feelings, and emotions . . . and then take our time to respond allows the executive brain to inhibit, organize, and modulate the hardwired automatic reactions programmed into the emotional brain'.[45] Self-regulation is the bedrock of resilience, allowing us to make a ready transition between intense emotional states and to maintain equilibrium and sanity.[46]

40 Levine, *Waking the Tiger*, 145.
41 Van der Kolk, *The Body Keeps the Score*, 47.
42 Van der Kolk, *The Body Keeps the Score*, 47.
43 Van der Kolk, *The Body Keeps the Score*, 68–70.
44 Van der Kolk, *The Body Keeps the Score*, 284.
45 Van der Kolk, *The Body Keeps the Score*, 62.
46 Levine, *Unspoken Voice*, 17.

Learning to strengthen our capacity for self-regulation means being able to face uncomfortable and frightening physical sensations and feelings without being overwhelmed by them.[47] This means learning to work with and trust our felt sense, which we do by learning to recognise the physiological sensations in our bodies that underlie our emotional reactions. As Levine observes, 'sensations come from symptoms, and symptoms come from compressed energy; that energy is what we have to work with in this process'.[48] Being open, curious, and kind towards ourselves as we learn to be aware of our sensations enables us just to notice them without judgement and without trying to change them or rush to attach meaning to them. Meaning will be important in the later stages, but just noticing our sensations brings them into awareness and frequently results in shifts and changes in them as tension is released and blocked energies can flow again, but always at their own pace.[49] For the traumatised person, getting in touch with the felt sense, and the awful sensations and feelings that have been defended against or split off, has to be a carefully calibrated process to avoid the person being overwhelmed again. This is similar to the process in chemistry where two opposing substances are gradually introduced to each other, drip by drip, to avoid an explosion.[50] So in a supported and well-contained environment, the traumatised person is invited to notice only so much as he or she can bear at each stage while being kept grounded in the present and resourced by the accompaniment of another.

How well we have learnt to recognise our inner feelings and needs, as well as how to regulate them in order to cope with life's ups and downs, depends very much on how well we have been nurtured and resourced in our development in our family and educational networks, or 'systems'. Experiences of neglect, abuse, horrific events, or witnessing the experience of others, can be traumatising for a child and can have an impact on their development and ability to be resilient in the face of future difficult and potentially traumatic experiences. Recent developments in neuroscience and epigenetics show that high levels of stress and anxiety in the mother can be passed on to the baby in the womb so that the baby is born with higher levels of adrenaline and cortisol, thus predisposing the baby to react more strongly to stressful stimuli.[51]

One method of exploring traumatic experience and memory, 'Systems Constellations',[52] uses people or tabletop objects to represent and map

47 Levine, *Unspoken Voice*, 15.

48 Levine, *Waking the Tiger*, 72–83.

49 Levine, *Waking the Tiger*, 72–83.

50 Levine, *Unspoken Voice*, 24.

51 Levine, *Unspoken Voice*, 91.

52 John Whittington, *Systemic Coaching & Constellations: The Principles, Practices and Application for Individuals, Teams and Groups* (2nd Ed.; London/Philadelphia, PA: Kogan Page, 2016). Systems constellations is an applied philosophy that enables people to explore webs

elements of an experience, enabling the person to look at that experience with the 'felt sense' and shift his or her bodily perception of the experience. They are then able to 'make sense' of it and integrate it so that it becomes a past memory rather than a repeating and fearful experience that dominates the present.

The process of *naming* sensations and feelings is a crucial step in self-regulation and resolving trauma. Although the brain expends huge amounts of effort trying to bury and keep at bay sensations and feelings to do with trauma, they still intrude on our lives and relationships, and we feel at the mercy of them and cannot understand where they come from. Sarah Peyton describes how, when emotional experience has not been named, 'it is still present in the body'.[53] 'Magic happens for our brains', she says, 'when we put precise words to what is happening for us'.[54] Magnetic resonance imaging scans reveal that naming what is happening soothes and regulates emotional alarm,[55] and calms the nerves that are firing in the amygdala.[56] It also allows the neuroplasticity of the brain to lay down new connections between the neurons and strengthen the self-regulating connections between the rational and emotional brain. The warm, resonant presence of another person is enhanced by helping the traumatised person to identify the sensations and name the emotions he or she is experiencing. When we can name our emotions precisely, they become available to work with so that we can begin to identify what they are telling us and what we need for healing.

Conversely, research has shown that the experience of not being received or believed, especially in relation to rape or sexual abuse, compounds the experience of trauma.[57] Van der Kolk states that '[t]rauma almost invariably involves not being seen, not being mirrored, and not being taken into account – treatment needs to reactivate the capacity to safely mirror, and be mirrored by, others'.[58] Conversely, it does not help to talk about our feelings if we feel judged, criticised, not taken seriously or believed or at the receiving end of someone else's 'fix-it' energy.[59] Levine underscores how important it is for therapists working with traumatised people to be fully present to the person, alongside them in the vulnerability of having attuned to their own process and engaged with 'their own traumas and emotional wounds'.[60] This stance of the 'wounded healer' as guide and collaborator in

---

of relationships and belonging in their systems and the impact of hidden dynamics within them.

53 Peyton, *Your Resonant Self*, 37.

54 Peyton, *Your Resonant Self*, 46.

55 Peyton, *Your Resonant Self*, 47.

56 Peyton, *Your Resonant Self*, 31.

57 Peyton, *Your Resonant Self*, 117–119, citing 2010 research into Nepalese boy soldiers.

58 Van der Kolk, *The Body Keeps the Score*, 59.

59 Peyton, *Your Resonant Self*, 47.

60 Levine, *Unspoken Voice*, 34–35.

the journey towards healing and wholeness is one very familiar to those in Christian ministry.[61]

'Made for relationship'

Human beings flourish in relationship with others – neurobiologists and theologians alike affirm this core principle of being and becoming.[62] We thrive and grow, from our earliest development onwards, if we are in the presence of those who genuinely care for us, believe in us, are solid and dependable, and are attuned to help us process and integrate difficult emotions and experiences. This is how humans learn resilience; through experiencing that bad things can happen but discovering that we can survive them and learn from them, drawing on our own resources and the resource of others alongside us – bad things will pass and good things also happen. However, for the traumatised person, the belief and experience tend to be 'It will always be like this'. The traumatised person is unable to imagine anything different and is stuck in confusing and frightening feelings that need to be kept at bay. As Levine says, '[t]he importance of the human ability to move through "bad" and difficult sensations, opening to those of expansion and "goodness", cannot be overstated: it is pivotal for the healing of trauma and more generally, the alleviation of suffering'.[63]

According to van der Kolk, the factor that makes the biggest difference in working with trauma in ourselves or others, either at the time of the traumatic event or subsequently, is the warm, resonant presence of another.[64] When we experience resonance and warmth from others, the natural flow of all the calming neurotransmitters increases and strengthens neural connections for bonding and self-regulation.[65] Resonance happens when we have a sense that the other person really 'gets us',[66] that we are truly heard and seen by them and held in their mind and heart. Simply being there alongside someone in a situation of trauma, showing your concern and warmth, not necessarily with words but through facial expressions, gestures, touch, a cup of tea, a blanket, staying with the person till help arrives, all this calms the nervous system and keeps the person grounded in him- or herself and in the present. The feeling of safety that this engenders is something that is felt in the body through the autonomic nervous system and helps us metabolise the stress hormones. In other words, 'people cannot relax until they know in

61 See, for example, Henri J. M. Nouwen, *The Wounded Healer* (London: Darton, Longman and Todd, 2014).

62 John Swinton, *Raging with Compassion: Pastoral Responses to the Problem of Evil* (Cambridge, UK: Wm. B. Eerdmans, 2007), 204; Peyton, *Your Resonant Self*, 47.

63 Levine, *Unspoken Voice*, 78–79.

64 Van der Kolk, *The Body Keeps the Score*, 79.

65 Peyton, *Your Resonant Self*, 45, 89.

66 Peyton, *Your Resonant Self*, 43.

their gut that they are safe'.[67] This applies not only to our physical environment but also in our social environment – the amygdala scans the scene, asking, 'Do I belong here? Do I matter? If I speak will people listen?'[68] Sensing the answer 'yes', from the warm attention of a person or a community of people who are truly present to us provides the safety and containment that we need to visit difficult experiences and emotions and to flourish and grow. Van der Kolk refers to numerous studies of disaster response around the globe that show that 'social support is the most powerful protection against becoming overwhelmed by stress and trauma'.[69]

The implications of this for congregations and pastoral care are immense, and Kate Wiebe explores them in her chapter on collective trauma. Congregations have in their 'DNA' the call to love one another, to bear one another's burdens, patterned on the relationship of love between God, Father, Son, and Holy Spirit (Gal 6:2). Physiological understandings of trauma help us to understand the significance and healing power of the way we are with one another. As van der Kolk observes, '[n]o doctor can write a prescription for friendship and love: these are complex and hard-earned capacities'.[70] The theologian John Swinton writes of love informing the telos of human beings and affirms that 'we are made to love, and all of our lives we seek after loving relationships'.[71] Richard Rohr, a Franciscan priest and teacher, reflecting on the Rublev Icon of the Trinity, writes that '[i]n the beginning was the relationship'. In the icon, Rohr suggests, the empty fourth place at the table is the invitation to each of us to find our place in a radical inclusivity of all creation.[72] Theologians such as Swinton and Miroslav Volf[73] emphasise that we become persons in community not as the result of a self-directed, autonomous project: 'Our personhood is constituted by our relationships with the other, and ultimately with God'.[74]

The experience of trauma strikes at the very heart of humans' capacity for relationship. Levine describes how the indigenous peoples of South America use the word *susto* to describe what happens in trauma, which translates as 'fright paralysis' or 'soul loss', experienced as 'the bereft feeling of losing your way in the world, of being severed from your very soul'.[75] This can be the result not only of a sudden traumatic experience but also of traumatising relationships, which 'are like slow poison, slowly but surely killing the soul

67 Peyton, *Your Resonant Self*, 153.
68 Peyton, *Your Resonant Self*, 153.
69 Van der Kolk, *The Body Keeps the Score*, 79.
70 Van der Kolk, *The Body Keeps the Score*, 79.
71 Swinton, *Raging with Compassion*, 198.
72 Richard Rohr with Mike Morrell, *The Divine Dance* (London: SPCK, 2016), 30.
73 Miroslav Volf, *After Our Likeness: The Church as the Image of the Trinity* (Cambridge, UK: Wm. B. Eerdmans, 1998).
74 Swinton, *Raging with Compassion*, 203.
75 Levine, *Unspoken Voice*, 31–32.

of the affected person'.[76] Sarah Peyton describes the experience of contempt or scorn as a 'discounting or dismissal of the other' that 'removes people from even existing as human'.[77] She continues: 'The dismissal of humans as not being worth the air they breathe is at the root of the worst evil that we can do to one another'.[78] Mariéle Wulf, a Dutch theologian, writes that '[t]he first principle of love is to *confirm existence*. It is good that you exist'.[79] For love to effect this, it must be unconditional, selfless, and trustworthy – I love you as you are, not for what you are, and this is true for all time. 'This is the essence of unconditional love – the love God gives eternally'.[80] It is the love embodied in the person of Jesus Christ through whom the trauma of sin, of broken connection and of broken relationship is restored and healed.

Conclusion

Levine writes, 'The paradox of trauma is that it has both the power to destroy and the power to transform and resurrect', depending on how we approach it.[81] For the cathedral community in the following days and weeks after the tragedy of the suicide, opportunities were provided on an individual and group level to facilitate the processing and integration of their experience. Information was given about the nature of trauma and, especially, about how the same event can impact people very differently. The importance of people's natural capacity to be alongside one another with kindness and warmth was affirmed. Practical learning about responding to such events was captured.

Personal and community resilience is built in the experience of 'coming through' such experiences while still sometimes bearing the scars of such experience. I am reminded of the Japanese tradition of 'Kintsugi', where a precious porcelain bowl or cup that has been broken is then pieced back together again with gold-infused resin, creating a differently beautiful item, with the experience of brokenness traced in its veins of gold.

Select references

Haines, Steve. *Trauma Is Really Strange*. London: Jessica Kingsley, 2016.

Levine, Peter A. *Waking the Tiger: Healing Trauma*. Berkeley: North Atlantic, 1997.

76 Mariéle Wulf, 'Trauma in Relationship – Healing by Religion: Restoring Dignity and Meaning After Traumatic Experiences', in *Lived Religion: Transcending the Ordinary*, ed. R. Ruard Ganzevoort and Srdjan Sremac (Cham, Switzerland: Palgrave Macmillan, 2019), 129–151, 129.

77 Peyton, *Your Resonant Self*, 209.

78 Peyton, *Your Resonant Self*, 209.

79 Wulf, 'Trauma in Relationship', 139.

80 Wulf, 'Trauma in Relationship', 139.

81 Levine, *Unspoken Voice*, 37.

Levine, Peter A. *In an Unspoken Voice: How the Body Releases Trauma and Restores Goodness*. Berkeley: North Atlantic, 2010.

Peyton, Sarah. *Your Resonant Self: Guided Meditations and Exercises to Engage Your Brain's Capacity for Healing*. London: W.W. Norton, 2017.

Whittington, John. *Systemic Coaching & Constellations: The Principles, Practices and Application for Individuals, Teams and Groups*, 2nd ed. London/Philadelphia: Kogan Page, 2016.

4 Toward a faith-based approach to healing after collective trauma

Kate Wiebe

This chapter employs Kai Erikson's sociological approach to identifying and observing the character of both collective trauma and collective healing in order to consider the role faith leaders, in particular, play in encouraging survivors as they (re)build trust amid a history of pain.[1] To begin, this chapter reviews Erikson's coining of the term *collective trauma* as well as the way in which he views traditional approaches to diagnosing and treating trauma as obstructing the possibility of more full understandings of how individuals and groups respond to adversity. This chapter highlights how few studies exist that focus primarily on how *community spirits*, too, can break and mend as a result of trauma as well as how groups (including families, schools, businesses, and church communities) participate effectively in expanding care and healing. Placing salient insights from psychologist Jack Saul in conversation with Erikson in order to gain further understanding of how communities innately can enact healing and restoration following catastrophic events, this chapter reviews key practices conducted by communities that prevail beyond tragedy including networks of collaborative response conducted through partnerships of Volunteer Organizations Active in Disaster (VOAD) in the United States. Finally, the chapter concludes with recommendations for clergy and ministry leaders to practically expand care and foster the rebuilding of trust among individuals, families, and their communities in order to encourage restoration and resilience in post-disaster settings.

Defining trauma: first, what broke?

Do all car accidents result in the same experiences for those who survive them? Do natural disasters cause the same levels of distress and destruction for those most directly affected? Why do some people appear to move beyond experiences of war and into vibrant relationships and careers, while others end up thoroughly debilitated and 'shell shocked'? These kinds of

1 Kai Erikson, *A New Species of Trouble: The Human Experience of Modern Disasters* (New York: WW Norton, 1994).

questions pique the curiosity of those – from esteemed scholars to ordinary neighbors – who finds catchall notions of pain or suffering unsettling. Such questions underscore the ways in which colloquial notions about how *time heals all wounds* or admonishments to *move on* fall short of lived experience and uphold the ways in which the residue of traumatic stress can linger with survivors across a lifetime and even across generations. What really gives way to a person or group enduring adversity *like water off a duck's back* while others seem to run around *like a chicken with its head cut off*? What does it mean to be witnesses of Jesus Christ amid a world of brokenness and heartache? To answer these questions best, one must first identify what of 'the heart' aches and what actually has broken.

Unfortunately, traditional approaches to treating trauma have inhibited effective curing practices by directing attention to what caused injury rather than the character of injury expressed by survivors. Why focus on the character of the result over the cause? It turns out that illness and healing both lie in the eye of the beholder. Put another way, the event does not necessarily dictate the result. Thus, in many cases, any approach that prioritizes the incident above the impact leads toward a dismissal of real claims of suffering, ultimately deeming them as either unwarranted or, worse, fictitious.

Through his pioneering mid-twentieth century examinations of the ways disaster affects groups, as well as how groups, and not only individuals, participate in restorative processes, sociologist Kai Erikson flips this archaic approach around and seeks instead to identify more useful routes toward healing by spotlighting how the impact of and response to trauma manifest within groups.[2] In so doing, he tips his hat toward his father, developmental psychologist Erik Erikson, as well as esteemed theorists such as psychoanalytic pediatrician D.W. Winnicott and self-psychologist Heinz Kohut, and charts an entirely new course that deftly depicts how forms of *broken trust*, rather than tragic incidents themselves, instigate what many today would call 'post-traumatic stress symptoms', essentially ailments that can linger and plague individuals and groups for years and even generations. Thus, according to Erikson, not every car accident is the same. In fact, the nature and character of a traumatic incident, or series of events, assume widely ranging meaning for survivors. Erikson further posits that by not focusing investigations on matters such as the ranging residual lack of confidence in a survivor's ability to manage adversity, for example, or how the reliability of care relationships following trauma may manifest with a survivor or group, practitioners risk varying misappropriation or even complete negation of care. After all, trauma, like art, is in the eye of the beholder and healing, like business, happens at the *speed of trust*.[3] Therefore, when at any level trust is perceived by survivor(s) to be broken, healing is thwarted. Thankfully,

2 Erikson, *A New Species of Trouble*.

3 See Steven Covey, *Speed of Trust* (New York: Free Press, 2006).

although trust can be broken, trust also can be built and reestablished. Christian communities know this reality at their heart, and being trust-building agents in their communities is just one of the ways they contribute to preparedness and effective disaster response.

Defining trauma: the manifestation of brokenness

From the start, Erikson found foundational language and methodological approaches for diagnosing and treating trauma mostly unhelpful for interpreting his sociological findings. Prior to his work, medical and psychotherapeutic practitioners tended to diagnose trauma primarily according to the event that causes injury rather than to what Erikson refers to as *the blow*. Yet, focusing on the event (such as a car accident, loss of limb, loss of livelihood, etc.) too often leads to misconceptions and judgments rooted in biased comparisons of events or presumed gradations of impact rather than within observations of affect. Thus, by not allowing or assisting a survivor to identify what he or she perceives has broken physically, mentally, emotionally, and/or spiritually, practitioners risk misappropriating care or, worse, entirely negating opportunities for effective care at all. This more cumbersome approach, as Erikson sees it, obstructs the view of how tragic adversity affects individuals and groups as well as how best they can cope.

For example, consider this more recent finding; curious about the patterns of gaining weight among severely obese people in his clinic, particularly how these patients mostly would gain weight quickly and then stabilize or, after losing large amounts of weight, would quickly regain the weight, internist Vincent Felitti decided to conduct subsequent interviews with his patients.[4] To ascertain further insight into the history of their behavioural patterns, Felitti asked patients a series of questions: How much did you weigh when you were born? How much did you weigh when you started first grade? How much did you weigh when you entered high school? How old were you when you became sexually active? and How old were you when you married?

One time, he misspoke and asked a female patient, 'How much did you weigh when you became sexually active?' She answered, '40 pounds.' He thought that maybe she had misheard his mistake, and so he repeated the misspoken question. She repeated her answer the same, and then cried, before going on to describe experiences of incest she had endured as a child. Felitti and his colleagues then interviewed more patients with questions about potential past experiences of sexual abuse and discovered that most of the patients in their study had been sexually abused as children, although some patients had experienced sexual abuse or violence as adolescents or young adults. In

4 Jane E. Stevens, 'The Adverse Childhood Experiences Study: The Largest Public Health Study You Never Heard Of', *The Huffington Post*, 2017, www.huffingtonpost.com/jane-ellen-stevens/the-adverse-childhood-exp_1_b_1943647.html

the course of more extended interviews, patients described, too, how weight functioned as a kind of protective barrier from further sexual advances. Eventually, the investigators saw that all their patients shared something in common. Overeating, for them, was not a problem – it had become a solution.

Felitti and his colleagues had stumbled on a complex challenge in treating trauma – one that other traumatologists, too, had observed; sometimes, seemingly taboo activities serve a purpose in providing a survivor with more adequate care than perceived as otherwise achievable. Similarly to the answer to Felitti's accidental question in 1985, practitioners such as Herman,[5] Hudson,[6] Fonagy,[7] Jones,[8] Felitti and Anda,[9] Levine,[10] Rambo,[11] and van der Kolk[12] also encountered curiosities in their research and discerned ways in which traditional approaches to defining and treating persons who had experienced trauma had proved unhelpful in meeting their clients, patients, and members' needs. Through their studies, eventually, the reality that survivors of childhood, adolescent, and young adult adversity lacked confidence they could adequately resolve mental, emotional, or spiritual wounds in any ways other than by 'self-medicating' through abusive, obsessive, or addictive methods, emerged for scholars, which begs the questions: Can Christian churches or ministries offer more effective solutions for care than the temporary relief some survivors experience through alternative and more abusive, obsessive, or addicting means of perceived relief? If so, then, in what ways?

An essential ingredient to healing: (re)building trust

According to Erikson, the experience of trauma involves a blow to the tissues of the body or to the structures of the mind resulting in lasting change:

> Something alien breaks in on you, smashing through whatever barriers your mind has set up as a line of defense. It invades you, possesses you, takes you over, becomes a dominating feature of your interior landscape, and in the process threatens to drain you and leave you empty.[13]

5 Judith Herman, *Trauma and Recovery: The Aftermath of Violence – From Domestic Abuse to Political Terror* (New York: Basic, 1997).

6 Jill Hudson, *Congregational Trauma* (New York: Rowman & Littlefield, 1998).

7 Peter Fonagy, 'The Transgenerational Transmission of Holocaust Trauma', *Attachment and Human Development* (1999): 92–114.

8 Serene Jones, *Trauma and Grace* (New York: Westminster, 2009).

9 Vincent J. Felitti and Robert F. Anda, 'The Relationship of Adverse Childhood Experiences to Adult Medical Disease, Psychiatric Disorders and Sexual Behavior: Implications for Healthcare', in *The Impact of Early Life Trauma on Health and Disease*, ed. Lanius et al. (Cambridge: Cambridge University Press, 2010).

10 Peter Levine, *In an Unspoken Voice* (New York: North Atlantic, 2010).

11 Shelly Rambo, *Spirit and Trauma* (New York: Westminster, 2010).

12 Bessel Van der Kolk, *The Body Keeps the Score: Brain, Mind and Body in the Healing of Trauma* (New York: Penguin, 2015).

13 Erikson, *A New Species*, 228.

More simply put, trauma breaks down your sense of trust in yourself, your relationships, and the world. Indeed, as Erikson says, traumatized people can stand out from the crowd. They

> scan the surrounding world anxiously for signs of danger, breaking into explosive rages and reacting with a start to ordinary sights and sounds, [and] at the same time all that nervous activity takes place against a numbed gray background of depression, feelings of helplessness.[14]

Despite needing or desiring more relational care, they simultaneously can exhibit 'a general closing off of [their personal] spirit as the mind tries to insulate itself from further harm'.[15] They struggle to participate in activities that previously gave them joy and often report feeling guilty for feeling happy. Survivors can feel the impacts of trauma 'radiating' through their days and nights, an experience that 'involves a continual reliving of some wounding experience in daydreams and nightmares, flashbacks and hallucinations, and in a compulsive seeking out of similar circumstances'.[16] Erikson succinctly summarizes how the echoes of tragedy can mar the lives of survivors in lasting ways: 'Our memory repeats to us what we haven't yet come to terms with, what still haunts us'.[17]

According to leading traumatologists, such as Erikson, Felitti and Anda, Levine and van der Kolk, trauma is a collection of physical, mental, emotional, and spiritual manifestations within the body of an individual or a group following an experience, or series of experiences, of stressful loss. While the collection of manifestations may transpire from a type of tangible loss (i.e., the loss of another person, of a limb, of a home), manifestations of trauma also can result from more intangible losses including, and not limited to, no longer feeling safe, no longer feeling confident in physical capacities, no longer feeling that others are reliable or caring, no longer feeling that one's personal space will be respected, or no longer feeling that leaders are trustworthy.

Trust in what is sensed physically, emotionally, mentally, and spiritually forms the undercurrent of what humans perceive as real. Human beings begin forming critical senses of *realness* in themselves, their relationships, and their world from birth. As babies, through practices of relational care, humans begin to trust in their personal value and the reliability of the care they experience from others, as well as the value of other persons and the value of the surrounding world. According to Erikson, 'human beings are surrounded by layers of trust, radiating out in concentric circles like the ripples in a pond',[18] and into their sense of relationship with God, family,

14 Erikson, *A New Species*, 228.
15 Erikson, *A New Species*, 228.
16 Erikson, *A New Species*, 228.
17 Erikson, *A New Species*, 228.
18 Erikson, *A New Species*, 242.

neighbors, co-workers, and leaders in their community, national, and the world. These bonds of belonging create forms of what Erikson calls *spiritual kinship*, or a sense of communal belonging, that humans rely on to varying extents for physical, mental, emotional, and spiritual nourishment throughout their lifetimes, both in times of peace and times of crises. The fact that 'the hardest earned and most fragile accomplishment of childhood, basic trust, can be damaged beyond repair by trauma' creates one of the greatest challenges for treating it individually or collectively.[19]

When trust breaks, survivors often struggle to know what remains reliable within themselves, their relationships, and in the world. Erikson notes how original medical and psychological approaches to treating either individual or collective trauma at times neglected the critical role of rebuilding these primary senses of trust in order to resolve health. 'The mortar bonding human communities together is made up, at least in part, of trust and respect and decency – and, in moments of crisis, of charity and concern. It is profoundly disturbing to people when these expectations are not met'.[20] Practitioners can further complicate the challenge survivors face by not naming 'the *state of mind* that ensues' following trauma. Instead, in these cases, *posttraumatic stress disorder* becomes a disorder 'named for the stimulus that brought it into being' rather than an acknowledgment of the 'persisting condition' of dis-ease related to a 'constellation of life experiences' for survivor(s).[21] In so doing, entire experiences of individual and collective trauma then go largely untreated:

> The experience of trauma, at its worst, can mean not only a loss of confidence in the self but a loss of confidence in the scaffolding of family and community, in the structures of human government, in the larger logics by which humankind lives, and in the ways of nature itself.[22]

Both tangible and intangible losses break down the bonds of belonging or attachment to one's self, family, previous friendships, and other groups, including social clubs, churches, schools, and places of work that make up the contours in which growth happens.

Unfortunately, for too long, too few heard Erikson's clarion call that trauma

> can issue from a sustained exposure to battle as well as from a moment of numbing shock, from a continuing pattern of abuse as well as from a single searing assault, from a period of severe attenuation and erosion as well as from a sudden flash of fear.[23]

19 Erikson, *A New Species*, 242.
20 Erikson, *A New Species*, 239.
21 Erikson, *A New Species*, 229.
22 Erikson, *A New Species*, 242.
23 Erikson, *A New Species*, 230.

Moreover, he would add, trauma can convert a single incident into an enduring state of mind, and survivors can relive the past to such an extent that the 'moment becomes a season; the event becomes a condition',[24] perhaps even far beyond whatever any bystander or practitioner may judge a stimulating event to imbue. Thus, for decades, various social service agents would struggle to fully recognize how experiences with adversity, including and not limited to intimate partner and domestic violence, sexual abuse, emotional neglect, or moral injury, could manifest in seemingly similar ways to experiences of losing a limb, surviving a car accident, or going to war. Unsurprising, practitioners also struggled to see how groups also could exhibit collective manifestations, like individuals, following experiences with shared trauma.

Defining trauma: collective experience

Following investigations of several community disasters, including devastating flooding and acts of violence, Erikson concludes:

> Sometimes the tissues of community can be damaged in much the same way as the tissues of mind and body, [and] even when that does not happen, traumatic wounds inflicted on individuals can combine to create a mood, an ethos – a group culture, almost – that is different from (and more than) the sum of the private wounds that make it up.[25]

Erikson coins this phenomenon *collective trauma*. He notes how 'one can speak of a damaged social organism in almost the same way that one would speak of a damaged body'.[26]

While collective trauma may result from a singular sudden and shocking event, Erikson makes clear post-traumatic stress occurs for many reasons, and collective trauma, in particular, can take two forms. For one, 'damage to the tissues that hold human groups intact', he observes as emerging as a shared sense that in some way the connectedness the group previously experienced has ruptured. For the second, following a shared critical incident, a new sense of community also may emerge, and 'the creation of social climates, communal moods' can 'come to dominate a group's spirit' as a result of trauma.[27] Church and ministry leaders do well to consider the multifaceted ways traumatic stress can manifest in complex forms among individuals, families, and groups, including these two forms of results from collective trauma. For example, approaching the existence of trauma from the view of how a blow to the tissues of an individual or corporate body manifests itself helps practitioners observe more effectively how collective trauma may

24 Erikson, *A New Species*, 230.
25 Erikson, *A New Species*, 231.
26 Erikson, *A New Species*, 234.
27 Erikson, *A New Species*, 237.

also emerge following a series of losses and the 'gradual realization that the community no longer exists as an effective source of support and that an important part of the [previous sense of group identity] has disappeared . . . "we" no longer exist' with the mutual sense of belonging as we once did.[28] Interestingly, a kind of spiritual kinship also can transpire among people who have shared common experiences of trauma, through a shared sense of identity.[29] Communal moods following shared adversity may be positive and generative, leading toward new growth, or they may prove detrimental and function to maintain a more pervasive sense of remaining stuck. In some cases, the incidents 'force open whatever fault lines once ran silently through the structure of the larger community, dividing it into divisive fragments'.[30] Common traumatic experiences can 'work their way so thoroughly into the grain of the affected community that they come to . . . govern the way its members relate to one another'.[31]

Psychologist Jack Saul, Director of the International Trauma Studies Program at Columbia University, largely concurs with Erikson's observations of how groups struggle through healing processes after trauma, create either new bonds or new forms of fragmentation, and, at times, prove unable to find their way through together.[32] In fact, he observes,

> On occasion, the aftermath of a traumatic event may cause more harm than the event itself. Social fragmentation at work and school, and the ensuing conflict, was more painful and destabilizing for many New York City residents than the events of September 11 itself, for instance.[33]

This phenomenon shows another example of why approaching the treatment of individual or collective trauma by what the survivor experiences as meaningful in the aftermath of overwhelming stress is critical to effective treatment. Otherwise, practitioners risk treating a presumed wound versus the actual, or more complex, wound(s).

Individual and collective trauma treatment: practical Christian care for constellations of affect

How best can the Christian community respond in the aftermath of trauma? If Christian churches and ministries embrace Erikson's view and focus their attention primarily on how the resulting experiences from adversity can manifest among congregants and surrounding community members in complex

28 Erikson, *A New Species*, 233.
29 Erikson, *A New Species*, 231.
30 Erikson, *A New Species*, 236.
31 Erikson, *A New Species*, 237.
32 Jack Saul, *Collective Trauma and Collective Healing* (New York: Routledge, 2014).
33 Saul, *Collective Trauma*, 105.

ways, how then does that approach lend itself to shaping effective ministries of care? How do Christian leaders best encourage a congregation or ministry group's practice of methods for resilience in the face of adversity? Granted, Christian leaders encounter forms of collective trauma ordinarily in several ways, including when families or ministry groups experience crises, when the whole congregation or ministry organization experiences crises, or when the greater community experiences a natural, structural, or human-caused disaster. In considering what role a particular congregation or ministry can play in responding to local adversity, leaders may find some of the following findings useful.

In the aftermath of trauma, expressions of personal and relational care prove to counter the impacts of post-traumatic stress.[34] Through acts of care, such intentional practices of nourishment help (re)build trust among individuals, group relationships, and the greater community. To further emphasize this critical point, Erikson notes how healthy organizations function like a communal store in which individuals invest individual energies together and then draw on the shared reserve supply in order to meet demands of everyday life.[35] As a result, individuals trust their community will be a source of care and nourishment when needed, and this trust enables survivors to weather adversity with fewer senses of harm. Christians, in particular, know the fruit of the Holy Spirit (Gal 5) with which to line the shelves of a healthy community storehouse: love, joy, peace, patience, kindness, goodness, faithfulness, gentleness, and temperance. These practices encourage calming or self-regulation, caring connection, and honest expressions, which all give way to the ability to navigate stress in healthier ways. As Erikson points out, ideally, it is 'the community that offers a cushion for pain, the community that offers a context for intimacy, the community that serves as the repository for binding traditions'.[36] For Christians, the cushion, content, and repository all are formed through acts of the Holy Spirit, which serve to enhance healthy community spirit.

Emerging studies in collective trauma further identify how individuals, families, and communities prevail beyond adversity. For example, through extensive observations of various types of groups striving toward healing and growth in New York City, particularly after 9/11 as well as within some refugee neighborhoods, Saul summarizes key practices that healthy groups exhibit following adversity.[37] He notes how the most resilient communities tend to have and make use of their access to biological, psychological, social, and spiritual resources within their local community. These relational sources of nourishment enable community members to make their way

34 Jones, *Trauma and Grace*; Levine, *Unspoken Voice*; van der Kolk, *Body*.

35 Erikson, *A New Species*, 234.

36 Erikson, *A New Species*, 234.

37 Saul, *Collective Trauma*.

through their pain together and sense together a more positive prevailing communal mood.

Saul underscores the following four specific practices as most likely to lead to community health:

- Mutual commitment to build community and enhance social connectedness among everyone affected;
- Identifying and practicing ways to tell the story of the whole community's experience and response;
- Mutual commitment to re-establishing ordinary rhythms and routines of life and engaging together in healing rituals; and
- Seeking to arrive together at a positive vision of the future with renewed hope.[38]

Saul observes how, for several different times of communities in New York City that had faced ranging forms of adversity, these practices created the mortar to begin rebuilding community together again, and, in turn, establish new senses of safety and vibrancy.

Many longitudinal studies have emerged following Felitti and Anda's initial reporting of how Adverse Childhood Experiences (ACEs) affect individuals, families, and groups across lifetimes.[39] For example, pediatrician and ACEs expert Nadine Burke Harris lists access to opportunities for practising mindfulness, practicing mental health and therapy, and access to caring relationships among six keys to overcoming adversity. The other three key practices are healthy sleep practices, regular exercise, and good nutrition.[40]

Especially in light of such findings, churches and ministry groups yield tremendous potential today to provide nourishment and healing in their communities and actively counter the impacts of trauma within and around them. As church and ministry leaders increasingly consider the ways their organizations can assist survivors more fully in rebuilding senses of trust, they can encourage their organizations to regularly review practices through this lens. Consider some of the following helpful practices:

- Child Safety Policy: If needed, find helpful examples and guides for creating and updating policies at Godly Response to Abuse in Christian Environments (GRACE.net).
- Fellowship: Consider hosting regular gatherings for prayer, worship, Bible study, sharing meals, and conducting ministry in the community at all times and especially following times of crises.

38 Saul, *Collective Trauma*, 105–106.
39 Felitti and Anda, *Relationship*.
40 Nadine Burke Harris, *The Deepest Well: Healing the Long-Term Effects of Childhood Adversity* (Basingstoke, UK: Pan MacMillan, 2018).

- Emergency Planning: Create clear and reliable communication plans and systems for keeping in touch with congregants and community members in times of peace and times of crisis. Consider having members fill out surveys for how they would like to keep in touch, including regular forms of post or electronic mail, and then, in cases where electricity, internet, or mobility may be challenged, how best they would like to confirm they are safe. Some may be eager to volunteer to assist members and neighbors in emergency. To help with communicating effectively with volunteers, consider creating a system to organize people and the skills or materials they can donate.
- Collaborative Partnerships for Response: To leverage better mutual response efforts, to avoid duplicating resources, and to better meet unmet needs, create multi-professional partnerships for response.[41]

While these forms of collaborations, guidelines, and mutually shared best practices have proved immensely helpful to communities across the United States, even so, the incessant hammering of events in recent years also leaves many organizations feeling stretched to their limits. These recent patterns of natural and human-caused disasters serve as a continual reminder, too, of the importance of adapting effective response efforts. Consider how the Director of Episcopal Relief and Development, Katie Mears, describes some of the organization's more recent experiences:

> We learned many things during the unprecedented disaster season in 2017. For many years, in the US and around the world, Episcopal Relief & Development has led trainings and provided critical resources to help dioceses determine how to build resilient systems and how to best respond to emergencies. The spate of disasters last fall truly tested all our own internal systems and processes.[42]

Moreover, take note of how the Associate for National Response of Presbyterian Disaster Assistance, James Kirk, describes the ministry's experience:

> More communities were impacted by more disasters with more severity in the past few years and the faith-based organizations that respond are feeling the pressure. For example, a 1000-year flood event should be

41 For example, in the United States, government agencies, non-government agencies, and faith-based agencies partner through membership in local or national Volunteer Organizations Active in Disaster (VOAD) groups, ministerial alliances, and other types of multidisciplinary partnerships. In turn, National VOAD committees and the Federal Emergency Management Agency provide guidelines to help communities navigate the chaotic terrain of the postdisaster trajectory.

42 Katie Mears, Director of Episcopal Relief and Development, July 2018, personal communication.

> extremely rare but in a five-month period during 2016 there were four 1000-year flooding events in the United States. More US citizens registered with FEMA for individual assistance in 2017 (4,800,000) than in the previous 10 years combined. In addition, the number of public mass shooting events continues to increase to the point that active shooter drills are as common as bad weather drills. All of this is taking place during a time when denominational giving is on the decline.[43]

Experiences of collective trauma or disaster are not new, and large Christian organizations in the United States actively seek to adapt to the ongoing challenges of evolving seasons of disaster. Some examples of how disaster response agencies in the United States are meeting ever-expanding needs following disaster, include the following:

> **Kate Mears, Director of Episcopal Relief and Development**
>
> Given the changing weather patterns and the increasing intensity and number of disasters, I have realized that in the impacted areas, *all* churches, no matter their size or capacity, are truly called to be a part of the response effort. Sometimes it's easy to see yourself as too small or too disconnected or too fill-in-the-blank, but we are all given gifts by God and are called to use them to serve those in need. This lesson has reinforced so much of what we do normally: to help churches see that call and to equip themselves to be more resilient and able to respond to their neighbors and communities in times of crisis.[44]
>
> **Kevin King, Director of Mennonite Disaster Service**
>
> Mennonite Disaster Service (MDS), a volunteer network of the Anabaptist churches in Canada and the U.S., has increased its response to the tremendous needs in light of the three major hurricanes and fires in 2017. In the backdrop of so many disasters while we are in an American moment notorious for dishonourable and divisive behavior, our volunteers are really stepping up and saying, 'we are somebody – we want to make a difference'. As a response, we have hired additional staff to leverage these hard working volunteers to come and let the hammer ring hope.

Those faith-based organizations that respond are learning ways to increase their ability to respond with fewer resources. One approach to this situation is to invest more resources and energy in preparedness and resilience strengthening. Preparedness does strengthen individual and community resilience. Individuals and communities that are resilient are

43 James Kirk, Director of Presbyterian Disaster Assistance, July 2018, personal communication.
44 Personal communication.

> better prepared. Preparedness and resilience does make individuals and communities less susceptible to the adverse impacts of a disaster and more capable to respond and recover with less outside intervention. We are relearning that an ounce of prevention is worth a pound of cure.[45]

Whether as a small or large faith-based organization, taking stock of how the organization or surrounding community have been impacted by critical incidents, as well as what assets the organization and neighboring organizations can bring through partnerships to potential future crises, helps prepare the organization well in trustworthy ways which members can rely on. Practices such as these ones prove to expand potential resiliency among widely ranging communities.

Conclusion

This chapter employed Kai Erikson's sociological approach to diagnosing and treating trauma, namely, to focus primarily on how the impacts of trauma manifest both in individual bodies and group systems and to what meaning survivors make of what they have endured in order to shape response efforts and inform ministry development. In so doing, this chapter identified key sociological and psychological understandings of collective trauma and healing to consider ways Christian congregations, in particular, can generate and enhance community-wide restoration following catastrophic events within their organizations or in their local regions. Erikson's observation of 'spiritual kinship' among groups with shared trauma experience and Jack Saul's recognition that human spirits prevail and perpetuate across generations when they have access to biological, psychological, social, and spiritual resources to cope and heal provided a helpful initial framework to begin considering the role that spiritual formation agencies can play in generating community healing. This chapter reviewed Erikson's coining of the term *collective trauma* as well as his depictions of past professional obstructions in order to more fully recognize the impacts of trauma and more functional treatment methods for groups. This chapter also placed salient insights from psychologist Jack Saul in conversation with Kai Erikson in order to explore further how communities innately can enact healing and restoration following catastrophic events. This chapter reviewed key practices conducted by communities that prevail beyond tragedy, including networks of collaborative response in the United States established through Volunteer Organizations Active in Disaster (VOAD), and provided recommendations for clergy and ministry leaders to practically expand care and, in turn, foster the rebuilding of trust among individuals, families, and within their communities in ways that can become contagious.

45 Personal communication.

Select references

Erikson, Kai. *A New Species of Trouble: The Human Experience of Modern Disasters*. New York: WW Norton, 1994.

Vincent J. Felitti and Robert F. Anda. 'The Relationship of Adverse Childhood Experiences to Adult Medical Disease, Psychiatric Disorders and Sexual Behavior: Implications for Healthcare'. In *The Impact of Early Life Trauma on Health and Disease*, ed. Lanius et al. Cambridge: Cambridge University Press, 2010.

Herman, Judith. *Trauma and Recovery: The Aftermath of Violence – From Domestic Abuse to Political Terror*. New York: Basic, 1997.

Jones, Serene. *Trauma and Grace*. New York: Westminster, 2009.

Saul, Jack. *Collective Trauma and Collective Healing*. New York: Routledge, 2014.

Van der Kolk, Bessel. *The Body Keeps the Score: Brain, Mind and Body in the Healing of Trauma*. New York: Penguin, 2015.

Part III

Theological explorations

Introduction to Part III

In the first part of the book, Elaine Graham and Carla A. Grosch-Miller reflected on theological method in the context of trauma. A strong emphasis in Grosch-Miller's chapter, in particular, was the primacy of *experience* in this form of practical theology. In this section, four authors apply the methods of practical theology to different contexts, in terms of content and confessional tradition.

First, Megan Warner draws inferences from her own expertise in biblical studies. Again, she draws very much on her own experience in living with Chronic Fatigue Syndrome in interrogating what resource biblical texts provide in the search for meaning when structures of meaning are profoundly challenged. Warner shows that traumatising contexts shaped much of the way biblical texts became the resource they are. Just as the canonical Gospels were formed in the crucible of the threat to and final fall of Jerusalem, so much of the Hebrew Bible reached its final form out of the experience of the Exile. Her inference is that the texts are robust; their re-performance in times of deep trouble offers to the traumatised words and narratives that endure.

Roger P. Abbott's theological journey is also formed strongly from experience – in his case of ministering at the Kegworth air crash of 1989. He has since done significant work in other contexts of disaster such as Haiti. Writing from an evangelical Protestant perspective, he poses the difficult question, How can the experience of great trauma sit within a strong confession of divine providence? In this essay, a robust framework of conviction as to the goodness and sovereignty of God sits alongside a confession that God works in the lives of believers to conform them to the likeness of Christ. Yet Abbott also acknowledges the difficulties of arriving at any easy interpretation of some events within this frame.

Christopher Southgate's chapter on theodicy acts in a sense as a complement to Abbott's. Southgate wants to push the question as to God's involvement in shock events beyond the parameters set down by Abbott, in particular in relation to those events where natural phenomena are the main cause. He draws on Hebrew Bible texts and Jewish thought to propose an expansion of the range of what Christian communities might pray and confess in contexts where God appears, at least in part, as the perpetrator. At the same time, Southgate offers a mode of Christian contemplation that includes both Passion and eschaton in the reading of natural phenomena.

The tension between Abbott and Southgate centres on whether an experience, however extreme, is to be incorporated into and understood within a system of belief or whether overwhelming experiences can and should lead to extreme expressions of anger, protest or disillusion with God. Either strategy, it seems, could be defended from Scripture.

In a further chapter, on narrative genre, Southgate draws on the seminal work of James Hopewell on genres of congregational narrative. Southgate considers the possibility that particular genres might be particularly vulnerable to certain types of traumatising events. He goes on to suggest that the performance, in preaching and liturgy, of different narrative genres in the Scriptures might help a congregation to develop resilience.

The section ends with Deanne Gardner's chapter from an Afro-Caribbean Pentecostal perspective. She reflects on the strongly collectivist character of such communities and the inheritance of experiences of shame and oppression. Gardner writes very movingly of communities accepting tragedy as within the sovereignty of God while uttering 'an eternal wail from our women and a difficult silence from our men'. These resources of endurance and 'always having a song to sing' are clearly strengths and yet may run the risk of reducing the element of righteous protest at what the community has to face.

As with the previous pair of essays, there are interesting links to be drawn between this last pair. It would be fascinating for Afro-Caribbean congregations to reflect on the genres Hopewell proposes and see how their interior narratives shape their responses to shock and tragedy.

5 Trauma through the lens of the Bible

Megan Warner

When I did my earliest formal biblical studies, one of the first things I learned about the four gospels in the New Testament (NT) was that scholars date them to the years immediately following the destruction of Jerusalem and the Temple by the Romans in 70 CE (or, in the case of Mark, during the years of tension and violence leading up to the destruction).[1] There was, we given were to understand, something about that experience of destruction and loss that acted as a kind of catalyst for the gospel writers. Later, when I started working more with the Old Testament (OT), I became interested in biblical writings that had either been composed or substantially edited during the period following the return of the Israelites from Babylonian exile in the 5th century BCE and later. Even so, it was not until I started working in the field of trauma studies that I began to put all the pieces together and realise – as others had done before me – that a surprisingly large percentage of the biblical text, in both testaments, was written in the context, or aftermath, of large-scale disasters.[2]

This insight could be thought to be obvious. Indeed, once I began to teach biblical studies to my own students I quickly recognised that it was not really possible to teach, or to understand, the OT without constant reference back to the events of its history. No class could begin without first drawing

1 'CE' (= AD) stands for Common Era and 'BCE' (= BC, see the later discussion) for 'before the Common Era'. These abbreviations are used by biblical scholars for reasons of hospitality to Jewish and Muslim colleagues.

2 The scholarly literature on this topic is growing at an impressive rate. See in particular, Elizabeth Boase and Christopher Frechette, *Bible Through the Lens of Trauma* (Semeia Studies 86; Atlanta: SBL, 2016); David M. Carr, *Holy Resilience: The Bible's Traumatic Origins* (New Haven, CT: Yale University, 2014); Mark G. Brett, *Political Trauma and Healing: Biblical Ethics for a Postcolonial World* (Grand Rapids, MI: Eerdmans, 2016); Kai Erikson, *A New Species of Trouble: Explorations in Disaster, Trauma, and Community* (New York: Norton, 1994); Jeffrey Kauffman, ed., *Loss of the Assumptive World: A Theory of Traumatic Loss* (New York: Brunner-Routledge, 2002). This work is essentially interdisciplinary in nature, and although the application of trauma theory to biblical interpretation owes its greatest debts to the fields of psychology, sociology and literary theory, other fields of study have also been influential.

a rough timeline of Israel's history – a mapping of slavery and conquest, military victories and defeats, exile, repeated destruction of Jerusalem and Temple, Crucifixion and the impact on ancient Israel of the relentless tides of empire.[3] The hard-won insight of the field of Biblical Theology – that it is impossible to distil a pure theology from biblical texts, free of the contamination of 'worldly' history and the influence of human beings – ought, perhaps, not to have been so hard won.[4] Theology is, and can only, be 'done' against the background, and in the context, of human history. This is a truth that has been rediscovered in recent decades as trauma theory has newly, but rapidly and influentially, come to be applied to biblical studies.

The violence of much of this history tends not to be foremost in the minds of biblical readers today partly because although biblical writings undoubtedly respond to it, they do not always describe it (being on the whole more interested in the theological interpretation of the events than in accurate reportage of them). Nevertheless, it is striking that the production of writings that made their way into the canon rose sharply after each of these primary disaster events. While it may go too far to say, as some scholars do, that nothing substantial was written in terms of biblical literature *prior* to the Babylonian exile, it is certainly the case that much, or even most, of the OT was written, or substantially edited, during or after the exile.[5] The same pattern can be seen in the NT; although Paul wrote in the years prior to 70 CE (itself a persecutory and violent period), the Gospels (probably other than Mark) were written after 70 CE so that the central Christian narratives of Jesus's words and deeds, life and death, were composed in the immediate aftermath of the destruction of Jerusalem and of the Temple.

3 For a study of the impact of the history of empires upon the Bible see Mark G. Brett, *Decolonizing God: The Bible in the tides of empire* (Sheffield: Sheffield Phoenix, 2008).

4 The distillation of such a 'pure' biblical theology had been the goal of Biblical Theology from its beginning, with Johann P. Gabler's 1787 lecture, 'An Oration on the Proper Distinction between Biblical and Dogmatic Theology and the Specific Objectives of Each'. For the text of Gabler's foundational lecture, and collected essays tracing the development of the field of Biblical Theology and its troubled relationship with 'history', see Ben C. Ollenburger, ed., *Old Testament Theology: Flowering and Future* (Winona Lake, IN: Eisenbrauns, 2004).

5 See, for example, the schemas of Konrad Schmid, *The Old Testament: A Literary History* (Minneapolis, MN: Fortress, 2012) and David M. Carr, *The Formation of the Hebrew Bible: A New Construction* (New York: Oxford University Press, 2011). It is important to note that despite (or perhaps because of) the high degree of anticipation of the exiles around their return to Canaan, the text suggests that the return, when it finally happened, was disappointing to the point of becoming a new source of trauma. The returners found not the golden Jerusalem of their memories and imagination but a small, dusty, cultural backwater that suffered from comparison with the sophistication of Babylon. There were no city walls, the Temple was in ruins and hopes for a new Israelite king were gradually dashed. The new reality was one of occupation – both the political occupation of Persia and the domestic and mercantile occupation of the lower-class Israelites who had not been taken into exile and who now lived in the returners' homes and worked their land and businesses. Books such as Ezra and Nehemiah tell the story of the tensions and disillusionment of this period.

Our Scriptures are, then, to a large degree, written out of the experience of trauma. The consequent question for us is a simple one: 'So what?' The remainder of this chapter considers possible answers to this simple question – looked at from a variety of angles. What difference, for example, does it make to reading the Bible with traumatised people, or congregations, that the Bible itself is the product of trauma? How can the Bible be a resource for responding to trauma? Should the Bible come with health warnings? Or is the Bible uniquely well placed to guide Christians through today's challenges and disasters?

I want to suggest four principal answers to the 'so what?' question. There are certainly others. These four answers are designed to help to kick-start imagination and questions around pastoral and theological use of the Bible. It is to be hoped that they will point not only to themselves but also to other answers, more profound and pastoral than these.

The biblical text is robust

I have written elsewhere about my experience of chronic illness.[6] I lived with ME (or 'Chronic Fatigue Syndrome') for 18 years – specifically, the years when I should have been busy establishing my career, marrying and having children. In the place of career and family, I had a 'syndrome' – and getting through it took up just about every ounce of my energy and creativity. At the time I often wondered what the point of it all was – what did it mean? ME is an apparently meaningless illness, so coming up with any kind of answer to this question was extremely challenging. After the first decade or so, for example, what lessons could this interminable experience possibly continue to have for me? One of the few answers that I could grasp at with any conviction was that my experience had been so awful, so protracted and so apparently devoid of meaning that I could have confidence about my capacity to sit alongside others experiencing suffering. I couldn't expect to know what *their* suffering felt like, but I could know that I understood suffering. I had earned some 'street cred', if you like.

I now think of the Bible in an analogous way. The biblical books are not in any sense trite or fragile. They come out of the experience of individuals and communities who have gone through the most painful and violent experiences that life can throw at human beings. They are written against a background of famines, wars, enslavement, political power struggles, natural disasters, forced migrations and apparent betrayal and desertion by God. The irreverent tags that we sometimes attach to the Bible – 'nice', 'conservative', 'boring' and 'irrelevant' – even when we do not mean to (for example, what images come to your mind in response to the phrase 'Bible stories'?) are mostly unwarranted and inaccurate. When understood against its own

6 Meg Warner, *Abraham: A Journey Through Lent* (London: SPCK, 2015).

contexts, the Bible is none of these things. It has street cred. It understands suffering. And that means that the biblical stories, letters, poetry etc. that make up the Bible are resources for ministering in the context of trauma in which we can have confidence. When read, sung, enacted, performed or prayed with sensitivity and imagination, these biblical writings can be the most profound resource for ministry with traumatised people and congregations. They meet traumatised people where they are.

It is worth emphasising at this point that the trauma lying behind the text is not always apparent on its face. Some books recount situations of violence or use inherently violent language and imagery. So, for example, the prophecies of Jeremiah and Ezekiel are particularly notable for their violence. The Book of Psalms is remarkable for its expressions of violence, cursing and generally unedifying human emotion.[7] Lamentations 2 speaks of YHWH as an enemy who has destroyed Israel and her palaces and strongholds, while violence between brothers begins as early as Genesis 4, with Cain's murder of Abel. The NT is generally less violent than the OT, but the Gospels nevertheless highlight the violence of Jesus's death, Acts recounts the sometimes-violent events following Jesus's ascension and Revelation presents images at once violent and surreal.

These are by no means, however, the only biblical books demonstrably influenced by experiences of trauma. Others betray the impact of traumatic experiences in a variety of other ways. The Book of Genesis, for example, despite telling the very beginning of Israel's story, reached its final form relatively late. A high proportion of Genesis was composed after the return from exile. The disappointments and tensions of this period are undoubtedly reflected in the narrative, even if that narrative is often described as 'eirenic'.[8] There is limited overt large-scale violence (Gn 14 and 34 are notable exceptions) and the ancestral narratives (Gn 12–35) depict a story of (relatively) peaceful coexistence that contrasts markedly with the suspicion, expulsion or destruction of foreigners that characterise the rest of the Hexateuch (Genesis–Joshua). That does not mean that relational tensions are absent from Genesis. In Genesis, the disappointments and tensions of the Persian period are domesticated in a story of ancient families, living long ago.[9] What appears to be an old, safe, family story is, in fact, a subversive political tract,[10] intelligible to certain groups but opaque to Persian occupiers and probably also to their Israelite supporters. Here is a resilient and subversive form of response to trauma but a response to trauma nevertheless.

7 In relation to the lament psalms, see my essay in Chapter Eleven of this volume.

8 For example, Norman C. Habel, *The Land Is Mine: Six Biblical Land Ideologies* (Minneapolis, MN: Fortress, 1995), 146.

9 I set this out in detail in *Re-Imagining Abraham: A Re-Assessment of the Influence of Deuteronomism in Genesis* (OTS 72; Leiden/Boston, MA: Brill, 2018).

10 See the essays in Mark G. Brett and Jakob Wöhrle, eds., *The Politics of the Ancestors* (FAT 124; Tübingen: Mohr Siebeck, 2018).

Other books display other forms of response to trauma. Lamentations and Psalms, for example, in addition to telling stories of violence, use the poetic form of lament to express the impact of trauma. The practice of lamentation, almost lost from contemporary Western language and culture, is increasingly understood as a therapeutic or pastoral response to traumatic experience, and recent scholarship has enthusiastically explored the lessons and examples it offers for therapeutic and pastoral response to traumatic experience today.[11] I write at greater length about the liturgical possibilities of lament in Chapter 11 in this volume, 'Teach to your Daughters a Dirge': Revisiting the Practice of Lament in the Light of Trauma Theory'.

The Bible tells us we are not alone

When we read biblical stories, we know that we are not alone and that our trials and tribulations are not unique. As unimaginable as some of today's disasters may seem, God's people lived through comparable experiences during the biblical period, and we have their stories. We can therefore read for the 'company' of others who understand the depth of the pain of our experience. We find this 'company' not only with the biblical characters whose stories are told in the text but also with the generations of Jews and Christians who have read and studied and taken solace from those stories over two millennia or more. Even if we may be physically, emotionally or spiritually isolated in our own lives, reading these stories tells us that we are not unique but that our individual story can be situated within a rich and thick history of the experience of God's people, all of whom are 'with' us through relationship with the text.

One of the practical ways in which we can experience this is to formulate and 'tell' our story in conversation with the biblical story (stories).[12] The accounts of the Passion in the Gospels offer a rich resource for this. To understand our own traumas and suffering in conversation, or in parallel, with Christ's suffering can help to bring to our experience dignity, meaning and a sense of Christ's presence and participation in *our* suffering. The fourfold character of the Gospels and the length and detail of the four Passion accounts mean that nearly everybody can find an aspect of the Passion that seems to speak directly and uniquely to their experience. Let me offer an example from my own. I talked earlier about my years spent living with ME and referred to the apparent meaningless of that experience. Over that time, finding meaning in what I was going through became more and more important to me, and I still see the making of meaning as central to the drive toward knowing God.[13] Much of the challenge, with ME, was to find

11 See, for example, Brent Strawn, 'Trauma, Psalmic Disclosure and Authentic Happiness', in *Bible Through the Lens of Trauma*, and the other references in Chapter 11 of this volume.

12 See, further, Warner, *Abraham: A Journey Through Lent.*

13 For a helpful discussion of the meaning-making literature, see Crystal L. Park, 'Making Sense of the Meaning Literature: An Integrative Review of Meaning Making and Its

meaning in a life that was almost entirely passive and in which opportunities to feel 'useful' to the world and to other people seemed hopelessly limited. In that context I found W.H. Vanstone's classic, *The Stature of Waiting*, unexpectedly helpful.[14] Vanstone had undertaken a study of the verbs in the Passion account and shown that once a certain point in the story is reached, the verbs that have Jesus as their subject are exclusively passive. Here was a story, I discovered, of the salvation of the world in which the agent of salvation is portrayed as mostly silent and wholly passive. It became possible for me to begin to believe that I could contribute to the world and to others simply by being who I was and by enduring the situation in which I found myself.

Others have found entirely other aspects of the Passion narratives to be pertinent to their lives and situations. This is not, of course, an innovation of the bringing of trauma theory to biblical interpretation. Nevertheless, scholars using trauma theory as a lens have demonstrated the value of bringing an awareness of the traumatic background of biblical stories to this practice of formulating one's own story in conversation with the biblical narrative. Prominent among these is Shelly Rambo, whose books *Spirit and Trauma: A Theology of Remaining* and *Resurrecting Wounds: Living in the Afterlife of Trauma*, explore the value of adopting Holy Saturday as a model of living with the impact of trauma and of recognising the focus of the post-resurrection Gospel narratives on wounds and the longevity and impact of wounds on post-resurrection life.[15]

The Bible offers us a language and literature of suffering

One of the stranger aspects of trauma is that it can have the effect of silencing its victims. It does this in two ways, as already noted in earlier chapters in this collection. Trauma can physically silence us; in disaster situations, the fight-or-flight reflex fuels those physical responses that aid physical speed and strength, while closing down other physical functions unnecessary to fight or flight, including the function of speech. When people get 'stuck' in the fight-or-flight response, this shutdown of the function of speech can

---

Effects on Adjustment to Stressful Life Events', *Psychological Bulletin* 136 (2010): 257–301.

14 W. H. Vanstone, *The Stature of Waiting* (London: Darton, Longman and Todd, 1982).

15 Shelly Rambo, *Spirit and Trauma: A Theology of Remaining* (Louisville, KY: Westminster John Knox, 2010); *Resurrecting Wounds: Living in the Afterlife of Trauma* (Waco, TX: Baylor University Press, 2017). See the treatments by Elaine Graham and Carla A. Grosch-Miller of Rambo's work in Chapters 1 and 2, respectively, of this volume. The Passion narratives offer a particularly fruitful resource for 'telling' one's own story in the shape of biblical narrative. Of course, they are by no means the only biblical resources in this regard. In my *Abraham: A Journey Through Lent* I model and encourage use of the Abraham story to shape the story of one's own life in the context of travelling the Lenten journey. In *Joseph: A Story of Resilience* (London: SPCK, forthcoming 2019) I use the Joseph story as a text for thinking about what resilient living might (or might not!) look like.

continue so that it continues to be physically impossible to speak. Trauma can also make it impossible to formulate or tell our experience as story. The essence of trauma is an experience of 'overwhelm' of the senses. The overwhelming nature of trauma can mean that the body is unable to 'experience' witnessed events – it cannot undertake processing of the event as experience or of experience as memory. The result can be dissociation, in which the body and mind distance themselves from the events – so that, for example, a person may report the experience of watching violence being done to herself from above. Because she never really 'experienced' that violence, she cannot process it as memory and therefore cannot tell it as a story. She has only jagged, unconnected pieces of recalled detail, awareness of which is painful and organisation of which into comprehensible narrative is impossible.[16]

Human beings are storytelling animals. We cannot know who we are without telling our stories. The inability to tell one's own story in the wake of a traumatic event serves to perpetuate the trauma response to that event. It has, in the recent past, been received wisdom that one will not recover from trauma until one has been able to tell one's story in the presence of a sympathetic witness. Scholars and practitioners are now learning that there are other ways of recovering from trauma (crucially, involving a range of physical practices as well as the use of the mind)[17] and that being encouraged to tell one's trauma story too early can, far from being necessary, instead be harmful. However, the telling of one's story remains the primary means of negotiating one's identity, and living without identity is intolerable for most people. The Bible provides resources that respond to both of these ways in which trauma silences people.

First, the Bible offers language to those who have no words. British OT scholar John Goldingay describes the Psalms as '150 things that God doesn't mind having said to him'.[18] When there are no words, the Psalms can step in and fill the gap.[19] They cover pretty much every human emotion (edifying and otherwise). Praying these words can be less confronting than trying to find one's own words to pray. The other important implication of Goldingay's description of the psalms is that they *authorise* expression, before God, of pretty much every human emotion (edifying and otherwise). The Psalms

16 Scholarship that explores the use of trauma theory as lens for reading the Bible makes use of this insight by arguing that trauma theory can help to make sense, and fill in the gaps, of trauma-influenced literature such as Jeremiah and Ezekiel: Boase and Frechette, *Bible through the Lens of Trauma*, 11.

17 These are explored in Van der Kolk, *Body Keeps the Score*.

18 Goldingay reportedly does not recall having said this. Generations of his students, however, witness to the fact that he did. For an account of Goldingay's personal and academic journey with the Psalms see John Goldingay, *After Eating the Apricot: (Inside Out Meditation)* (Carlisle: Solway, 1996).

19 According to Claus Westermann ('The Role of Lament in the Theology of the Old Testament', *Union Seminary Review* 28 [1974]: 20–38, 31), 'The lament is the language of suffering; in it suffering is given the dignity of language: it will not stay silent!'

tell us that it is OK, and even an expression of faith, to bring our most raw, disillusioned, angry, doubtful or vengeful thoughts and feelings to God and lay them at God's feet.[20]

Second, the Bible offers literature to those who have no stories. I suggested earlier that trying to live without stories can be excruciating and that trauma can make storytelling difficult or impossible. Here is a set of stories (robust, pre-loved and authorised) that can become our own stories and function as a foundation for our identity building, even after the most disorienting and destructive experiences. One may choose to use biblical stories as a kind of framework to assist in the construction of one's own story, as I was suggesting earlier, or might, alternatively, simply adopt a story or stories as one's own.

I have said quite a bit about stories and Bible stories, in particular. Some readers may find the concept of 'story', particularly in connection with Scripture, a little disconcerting, and fear that I may be trivialising biblical narrative. I should say that I have a very 'high' view of story. I believe that we human beings are constituted by stories and that stories are capable of containing and reflecting the most profound truths – including truths that are internally paradoxical or conflicting. Jesus chose a particular kind of story, the parable, as his principal teaching vehicle. Parables enabled him to respond to trick questions – simultaneously instructing his followers and exposing the hypocrisy of his opponents. They also enabled him to say several crucial, or subversive, things at the same time, and to say them, to some degree, under the radar. We still read Jesus's parables today and find not only that they speak fresh truths into our own conflicts and situations but that over our lives, these truths and our perspectives on them change. A story can be like a diamond in this respect – its appearance depends on where you happen to be standing and what the light is like on any given day.

Furthermore, Jesus was following his Jewish heritage in using stories in his teaching. The OT is full of stories that weigh possibilities, balance alternatives and bring together unexpected and unrelated ideas – generally without expressing hard or fixed opinions.[21] For example, how should the daughters of Lot have acted in the aftermath of the destruction of the world as they knew it in Sodom? Which would have been worse, the incest they committed with their father or allowing their father's line, and his name, to die out without taking steps to 'preserve offspring' for him (Gn 19:30–38, 32 and 34)?[22] We are still arguing about stories like this one and finding that even our own views and responses change over time. Stories hold meaning

20 See Chapter 11 for more detailed discussion of the lament psalms and their use with traumatised people and groups.

21 I develop this further in Megan Warner, 'What if They're Foreign?: Inner-Legal Exegesis in the Ancestral Narratives', in *The Politics of the Ancestors*, 67–92.

22 The answer to this conundrum is by no means clear – the story sets it out, but does not attempt to answer it. The heading to the passage in the New Revised Standard Version,

and reflect truth far more efficiently, effectively and suggestively than do rules or statements of dogma.

The Bible models resilience

The books of the OT and NT respond to the traumas experienced by early Israelites and Christians in a wide range of ways. In light of recent research, it is possible to see that many biblical books model resilience, both of individuals and communities. I would like to offer you some examples.

Storytelling is an important element of building resilience. Specifically, what is important for resilience is preparedness to be flexible in the telling of one's story, allowing it to shift and develop with changing experiences. If you have lived through an experience of suffering, perhaps like the years I spent with ME that I mentioned earlier, you may have found that the story you told about yourself before the experience was not one you could tell afterwards. Perhaps the story did not allow space to acknowledge the reality or pain of the experience of suffering, or you might have felt that you were a completely different person afterwards so that your early stories no longer fit you. This was my experience of having ME. My early stories were full of striving for successes and achievements, but my new story had to include an account of finding meaning in the face of incapacity and passivity. Hospital chaplains tell me that their ministry is all about encouraging and helping people to tell their story in a new way – a way that not only takes account of illness and suffering as well as wellness but that also sees a way ahead to some form or peacefulness and acceptance of what the present is and what the future may or may not bring.[23] This retelling of one's story need not involve dramatic change. It is best when the resulting story resembles a tapestry or carpet, into which new experiences are woven, influencing the colour and pattern of the whole but without making it an entirely new carpet.

This kind of resilient retelling, or reframing, of stories is a feature of the OT. Communities, as well as individuals, develop and build their identities through the telling of stories, and this was particularly true of Ancient Israel. Prior to Babylon's defeat of Jerusalem and the destruction of the Temple, Israel's story was the story of Mosaic Yahwism – Israel lived out its destiny as YHWH's chosen people, under YHWH's appointed king. During the years of the exile, however, this story stopped working. The unthinkable had happened, and the Yahweh who had previously gone out with Israel's armies,

'The Shameful Origins of Ammon and Moab', does both the story, and its readers, a serious disservice. See my 'What if They're Foreign' for a fuller discussion.

23 Helpful in this regard is the work of gerontologist William L. Randall on the therapeutic application of narrative in ageing. See, for example, William L. Randall, 'The Importance of Being Ironic: Narrative Openness and Personal Resilience in Later Life', *The Gerontologist* 53 (2013): 9–16, 14.

assuring their military success, had now allowed the sacking of Jerusalem and the Temple. For the exiles, the old story raised too many uncomfortable questions. Was YHWH not the strong God they had imagined, or did YHWH just not like them anymore? Had they, perhaps, backed the wrong 'god' from the beginning? The new story eventually developed by the exiles represented a strong response to these questions – YHWH was neither weak nor fickle but had arranged for Israel to be punished (through the agency of her enemy Babylon) for its failure to keep the Torah. This new story allowed the exiles to affirm YHWH's power (indeed, it allowed them to insist that YHWH could direct the actions not just of Israel but of the nations also) *and* YHWH's continued faithfulness (YHWH had not abandoned Israel but had punished it for its own sake). Following the return from exile, however, the returners had to 'retell' their story yet again. The story of punishment by a strong God functioned differently in the new context of return to the promised land, suggesting a future that was uncertain at best – if Israel had been poor at keeping Torah in the past, what guarantee was there that Israel would now do better? When would YHWH next rip Israel from its land and exile it, ostensibly for its own good? Israel's new retelling of its story following the return from exile emphasised the everlasting nature of God's relationship with Israel and the possibility of forgiveness.[24] This process, of development and 'retelling' of Israel's national story continued, over the years, influenced by changing circumstances. The Shoah, or Holocaust, was the trauma event that has most necessitated Israel's retelling of its story in the modern era. It was so devastatingly horrific that in its wake, it became obvious that a theology (or story) of punishment of the victim of aggression could no longer be maintained in any form.[25]

One of the ironies of Christian attempts today to 'follow the Bible' and to do what 'it' says, is a tendency to overlook the Bible's own inner processes of development and revision, which ensured that the revelation of YHWH to the Israelites continued to speak to successive generations. The Bible is

24 The development of Israel's story, charted here, is perhaps best illustrated in a comparison of the books of Samuel and Kings with Chronicles. Chronicles repeats long portions of Samuel and Kings verbatim. It tells the same story all over again. However, Chronicles, which was written considerably later than (most of) Samuel and Kings, does not tell *exactly the same* story: some bits are left out; some bits are changed; some bits are added. What becomes really interesting, then, in reading Chronicles, is to notice what is *different* from Samuel and Kings. This process, of repeating the monarchic story from Samuel and Kings, but differently, is an unusually graphic example of what I mean by retelling. I have argued elsewhere that Genesis participates in this process of retelling, 're-imagining' Abraham as a new David, albeit one who lived in the distant past; see *Re-Imagining Abraham*. For a fascinating study of the techniques by which this re-telling was achieved see Bernard M. Levinson, *Legal Revision and Religious Renewal in Ancient Israel* (New York: Cambridge University Press, 2008).

25 See, for example, Marvin A. Sweeney, *Reading the Hebrew Bible After the Shoah: Engaging Holocaust Theology* (Minneapolis: Fortress, 2008).

profitably understood as modelling, across its various books and genres, a practice of retelling that has proved remarkably resilient.

Conclusion

I have outlined recent scholarship that recognises the influence of ancient traumas on the biblical text and asks what difference a sensitivity to this history of influence makes to interpretation and to the use of the Bible as a resource for ministering with traumatised people and church communities. I have argued that the Bible's traumatic heritage fits it remarkably well to be a resource in this context and outlined a variety of respects in which this is so. It is always the case that pastoral use of the Bible as a resource should be undertaken with great care. The very history that fits biblical writings to be resources for pastoral use with traumatised people and congregations also makes its potential for doing harm, including retraumatization, very real. Biblical texts, and, in particular, personal interpretations of those texts, should never be forced and, in particular, should never be forced on the already traumatised. Those readers who wish to follow the thoughts and directions of travel pursued here may wish to read also Chapter 11 of this volume in which I discuss the liturgical use of lament psalms in more detail.

Select references

Boase, Elizabeth and Christopher Frechette, eds. *Bible Through the Lens of Trauma*. Semeia Studies 86. Atlanta: SBL, 2016.

Brett, Mark G. *Political Trauma and Healing: Biblical Ethics for a Postcolonial World*. Grand Rapids: Eerdmans, 2016.

Carr, David M. *Holy Resilience: The Bible's Traumatic Origins*. New Haven: Yale University Press, 2014.

Levinson, Bernard M. *Legal Revision and Religious Renewal in Ancient Israel*. New York: Cambridge University Press, 2008.

Vanstone, William Hubert. *The Stature of Waiting*. London: Darton, Longman and Todd, 1982.

Warner, Megan. *Re-Imagining Abraham: A Re-Assessment of the Influence of Deuteronomism in Genesis*. OTS 72. Leiden/Boston: Brill, 2018.

6 An evangelical practical theology of providence in the light of traumatic incidents

Roger P. Abbott

The doctrine of providence is a massive topic that has interested not just theologians and pastors but also philosophers and ethicists. An associated doctrine, 'theodicy' – the justification of God's providential care or apparent lack of it – carries an equal interest. This chapter restricts its focus to be that of an evangelical practical theology of providence. The major influences in this approach to the doctrine of providence have come from the evangelical constituency, with their particular interest in, and sympathy towards, both the Bible and the sovereignty of God. This is not to suggest there are no alternative perspectives. Indeed, in this chapter I hope I have been able to cast a critical eye at certain places over the evangelical views and the practices relating to the doctrine of providence.

Definition

Because of this particular focus on an evangelical perspective, some definitions are important at this early stage.

Evangelical theology has been defined, sociohistorically, in David Bebbington's classic work on evangelicalism,[1] as 'conversionism, activism, Biblicism, and cruciocentrism', a definition we shall take as foundational for this chapter. Evangelical theology is also characterised by two main themes: the *reality* of life, often fraught with suffering and bad news, being the sphere in which divine providence operates, and the *hope* of transformation by way of the *evangel*, the good news of the Gospel of Jesus Christ, a theology 'which is evoked, governed and judged by the gospel.'[2]

The reality theme informs us of our vulnerability in life to tragedy in a world where life is not what it is supposed to be.[3] Part of the 'mystery of

1 David W. Bebbington, *The Dominance of Evangelicalism: The Age of Spurgeon and Moody* (Downers Grove, IL: InterVarsity, 2005).

2 John Webster, 'The Self-Organizing Power', *International Journal of Systematic Theology* 3 (2001): 69. Note that Webster uses 'evangelical' here as an adjective, rather than as a proper noun.

3 I borrow this phrase from Cornelius Plantinga's *Not the Way It's Supposed to Be: A Breviary of Sin* (Grand Rapids, MI: Eerdmans, 1996).

providence' is that God is sovereign, and yet life is not what it is meant to be. Tragedy is writ large in the evangelical reading of the Bible.[4] Tragedy in the Bible is encountered in historical records, in wisdom literature, in poetic psalms of lament, and in prophetic announcements. It is impossible to read Old and New Testaments without encountering tragedy of some form in every book. Although never voyeuristic in the depiction of tragedy, the biblical representation is realistic and, at times, horrific. No one can justifiably protest that the Bible does not warn him or her of what life can be like, and, likewise, what the Bible shows us must ensure, as Professor David Bentley Hart warns, 'words we would not utter to ease another's grief we ought not to speak to satisfy our own sense of piety'.[5]

On the other hand, however, the hope theme assures us of the promise of our transformation and ultimate redemption, irrespective of the degree of tragedy we have endured. Unlike other Ancient Near Eastern myths, the Bible does not seek to normalise tragedy and suffering; it does not construct for us a deity who celebrates the reality of evil and suffering but a God who has promised an ultimate redemption that will banish both, precisely because they do not 'fit' with life as it is supposed to be (Rv 21:4). This transformative hope is grounded, exclusively, in the life, death, and Resurrection of the person of Jesus Christ, the Son of God, and it forms the foundation for an evangelical doctrine of providence.

As the name suggests, the doctrine of divine providence is about the *provision* a personal God makes in terms of his loving and compassionate care for people caught up in such tragedies. Thus, in evangelical thought, providence is fundamentally rooted in the loving Trinity of God. It is because God is loving Trinity he creates, governs, responds to evil and suffering, has common grace and compassion, reveals himself in Christ to redeem, and will restore all things unto himself. As Trinity, God can relate to, and with, humankind. Perhaps the passage of Scripture where this doctrine is expressed most eloquently and comprehensively is Rom 8:17b–30. This passage unfolds with the bold affirmation of the Apostle Paul, 'For I consider that the sufferings of this present time are not worth comparing with the glory that is to be revealed to us' (Rom 8:18). The reality of suffering that is stated in that affirmation is accompanied by the disclosure of the creation – both animate and inanimate – experiencing tragedy in the form of futility, bondage, and groaning. However, the Spirit of God within the Christian creates and sustains hope in a final redemption. As this final redemption is

4 Some contemporary scholars are suggesting that the theme of trauma is foundational to understanding the Bible, a necessary lens through which the Bible needs to be read. See Elizabeth Boase and Christopher G. Frechette, *Bible Through the Lens of Trauma* (Atlanta, GA: Society of Biblical Literature, 2016); David M. Carr, *Holy Resilience: The Bible's Traumatic Origins* (London: Yale University Press, 2014).

5 David Bentley Hart, *The Doors of the Sea: Where Was God in the Tsunami?* (Grand Rapids, MI: Eerdmans, 2005), 99.

awaited, the Spirit provides hope through intercession for us, and through assurance that 'for those who love God all things work together for good' (Rom 8:26), because a *sovereign* God is managing the redemptive process. Those 'he foreknew he predestined to be conformed to the image of his Son . . . those whom he predestined he also called, and those whom he called he also justified, and those whom he justified he also glorified' (Rom 8:29–30).

It is important to understand that the theology so eloquently expressed and affirmed in that passage of Scripture was not composed within the secure, safe, cloistered environment of academia but from within the context of the Apostle's own suffering as he wrote pastorally to a Christian community also facing tragedy. Here, realism and hope combined to issue a profound evangelical theology of providence. This was a theology crafted out of Paul's own experience of suffering and tragedy, concurring with that which is narrated more fully elsewhere in the New Testament, especially in the Acts of the Apostles and in the Pauline letters.

However, it is one thing to read the theology, especially when bound up as a neat theological 'package', such as Rom 8:17b–30, can appear to be. It is another thing altogether to make sense of it when tragedy strikes and leaves you in emotional/psychological shreds.

The doctrine of providence is crucial to pastoral care in a context of trauma, providing a pastoral base for helping survivors of, and the bereaved and the traumatised from, tragedy. A traumatic incident can often deconstruct cherished assumptions, leaving attendant despair and meaninglessness. Providence is a repository, storing pastoral resources for responding to the 'Why?' 'What?' and the 'Help me!' questions, which are frequently instinctive to the traumatised human psyche. I do not mean that the doctrine provides complete answers, but it supplies a hermeneutic to events that overwhelm the epistemology of common sense.[6] So, for John Calvin, ignorance or unbelief of providence represents 'the ultimate of all miseries.'[7] However, the hermeneutical exercise is a learning process: reconciling horrors and providence is a task undertaken from within our fellowship with God; outside of such, there is no reconciliation.[8]

6 I concur with Hans Reinders, Hans S. Reinders, 'Why This? Why Me? A Theological Reflection on Ethics and Providence', in *The Providence of God*, ed. Francesca Aran Murphy and Philip G. Ziegler (London: T&T Clark, 2009), 296, when he states, 'The "why?" question is a lament, indicating that people long to be comforted; they are not trying to find out who did it'. I am indebted to Professor Reinders for sending me a copy of his conference paper. All citations are from this version of his paper.

7 John Calvin, *Institutes of the Christian Religion*, ed. John T. McNeill and trans. Ford Lewis Battles (Philadelphia, PA: Westminster, 1967), Book 1, Ch. xvii, Section 11. (Citations from the *Institutes* are made in this format in this chapter to facilitate finding the references in other editions.)

8 See John Webster, 'On the Theology of Providence', in *The Providence of God*, 158.

Challenges to the doctrine of providence

The doctrine of providence encountered many challenges as the twentieth century progressed. Earlier, it had been accepted tradition in the church, albeit latterly overstimulated by the optimism of the eighteenth and nineteenth centuries. However, the fact of two World Wars and the occurrence of disasters, along with major technological advances in emergency response and healthcare, brought serious intellectual and emotional questioning of the doctrine of providence to a public already weakened religiously by secular modernist thinking and ill-equipped to fathom the evils of the two World Wars.[9] Instead of a firm belief in providence, despair, flippancy, and nihilism took over. Ironically, the late twentieth century saw the rise, throughout the United Kingdom, of secularism not only infused with spirituality, evidencing fascination in spiritism, astrology, and New Age strands, but also more given to trusting in chance, fortune, or fate than in divine providence. Today, one finds a public very willing openly to display reflections upon tragedy and suffering through floral tributes and notes, which are laid at scenes of tragedy. These frequently evoke themes of angels, hopes of being re-united with loved ones after death, and prayers of hope that God's care will rest on the departed.[10] These reflections of spirituality are displayed by persons, and in the memory of persons, who may not identify as possessing any particular faith whatsoever. Spirituality, if not religion, is never absent from tragedy in even the most secular of societies![11]

Traumatic incidents, therefore, tend to reveal a metaphysical, even sentimental, cocktail of spiritualities that today informs the lives of so many, presenting the Church with a real mission. As Berkouwer stated,

> [y]et there is a strong warning for the Church not to lift herself out of contact with those who, in storm and night, in distress and fear, feel the ground shaking under their feet, a warning for the church to witness, not to the night, but in the night.[12]

9 The Lisbon earthquake of 1755 is often credited with the disillusionment in Christianity. In academic circles, this might have been so. However, belief in the doctrine of providence continued, at least in the churches, long after this event. More significant, in my view, in influencing the church, were the two World Wars in the twentieth century, coming as they did at a time of evolutionary cultural optimism, and what I would describe as the church's 'sell out' to liberalism and secularism. For an evangelical theodicy written out of the First World War, see Peter Taylor Forsyth, *The Justification of God: Lectures for War-Time* (Studies in Theology; London: Duckworth, 1916).

10 See Anne Eyre, 'In Remembrance: Post-disaster Rituals and Symbols', *The Australian Journal of Emergency Management* 14, no. 3 (1999): 23–29.

11 There is by now an assumption among sociologists and theologians that spirituality and religion are distinctly separate concepts, a distinction I do not necessarily hold to.

12 Gerrit Cornelis Berkouwer, *The Providence of God* (Studies in Dogmatics; Grand Rapids, MI: William B. Eerdmanns, 1972), 17.

After all, Jesus asked the Father not to take his disciples out of the world, but that he would keep them from evil while in the world (Jn 17:15).

Providence and interpretation

Incidents of tragedy concentrate the mind and instil an insatiable inquisitiveness even in those normally most sanguine. The questions that arise range from the basic 'Why?' to 'What was I meant to learn?' and even 'Was God telling me something?' However, for victims of tragedy questions such as these can be traumatic and crippling in themselves, and without due care and attention to language and timing, the responses carers bring can risk only further traumatisation.[13]

Believing in sovereign providence is just one part of the response of theology and of pastoral care. *Reading or interpreting* providence is another part, the more difficult, and the more controversial of the two.[14] Providence is not simply a descriptor; it should also be an *evaluator*, if it is to be much more than fate or fortune.[15] Because God states that all that happens to us is for our good (Rom 8:28), then we are justified in evaluating how an incident can contribute to our/others' good and our knowledge of God. Some principles for such evaluating may serve helpful. I offer the following.

The good purpose of providence is to conform those who love God to the image of Christ

Even though providence may permit us to achieve favourable consequences by certain actions or events, we cannot presume this to be divine approval for all that is permitted (Jonah, in running away from his explicitly divinely

13 For those interested in pastorally addressing themes of divine judgement, see my *Sit on our Hands, or Stand on our Feet?: Exploring a Practical Theology of Major Incidence Response for the Evangelical Catholic Christian Community in the UK* (West Theological Monograph Series; Eugene, OR: Wipf and Stock, 2013), 303–323.

14 One might add 'even notorious' given some of the Puritan enthusiasm to read the meaning of providence in everyday events. See, for Puritan interpretations, Keith Thomas, 'Providence: The Doctrine and Its Uses', in *Seventeenth-Century England: A Changing Culture* (ed. W. R. Owens, Vol. 2 Modern Studies; Ward Lock Educational in association with The Open University, 1984 reprint); also Philip Ziegler, 'The Uses of Providence in Public Theology', in *The Providence of God*, 307–325. Thomas comments on the way the clergy in the seventeenth and eighteenth centuries saw 'providences' as frequently as their Puritan predecessors, in terms of famines, epidemics, fires, and earthquakes, being divine judgements. The poor, in particular, were encouraged to see their plight in terms of an inscrutable providence that had promise in a life to come. Reactively, the poor turned to other things that promised more immediate help. Taylor, in light of clergy on the Pacific Cook Islands placing immediate blame for volcanic disasters on the moral transgressions of the islanders, suggests this hermeneutic had been passed down to them from the eighteenth-century missionaries.

15 Paul Helm, *The Providence of God* (Contours of Christian Theology; Downers Grove, IL: InterVarsity, 1994). Also N.T. Wright, *Evil and the Justice of God* (London: SPCK, 2006), 56.

revealed mission, e.g., 'conveniently' found a ship in Joppa ready to take him to Tarshish [Jon 1:3]). To do so could be tantamount to calling evil good, which Scripture condemns (Isa 5:20; cf. Rom 6:1). That God cannot do evil is fundamental to Scripture. However, he permits what he does not will and what he forbids by command in order to achieve his good purposes.[16] Thus, while the *events* of providence are not our guide to a constructive interpretation, the commands and grace of God are. The Apostle Paul indicates that the good for which God works all things is our conformity to Christ (Rom 8:29). All that providence permits is not necessarily morally justified. Indeed, at times, providence can appear morally moot, leaving us with the responsibility for the right interpretation for a virtuous action. An example would be when the storm threatened to wreck the ship carrying the Apostle Paul and others (Acts 27). Some crew decided for abandoning ship and the other passengers, while Paul viewed remaining as God's special providence for saving both crew and passengers. How much an event of tragedy helps conform us to the image of Christ is one guideline for reading the mystery of providence.

An immediate hint to providence can be obtained if there is an element of unexpectedness, undeservedness, or disproportion about the events, and the outcome is beneficial

However, such hints are only immediate and should be subject to further evaluation as time goes on and situations change. The doctrine encourages observation of coincidences and linkages in life, even though we may, initially at least, just keep these things in mind or suspend firm judgement (Gn 37:11; Lk 2:19).[17] However, the danger that the personal preferences of one individual concerning what constitutes 'unexpectedness', 'undeservedness', and 'disproportion' influencing our perceptions needs to be wisely discerned and acknowledged.

Hinton, in his discussion of the role of providence in historical evangelical social thought, reflects on the division of views between 'moderates' and 'extremists'. 'Extremists' tended to look on any sudden or dramatic event as possessing special, divine meaning, usually as judgement for individual or national sins. For the 'moderates', providence was more a system of government God had set in motion, to which one resigned oneself and which one did not question or seek to change. Hinton's analysis is instructive,

16 Hart, *Doors of the Sea*, 82–83. In arguing the 'no-risk' case – that God's permission of evil does not necessitate God being responsible for evil – Helm states it thus: 'Then God controls an evil action by permitting it – by deciding not to prevent it – and the evil action occurs because it is caused by the natures and circumstances of those who perpetrate it.': Paul Helm, 'Evil, Love, and Silence', http://paulhelmsdeep.blogspot.com/2008/02/evil-love-and-silence_01.html.

17 On the other hand, the Corinthian congregants at the Lord's Supper were meant to interpret the disproportionate action of God (rendering some weak, sick, and dying) to indicate divine discipline (1 Cor 11:30).

commenting that 'moderates', with their more passive concept of providence, undertook less self-examined systemic failure and resisted mitigating risk. I believe there has to be a mid-place between both these extremes, and the principle I am endorsing here steers us in that direction.

Some aspects of traumatic incidents cry out for systemic change, if not personal change, and to deny this would be cruel and could continue the high risk of further disaster.[18] The New Zealand psychologist Anthony Taylor argues that passivity, and the failure to read from the perspective of secondary causes, prevented significant systems mitigation work being implemented for Pacific Islanders to reduce disaster risk.[19] In the aftermath of Hurricane Katrina's devastation of New Orleans, Peter Steinfels argued, in *The New York Times*, that, even though this was a catastrophe involving so many human factors, it still demanded some interrogation of God, because, '[f]or believers, humanity, with all its faults and contrivances, is no less God's creation than hurricanes and ocean surges and the law that water seeks its own level'. Two days earlier, Edward Rothstein had argued that

18 See Boyd Hinton, 'The Role of Providence in Evangelical Social Thought', in *History, Society and the Churches: Essays in Honour of Owen Chadwick*, ed. Derek Beales and Geoffrey Best (Cambridge: Cambridge University Press, 1985), 215–233. Hinton reflects on the way that Thomas Chalmers and other evangelicals at the time reacted to the Irish Famine, opposing legislation for the compulsory relief of the poor, 'partly because the certainty of such relief interfered with the machinery of suffering and judgment which God had devised for the poor, but also because relief had to be provided voluntarily if it was to count in the credit column of the rich man's spiritual balance sheet' (231–232). In fairness to Chalmers, he was dismayed when voluntary donations were not forthcoming from the rich English, but he resisted any moves for government intervention as 'coming between providence and the individual sinner' (232). Because of this kind of thinking and practice, some came to view the Irish Famine as God's judgement on a *mean* England more than on poor Ireland.

19 See Antony James William Taylor, 'Value Conflict Arising From a Disaster', *Australasian Journal of Disaster and Trauma Studies* (1999): n.p.; David K. Chester, 'Theology and Disaster Studies: The Need for Dialogue', *Journal of Volcanology and Geothermal Research* 146 (2005): 319–328. Lee Bosher's research in South India, *Social And Institutional Elements of Disaster Vulnerability: The Case of South India* (Bethesda, MD: Academic, 2007), 132–140, 177, concluded that the Hindu caste system played a key role in how disasters were interpreted and accepted there. Disappointingly, he also found that social networks of Hindu and Roman Catholic priests gave no access to resources and that they 'are of little support when it comes to helping people cope' other than performing funerals. See also Russell R. Dynes, 'Noah and Disaster Planning: The Cultural Significance of the Flood Story', Preliminary Paper 265, University of Delaware Disaster Research Centre (1998). Hunter Thompson referred to hazard mitigation as, calling on God but rowing away from the rocks! (In Amanda Ripley, 'How to Survive a Disaster', *Time* in partnership with CNN, June 13, 2008, http://content.time.com/time/magazine/article/0,9171,1810315,00.html, accessed June 13, 2008). Owen Chadwick, *The Victorian Church: Part One 1829–1859* (3rd Ed.; London: SCM, 1971), 490, in reflecting on a cholera outbreak, in Edinburgh, in October 1853, comments that whereas the presbytery of Edinburgh requested Home Secretary Lord Palmerston to appoint a day of national fast and supplication, Palmerston replied that what needed to be addressed, *before* such prayer and fasting, was the overcrowding and the insanitary habits of the poor.

the Katrina incident was notable for the lack of any public interest in divine interrogation since it could be wholly explicable in terms of human errors.[20] Lance Marrow argues that nature has 'clean hands' as far as contemporary evil is concerned compared to humankind. The 'developed world' regards nature as the 'vulnerable innocent' and humans as the enemy.[21]

- All our evaluations need to be tentative, recognising that the best perspective on Providence is often retrospective[22]

As Helm observes, at the time of a tragedy, '[o]ften Christians are left to affirm that their lives are governed by divine providence while lacking the data to demonstrate this'.[23] Reading providence is often, at best, exploratory – a process of learning how to believe (Phil 4:11). Thus, Berkouwer, commenting on discerning the 'finger of God' in events, concludes that no event 'speaks so clearly' that God is of a particular disposition unless God clearly reveals such a disposition in the given event. He also doubts that God does reveal such a precise disposition.[24] Tragic events only speak clearly when God speaks clearly of those events out of his word. Sadly, today, all too often one finds Christians feeling spoken to by God or receiving prophetic words from God that such-and-such a tragedy was caused by some specific providential action, despite Jesus's own warnings against such methods of interpretation (Lk 13:1–5; Jn 9:1–5). Sadly, the history of Evangelicalism records a long list of instances of Jesus's words being ignored and survivors being left to carry burdens of guilt that such 'prophets' have needlessly loaded onto them in God's name.[25] Whether when it comes to major incidents or to personal trauma, the

20 Peter Steinfels, 'Scarcely Heard Question: How God Could Have Allowed Catastrophe to Occur', *The New York Times* September 8, 2005, www.nytimes.com/2005/09/10/us/nationalspecial/scarcely-heard-question-how-god-could-have-allowed.html, accessed June 2008. Edward Rothstein, 'Seeking Justice, of Gods or the Politicians', *The New York Times* September 8, 2005, www.nytimes.com/2005/09/08/books/seeking-justice-of-gods-or-the-politicians.html, accessed June 2008. Also black faith, as identified by Michael Eric Dyson, *Come Hell or High Water* (New York: Basic Civitas, 2006), 179–201, holds this balance.

21 Lance Marrow, 'Evil', *Time* 137, no. 23 (1991), cited in in J. Clinton McCann, *A Theological Introduction to the Book of Psalms: The Psalms as Torah* (Nashville: Abingdon, 1993), 94.

22 For both these points, I am indebted to Helm, *The Providence of God*, 122–130.

23 Helm, *The Providence of God*, 128.

24 Berkouwer, *The Providence of God*, 170.

25 During my fieldwork in Haiti and New Orleans I listened to survivors tell me of Christians, who possess celebrity status among their circles, specifically stating that Hurricane Katrina, which devastated the city of New Orleans, Louisiana, in the United States, and the Haitian earthquake, January 12, 2010, which killed more than 220,000 people and made a million Haitians homeless, were events sent deliberately by God to punish the inhabitants for their sins. These perspectives carried on an historical trend in Evangelical tradition, for example, Thomas Vincent's writing about the great plague and fire of London (1665–1666) as a judgement on London's sins, although he, at least, remained in London, offering succour throughout the disaster (Thomas Vincent, *God's Terrible Voice in the City* [London: George Calvert, 1667; Reprinted Morgan, PA: Soli Deo Gloris, 1997]). John Wesley and

church community needs to refrain from such declamations in God's name, even more so in speculative gossip behind the backs of the bereaved and the survivors. This is because, as Hart asserts of the 2004 Asian tsunami,

> [u]nless one can see the beginning and end of all things, unless one possesses a divine, eternal vantage upon all of time . . . one can draw no conclusions from finite experience regarding the coincidence in God of omnipotence and perfect goodness.[26]

- Evaluation must take into account the complexities in discerning the will of God

Evangelical theologians have explained this in terms of the two aspects of the will of God – his secret and revealed (or permissive) will.[27] Conceptually this duality arises originally from Deuteronomy 29:29: 'The secret things belong *to the LORD* our God, but those things which are revealed belong *to us and to our children* forever, that we may do all the words of this law.' There are difficulties, however, with this concept, which can bring confusion to the traumatised in tragic incidents. It creates a divine 'get-out clause' for whatever happens; God always has his 'other' will as an excuse! For some, this gives the impression of a secret 'dark side', with God's 'good' side being just half the story. Theologically, this cannot be justified of course, as 'God is light, and in him is no darkness *at all*' (1 John 1:5), but this does not prevent the concept worrying confused and traumatised minds unnecessarily.[28] Hans Reinders rejects the two wills idea, preferring an understanding of

---

George Whitefield declared the Lisbon earthquake (and tsunami) of 1755 to be an act of divine judgment against popery: George Whitefield, *Whitefield at Lisbon: Being a Detailed Account of the Blasphemy and Idolatry of Popery . . . With Mr. Whitefield's Remarks Thereon* (London: R. Groombridge and Sons, 1851), 19–32; John Wesley, 'Serious Thoughts Occasioned by the Late Earthquake at Lisbon', in *The Works of the Rev. John Wesley A.M.* (5th Ed., Vol. 11; London: Wesleyan Conference Office). Islamic condemnations can outdo those of Christians at times, such as the condemnatory proclamations to the survivors in Banda Aceh, Indonesia, following the Asian tsunami, and the Iranian earthquake of 2003 in Bam. See 'Iranian Cleric Blames Quakes on Promiscuous Women', *BBC News*, Tuesday, April 20, 2010, http://news.bbc.co.uk/1/hi/world/middle_east/8631775.stm.

26 Hart, *Doors of the Sea*, 13–14.

27 Both Helm and John Piper discuss the idea of God having two wills, not just aspects of one will. See Helm, *The Providence of God*, 131–133; John Piper, 'Are There Two Wills in God?', in *Still Sovereign: Contemporary Perspectives on Election, Foreknowledge and Grace*, ed. Thomas R. Schreiner and Bruce R. Ware (Grand Rapids, MI: Baker, 2000), 107–131.

28 One must bear in mind that traumatic situations often create paranoia. This is because of the suspicions incidents cause to arise between victims and those suspected of culpability in some way. Kettler opposes Helm's concept of the two wills of God, suggesting that it implies divine 'double-mindedness.' See Christian D. Kettler, 'He Takes Back the Ticket . . . For Us: Providence, Evil, Suffering, and the Vicarious Humanity of Christ', *Journal of Christian Theological Research* 8 (2003): 32–57. In view of Helm's concept of compatibilism, however, Kettler's perception seems invalid.

God having one will in which, 'there is wisdom that is known to God alone, and there is "a portion of wisdom prescribed for men." The aim of the distinction is no other than to "humble our minds."'[29]

Therefore, all our legitimate reading of God's will is limited and open to correction, but nevertheless, as long as we are acting within revealed boundaries of Scripture, we are bidden to seek to understand the will of the Lord (Eph 5:17), whilst trusting his integrity (Rom 11:33). Hence, our means of reading providence must be from what has been revealed in the word of God, understood using the hermeneutical tools available to us. This exercise is far from easy. Hermeneutical challenges aside, life's complexities can seem to exceed the details Scripture's answers serve to us in this messy world.[30] There is a limit to reading providence, and we must resist the appetite for detailed answers that we think will resolve all our dilemmas. An important pastoral consequence of applying the doctrine of providence is patient endurance, the capacity to keep on keeping on.

- Reading providence must take into account the perspectives of primary and secondary causes, with the limited understanding primary causes give

By this I mean that due acknowledgement of God as the prime cause – his sovereignty ordains all actualities – may yield us very little more in terms of explanation of a traumatic incident than does chance or bad luck. What has happened has happened.[31] There is often nothing self-evident about providential purpose at the level of human experience, which is why events can appear to us as fortuitous. Calvin acknowledged:

> Since the sluggishness of our mind lies far beneath the height of God's providence, we must employ a distinction to lift it up. Therefore, I shall put it this way: however all things may be ordained by God's plan, according to a sure dispensation, for us they are fortuitous . . . But since the order, reason, end, and necessity of those things which happen for the most part lie hidden in God's purpose, and are not apprehended by human opinion, those things, which it is certain take place by God's will, are in a sense fortuitous. For they bear on the face of them no other appearance, whether they are considered in their own nature or weighed according to our knowledge and judgment.[32]

29 Reinders, 'Providence and Ethics'.

30 Helm, *The Providence of God*, 134–135.

31 For Calvin on primary and secondary causes, see Calvin, *Institutes*, Book I, Ch. 17, Sections 6 & 9. As one Haitian survivor of the catastrophic earthquake was heard to say during a group therapy session for her trauma, 'the one who made the shoulders, it is the same who distributes the crosses'.

32 Calvin, *Institutes*, Book I, Ch. vi, Section 9.

Therefore, it is not wrong to conclude that a tragic incident, with all its attendant coincidences and timings, was just fortuitous, an accident, or what *Time* magazine described as 'the whimsey of the devastation'.[33] We do not have to prove our spiritual discernment by presenting some theological interpretation. Better for the traumatised to learn to live at peace with a certain amount of uncertainty from providence than to think they have something more accurate but which is actually wrong. The evaluation that you were just in the wrong place at the wrong time is not pastorally awry. Yes, primarily, God ordained it and therefore has a purpose in it for both victim and responder, but at least for the moment, that is all hidden, inscrutable. For the moment, it was just bad luck![34] The very closest, it seems to me, the doctrine of providence brings us to any understanding of a divine purpose for each and every tragedy is that which Jesus challenged his inquirers with when they confronted him with the two tragedies, in Luke 13:1–5. Jesus addressed various 'spectators' to these tragic events, people who had heard of them but who had not actually been involved in them. This aspect should not be overlooked. Therefore, it was to them, not as being traumatised by bereavement or as having survived tragedy but as *spectators* of such, that Jesus said the purpose, *for them*, was to lead them to repentance before God. Further than that, we are forbidden to venture opinion on the divine intention.

- In our reading of providence, the eschatological purpose of Christ's return is an important hermeneutic

Evangelical theologian Carl Henry averred, 'Divine Providence is not only ethical and purposeful; it is also eschatological'.[35] Since interpreting God's providence requires hermeneutical horizons,[36] there will be purposes in God's ordaining of events that may be immediate, intermediate, and long term. The case of Joseph exemplifies this:

- *Immediate = his visit to the brothers, dressed in the provocative coat; the plot for murder being changed to that of a sale; his conveyance to Egypt (Gen 37).*
- *Intermediate = Joseph's favour with Potiphar; his prolonged imprisonment with the butler and baker; the famine; Joseph's promotion to*

33 Amanda Ripley, 'How to Survive a Disaster', *Time*.

34 See Berkouwer, *The Providence of God*, 170. Guinness' counsel, Os Guinness, *Unspeakable: Facing Up to the Challenge of Evil* (New York: Harper San Fransisco, 2006), 205, seems wise: 'False accounting for evil always ends in falsely accusing someone, whether someone else, ourselves, or God. When we are with anyone who is suffering, we should never give words without love, and we should never give answers without knowledge'.

35 Carl F.H. Henry, *God Who Stands and Stays* (Carlisle: Paternoster, 1999), 457.

36 See Anthony C. Thiselton, *New Horizons in Hermeneutics: The Theory and Practice of Transforming Biblical Reading* (Grand Rapids, MI: Zondervan, 1997).

prime-minister; the visit of the brothers to Egypt; Joseph's revelation; Israel's settlement in Egypt (Gen 39–50).

- *Long term = the Exodus; law-giving; Canaan; and the Christ.*

These are just a few of the possible eschatological horizons of providence. Ultimately, God's acts are steered toward the final revelation of God in Christ. Ray Anderson reflects,

> While the first century of the church is normative for the revelation of Christ as the incarnation of God and the redemption of humans from sin and death, the return of the same Christ and the resurrection from the dead constitute the normative praxis of the Spirit.[37]

The fuller understanding and meaning are grasped only from the vantage point of this perspective (1 Cor 4:4–5). Much of providence cannot be understood until we arrive, and, meanwhile, we must not forget to read providence in terms of where God is willing us to go – into the future, not the past.

Providence and compassion

A final, and essential, contribution to an evangelical practical theology of providence must be a theology and praxis of compassion. In the context of responding to traumatic incidents, great or small, the doctrine of providence is about bringing clarity, or at least comfort and composure of faith, where there is enormous uncertainty and heartbroken confusion. Into the often very cognitive and emotional messy 'mix' trauma creates, one action an evangelical theology of providence demands is provided is compassion. Not only a theology in itself but also an aspect of divine providence, compassion forms the basis for a pastoral response to traumatic incidents.

According to Scripture, compassion is a powerful fusion of feeling and action. The Greek term often used for compassion in the New Testament expresses the emotional component vividly. The Greek *splagchnizomai* was used by Jesus to express his compassion towards crowds of people who came to hear him (Mt 9:36; 14:14; 15:32, etc.). Literally, the word translates as 'innards,' because the emotions of compassion are felt bodily, 'in the guts'. However, compassion does not remain only in such feelings. Compassion also involves action, or a driven response to try to do something to relieve the state of the suffering other. In the words of Andrew Purves, '[c]ompassion is not caring from a distance. It has a face-to-face quality, and

37 Ray S. Anderson, *The Shape of Practical Theology: Empowering Ministry with Theological Praxis* (Downer's Grove IL: InterVarsity, 2001), 106.

something of the sense of presence and involvement'.[38] Compassion is the assured expression of divine providence towards those who suffer in this earthly life.

What is this compassion when it is feeling in action? Kathleen O'Connor expounds this brilliantly in her commentary on the Old Testament Book of Lamentations. She describes the movement of perspective found in the change of narrator from the third-person objectivity of chapter 1 to the intensely personal first-person perspective of chapter 2. The spectator to the suffering in chapter 1 becomes the co-suffering witness in chapter 2. Thus, she describes compassion in terms of being a witness of a very particular kind:

> In Lamentations the afflicted need a comforting witness, neither the evangelist who announces messages from outside suffering nor the legal witness in a court of law who 'objectively' states the facts, but something at once simpler and more difficult. The witness sees suffering for what it is, without denying it, twisting it into a story of endurance, or giving it a happy ending. The witness has a profound and rare human capacity to give reverent attention to sufferers and reflect their truth back to them. And in the encounter with those who suffer, the witness undergoes conversion from numbed or removed observer to passionate advocate.[39]

At the very least, an evangelical theology of providence must bring carers to such a position of compassion, from which they will be most effectively positioned to assist the traumatised bring the principles of interpreting providence to bear on their experiences.

Conclusion

In conclusion, out of a disposition of compassion, the principles outlined can aid the attempt to interpret providence, to form a praxis for 'understanding what the will of the Lord is'. They are a valid toolbox for sufferers to use in trying to interpret situations that can seem beyond repair. Working with these principles can be a way of post-traumatic empowerment for survivors to address an event that threatened disempowerment whilst recognising it will not provide all the answers. These principles also provide tools for

38 Andrew Purves, *Search for Compassion: Spirituality and Mission* (Louisville: John Knox, 1989), 125. For additional reading on compassion, see Oliver Davies, *A Theology of Compassion: Metaphysics of Difference and the Renewal of Tradition* (London: SCM, 2001), and Roger Philip Abbott, *Sit on our Hands, or Stand on our Feet: Exploring a Practical Theology of Major Incident Response for the Evangelical Catholic Christian Response in the UK* (Eugene, OR: Wipf & Stock, 2013).

39 Kathleen O'Connor, *Lamentations: The Tears of the World* (Maryknoll, NY: Orbis, 2002), 100.

Christian carers to work with in a proactive way in the interests of providing a pastoral response for the traumatised.

Select references

Abbott, Roger P. *Sit on Our Hands, or Stand on Our Feet?: Exploring a Practical Theology of Major Incidence Response for the Evangelical Catholic Christian Community in the UK*. West Theological Monograph Series; Eugene, OR: Wipf and Stock, 2013.

Berkouwer, Gerrit Cornelis. *The Providence of God*. Studies in Dogmatics. Grand Rapids: William B. Eerdmanns, 1972.

Davies, Oliver. *A Theology of Compassion: Metaphysics of Difference and the Renewal of Tradition*. London: SCM, 2001.

Helm, Paul. *The Providence of God*. Leicester: InterVarsity, 1993.

Murphy, Francesca Aran and Philip G. Ziegler. *The Providence of God*. London: T&T Clark, 2009.

7 'In spite of all this, we will yearn for you'

Reflections on God's involvement in events causing great suffering

Christopher Southgate

'What was God's involvement in the horrific event?'

This question naturally arises in the minds of victims and their supporters alike – be the event an act of terrorism, such as the London Bridge attack of 2017, or disastrous negligence, such as the fire at Grenfell Tower in the same year, or a great natural disaster, such as the Indian Ocean tsunami of 2004. Two famous responses to that question, both in response to human cruelty that caused great suffering, are first, that of Elie Wiesel in his concentration camp recollections in *Night*:

> Then the march past [the victims hanged by the SS] began. The two men were no longer alive. Their tongues hung swollen, blue-tinged. But the third rope was still moving; being so light, the child was still alive . . .
>
> For more than half an hour he stayed there, struggling between life and death, dying in slow agony under our eyes. And we had to look him full in the face. He was still alive when I passed in front of him. His tongue was still red, his eyes were not yet glazed.
>
> Behind me, I heard the same man asking:
>
> 'Where is God now?'
>
> And I heard a voice within me answer him:
>
> 'Where is He? He is here – He is hanging here on this gallows . . .'[1]

Second, Rowan Williams's response to being challenged in a New York street at the time of the 9/11 attacks on the World Trade Center:

> What do you say? The usual fumbling about how God doesn't intervene, which sounds like a lame apology for some kind of 'policy' on God's part, a policy exposed as heartless in the face of such suffering. Something about how God is there in the sacrificial work of the rescuers, in the risks they take? . . . Any really outrageous human action tests to the limit our careful theological principles about God's refusal to

1 Elie Wiesel, *Night*, trans. Stella Rodway (New York: Bantam, 1982), 61–62.

> interfere with created freedom. That God has made a world into which he doesn't casually step in [sic] to solve problems is fairly central to a lot of Christian faith. He has made the world so that evil choices can't just be frustrated or aborted . . . They have to be confronted, suffered, taken forward, healed in the complex process of human history, always in collaboration with what we do and say and pray.[2]

Williams's interlocutor 'was a lifelong Christian believer, but for the first time it came home to him that he might be committed to a God who could seem useless in a crisis'.[3]

In both cases the response stems from a profound spiritual reflex in a deep thinker. But it necessarily begs the question: Why is the God who is confessed as present seemingly so powerless to prevent cruelty inflicting great suffering?

A very tempting explanation, arrived at independently by two important Jewish thinkers, is that God *cannot* effect any change in such situations. God, for whatever reason, has entrusted Godself to humanity. Hans Jonas, whose mother died in Auschwitz, took the view that God empties Godself of mind and power in giving the creation its existence and then allows the interplay of chance and natural law to take its course. God's only further involvement is that God holds a memory of the experience of the creation – God receives God's being back 'transfigured or possibly disfigured by the chance harvest of unforeseeable temporal experience'.[4]

For a more first-hand, up-close theological response to Nazi tyranny, we may turn to Etty Hillesum, the young Dutch intellectual whose diaries and letters in the last two years of her life (1941–1943) have had such an impact on so many readers.[5] Etty comes to conclude that God will not, cannot, help those in the camp. All they can do is 'safeguard that little piece of You, God, in ourselves'.[6] Her God has handed Godself over to the world, entering the human heart and being 'guarded' by those with the least worldly power. She writes: 'there must be someone to live through it all and bear witness to the fact that God lived, even in these times'.[7] Her concern is 'if we just care enough, God is in safe hands with us despite everything'.[8]

2 Rowan Williams, *Writing in the Dust: Reflection on 11th September and Its Aftermath* (London: Hodder and Stoughton, 2002), 7–8.

3 Williams, *Writing in the Dust*, 8.

4 Hans Jonas, *Morality and Morality: A Search for the Good After Auschwitz – A (Posthumous) Collection of Essays Edited by Lawrence Vogel* (Evanston, IL: Northwestern University Press, 1996), 125.

5 English speakers will be helped in studying Hillesum by Patrick Woodhouse's sympathetic study, *Etty Hillesum: A Life Transformed* (London: Bloomsbury, 2009).

6 Etty Hillesum, *Etty: The Letters and Diaries of Etty Hillesum 1941–1943*, ed. Klaas A.D. Smelik, trans. A.J. Pomerans (Grand Rapids, MI: Eerdmans, 2002), 488.

7 Hillesum, *Etty*, 506.

8 Hillesum, *Etty*, 657.

Such strategies for characterising God as a vulnerable co-victim emerged with great integrity out of reflection on intolerable suffering. But they seem a far cry from the more usual confession of God as transcendent creator. This chapter considers communities' possible answers to questions of God's involvement in shock events, if those strategies, based on God's voluntary self-disempowerment, are not adopted. Different arguments are needed in the case of moral and natural evil, as defined in the following two sections.

Moral evil

I differentiate between harms and suffering caused by acts by freely-choosing self-conscious agents (usually called 'moral evil') and other harms and sufferings ('natural evil'). I am not suggesting that any given human action is completely free. I acknowledge how much of our activity results from our neurological wiring and our familial and cultural conditioning. I also acknowledge that our self-consciousness is likewise limited and conditioned. I nevertheless hold that human experience suggests compellingly that within those constraints is a real, if partial, freedom and that the scientific evidence does not rule that out.[9]

I write this as the first anniversary of the terrorist attack on a concert in Manchester is rapidly followed by that of the further terrorist attack on London Bridge and Borough Market and then by that of the terrible fire in Grenfell Tower. Two of these events clearly demonstrated malice, indeed the intention to harm those completely unknown to the perpetrators. There is substantial evidence that the extent and horror of Grenfell reflected not only an accidental start to the fire but also a negligent approach to the building, especially the external cladding of the tower.

When we contemplate such harm-infliction and negligence caused by humans, I hold that we cannot expect to see signs of God *in those causes*. God gave the humans concerned freedom, and the causes of the harms and suffering were to be found in the misuse of that freedom. I return later to the question of God's involvement in the causes of natural disasters.

Ruard Ganzevoort is surely right to draw an important distinction between responses to malicious action, on one hand, and to events that seem rather to connote tragedy, on the other, including harmful actions committed without intent to harm.[10] This distinction is necessary for a healthy response to

9 For a painstaking analysis giving the scientific account the utmost purchase, see Philip Clayton, *In Quest of Freedom: The Emergence of Spirit in the Natural World: Frankfurt Templeton Lectures 2006*, ed. M. G. Parker and T. M. Schmidt (Göttingen: Vandenhoeck and Ruprecht, 2009).

10 R. Ruard Ganzevoort, 'Coping with Tragedy and Malice', in *Coping with Evil in Religion and Culture*, ed. N. van Doorn-Harder and L. Minnema (Amsterdam: Rodopi, 2008), 247–260; 'Scars and Stigmata: Trauma, Identity and Theology', *Practical Theology* 1, no. 1 (2008): 19–31.

a traumatising event, as is eventual separation from the event, so that the victims no longer derive their identity solely from it. It does not, however, seem to me that Ganzevoort has quite addressed that other category of moral evil – *negligent* action or inaction, which while having no direct intent to harm is nevertheless culpable and can and should provoke powerful protest from victims and supporters.

Response to traumatising events within a Christian community caused by malice or negligence may reasonably include worship of God, protest, lament, and practical assistance. This is, indeed, the same combination of responses as would be elicited by a natural disaster. But the balance of the response must be different in the case of moral evil. The *dominant* dimension of response to moral evil must be making the community safe against further perpetrators, protest against all injustice and culpable negligence, and rejection of all gratuitous harming, followed, ultimately, when possible, by the exploration of the possibility of reconciliation. But always the victims and their narratives must be attended to; always, as is proverbial in trauma theory, 'the survivor is the expert'. Arguably, theodicy has been much too preoccupied with the stories of the causes of great harm and suffering. The stories of victims and their supporters are coming to be recognised as of prime importance. So, remarkably, the public enquiry into the Grenfell fire began with days of testimony from survivors and relatives of victims (two importantly different groups in the immediate aftermath of a tragedy but brought together at the enquiry in a common act of re-telling).

Caution needs to be exercised, however, in fastening too firmly onto these stories, both because of the very fluid character of narratives of recollection in trauma[11] and also because of the risk of scapegoating. Here, the analysis of Hauerwas and Burrell as to what constitute 'good' stories is helpful.[12] They claim that any story that is adopted by a community will have to display (1) power to release from destructive alternatives (2) ways of seeing through current distortions (3) room to keep the community from having to resort to violence and (4) a sense of the tragic – how meaning transcends power. I return to these criteria later.

Where perpetrators (and the negligent) are culpable, the protest and desire for justice may eventually lead to an effort to reach for the sort of love and empathy that Jesus is recorded as having evinced when he said of his executioners, that 'they know not what they do' (Lk 23:34). Even the enemy is to be loved as a fellow creature, in imitation of God's love that never lets the creature go. But reaching anything like that position is a long labour of love,

11 Especially in the 'disillusionment' phase, see Laurie Kraus, David Holyan, and Bruce Wisner, *Re-Covering From Un-Natural Disasters: A Guide for Pastors and Congregations After Violence and Trauma* (Louisville, KY: Westminster John Knox, 2017), see esp. Ch. 4.

12 Stanley Hauerwas and David Burrell, 'From System to Story: An Alternative Pattern for Rationality in Ethics', in *Why Narrative?*, ed. Stanley Hauerwas and L. Gregory Jones (Grand Rapids, MI: Eerdmans, 1989), 158–190.

which perhaps few may attain. Sometimes a 'staged' version of reconciliation may be necessary, as in the work of the Truth and Reconciliation Commission in South Africa after the apartheid era.

Natural evil

What will concern us in the rest of this chapter are those shocking events where the main cause is not human malice or human negligence or even a very rare combination of chances but the fabric of the physical universe as God has created and sustained it. A familiar defence of God in respect of moral evil is that the gift of freedom to freely-choosing creatures conscious of themselves and others necessarily implies the possibility of the misuse of that freedom (and that, as was noted earlier in the quotation from Rowan Williams, God would render that gift incoherent by continually intervening to mitigate bad human choices). In the case of shock events occasioned by the way the world is, rather than the particular choices of conscious choosers, that defence can no longer operate in quite the same way.[13] God seems, rather, to be directly responsible for the creation containing the violence of earthquakes, hurricanes, forest fires caused by lightning strikes, flash floods, and volcanic eruptions.[14]

Some scholars want to insist on denying this responsibility of God's. For discussion of theological moves behind such denial, either in the form of a fall event or some variety of what I have termed 'mysterious fallenness', and my reservations about such moves, see the exchanges in the journal *Zygon* in the issue for September 2018.[15] But there are also more practical denials

13 Though see Christopher Southgate, '"Free-Process" and "Only-Way" Arguments', in *Finding Ourselves After Darwin: Conversations on the Image of God, Original Sin, and the Problem of Evil*, ed. Stanley P. Rosenberg, Michael Burdett, Michael Lloyd, and Benno van den Toren (Grand Rapids, MI: Baker Academic, 2018), 293–305, for an evaluation of those theodicies that appeal to the good of freedom of natural processes.

14 And also, thinking of Karen O'Donnell's powerful testimony in her *Broken Bodies: The Eucharist, Mary and the Body in Trauma Theology* (London: SCM Press, 2018), the familial tragedy of unwanted miscarriage. Note also Deanna A. Thompson's recent study, *Glimpsing Resurrection: Cancer, Trauma and Ministry* (Louisville, KY: Westminster John Knox, 2018) on cancer diagnoses in apparently healthy people in midlife. B. Jill Carroll, writing of the work of the nature-contemplative Annie Dillard, B. Jill Carroll, *The Savage Side: Reclaiming Violent Models of God* (Lanham, MD/Oxford: Rowman and Littlefield, 2001), 45, goes as far as to say this: 'It is because of the conditions of human existence in the world – conditions which have God's full blessing – that people suffer what they like to call "freak accidents." In truth, there is no freak accident, because such accidents are inevitable given the conditions of time, space, matter and freedom.'

15 Neil Messer, 'Evolution and Theodicy: How (Not) to Do Science and Theology', *Zygon: Journal of Religion and Science* 53 (2018): 821–835; Nicola Hoggard Creegan, 'Theodicy: A Response to Christopher Southgate', *Zygon: Journal of Religion and Science* 53 (2018): 808–820; Celia Deane-Drummond, 'Perceiving Natural Evil through the Lens of Divine Glory? A Conversation with Christopher Southgate', *Zygon: Journal of Religion and*

such as that of Robert White.[16] It is indeed possible, as White holds, to identify areas of human hubris and negligence contributing to the extent of suffering from natural disasters. For example, the loss of life from the Indian Ocean tsunami of 2004 was exacerbated by a civil war, the cutting down of mangrove swamps on coastland, and the lack of the early-warning system that was already present in the Pacific. The suffering caused by the Haiti earthquake of 2010 was greatly enhanced by the poverty of a country that is a close neighbour of the world's wealthiest nation. Yet to exclude God from all responsibility for natural evil is a hard task. (What, for example, about that famous case in the history of theodicy – the Lisbon earthquake and tsunami of 1755, of which there could have been no possible warning? Are we to return to Charles Wesley's view, five years earlier, when he began a sermon with the statement that '[o]f all the Judgments which the righteous God inflicts on Sinners here, the most dreadful and destructive is an Earthquake'.)[17] In the end, diversion of all culpability for catastrophic natural events from God to humans can only rest on a prior theological commitment to radical human corruption resulting from primal sin. On such a view, even a young baby falls rightly under divine judgement. It seems much more natural to concede that God has underlying responsibility for the way the violent processes of the world occasion human suffering.[18]

So we now find ourselves beginning to answer our starting question – about God's involvement in the shocking event – with the disturbing thought that in instances of natural evil God is the major responsible agent, the creator of the forces behind the most harm-producing manifestations of nature, be they floods, eruptions, typhoons, genetic diseases, or epidemics of natural pathogens. Christian theology has been very shy of this conclusion, though it is in a way a logical route to follow once Marcion's distinction between the Gods of the two Testaments is abandoned, and *creatio ex nihilo* becomes the orthodoxy of the Church.

Wesley Wildman has tackled this subject with characteristic clarity. He gives a skilful critique of 'determinate-entity theism' (belief in a personal God, such as the Christian conviction that God is creator and redeemer and can be known through God's Son and the work of the Holy Spirit) and goes on to show the weaknesses of process theism. Wildman's solution is to

---

Science 53 (2018): 792–807; Christopher Southgate, 'Response with a Select Bibliography', *Zygon: Journal of Religion and Science* 53 (2018): 909–930.

16 Robert S. White, *Who is to Blame: Disasters, Nature and Acts of God* (Oxford: Monarch, 2014).

17 Charles Wesley, quoted in Ryan Nichols, 'Re-Evaluating the Effects of the1755 Lisbon Earthquake on Eighteenth-Century Minds: How Cognitive Science of Religion Improves Intellectual History with Hypothesis Testing Methods', *Journal of the American Academy of Religion* 82, no. 4 (2014): 970–1009.

18 And non-human suffering in wild nature, on which see, for example, Christopher Southgate, *The Groaning of Creation: God, Evolution and the Problem of Evil* (Louisville, KY: Westminster John Knox, 2008).

regard God as the ground of being, whose nature is glimpsable not only in the beauty but also in the violence of the cosmos. His God is not a personal entity, let alone a benevolent entity. Wildman writes, 'Suffering in nature is neither evil nor a by-product of the good. It is part of the wellspring of divine creativity in nature, flowing up out of the abysmal divine depths like molten rock from the yawning mouth of a volcano'.[19]

But this will be too big a step for most Christians, who will want to insist, even in this difficult territory, on the personal nature of God, revealed especially in the person of Jesus. How to combine this with God's accountability for the disvalues of creation? Veli-Matti Karkkainen, reporting on the Finnish school of Lutheran studies, writes this of the thought of Luther:

> God's alien work [*opus alienum Dei*] means putting down, killing, taking away hope, leading to desperation, etc. God's proper work means the opposite: forgiving, giving mercy, taking up, saving, encouraging, etc . . . Luther in fact says that God's proper work is veiled in his alien work and takes place simultaneously with it . . . God's works are not just veiled in their opposite but they also sometimes create bad results . . . God makes a human being a *nihil* . . . to make him/her a new being.[20]

Karkkainen concludes finally that 'God is not to be excused, but is to be trusted'.[21]

So there is thinking from a major element of the Christian tradition that accepts God's responsibility for the violence in creation as part of the paradox of God's ways with the world. The key element in that last quotation is that second half 'but is to be trusted'.

This is surprisingly close to a famous passage in contemporary Jewish theology, from David Blumenthal's book on Holocaust theology *Facing the Abusing God*. In the extraordinary coda to that book he writes to God as follows:

> I do not deny You or Your Torah. You denied us, for we were innocent. You crushed us, yet we were guiltless. You were the Abuser; our sins

19 Wesley J. Wildman, 'Incongruous Goodness, Perilous Beauty, Disconcerting Truth: Ultimate Reality and Suffering in Nature', in *Physics and Cosmology: Scientific Perspectives on the Problem of Natural Evil*, ed. N. Murphy, R. J. Russell and W. R. Stoeger, SJ (Berkeley, CA: CTNS and Vatican City: Vatican Observatory, 2007), 267–294, at 294. See also Wesley J. Wildman, *In Our Own Image: Anthropomorphism, Apophaticism and Ultimacy* (Oxford: Oxford University Press, 2017).

20 Veli-Matti Karkkainen, 'Evil, Love and the Left Hand of God: The Contribution of Luther's Theology of the Cross to an Evangelical Theology of Evil', *Evangelical Quarterly* 74, no. 3 (2002): 215–234, at 222–223. On the 'violent side of God', in Christian reflection see also Carroll, *Savage Side*; Charlene P.E. Burns, 'Honesty About God: Theological Reflections on Violence in an Evolutionary Universe', *Theology and Science* 4, no. 3 (2006): 279–290.

21 Karkkainen, 'Evil', 232.

> were not commensurate with Your actions. The responsibility is Yours, not ours . . . In spite of all this, we will gather our strength and support one another. We will build our world. We will love one another. We will defend our people and our land. We will believe in You, we will place our hope in You. We will yearn for You, we will wait for You, and we will anticipate the time when we will see Your Face again.[22]

As with Karkkainen's conclusion about the theology of Luther, God is not excused (rather the reverse!) *but* in spite of all, God is the one in whom ultimate trust will be placed.

Blumenthal is addressing the extreme moral evil of the Holocaust. It draws from him, very understandably, a conviction that God's apparent abandonment of the chosen people of God amounts to abuse. This conviction and Blumenthal's analogy with child abuse have been much criticised, not least by Wendy Farley in her dialogue with the author within *Facing the Abusing God*.[23] And it may also be criticised for blurring the distinction noted earlier between malice and negligence. God did not, on most accounts, actually *commit* the moral evils of the Holocaust, although God did not, apparently, intervene to prevent or even mitigate them.[24] Hence the responses of Wiesel and Williams with which we began this chapter.

Our concern in this section is possible Christian responses to events of massive natural evil, events causing great harm and suffering through the operation of causes that God created and which did not operate through the choices of other moral agents. The response of holding God accountable, I suggest, is truer to the origins of Judaism and Christianity than either the hyperkenotic position of Jonas or the powerless power of Etty Hillesum's God, whom she could still call her 'high tower',[25] even though that God not only would not, but also could not, rescue her from oppression or execution. I also hold that a God accountable for natural evil is truer to a biblical faith than philosophical theodicies that 'square the circle' of God's moral perfection and God's involvement in harms and suffering.[26] The shortcomings of

22 David R. Blumenthal, *Facing the Abusing God: A Theology of Protest* (Louisville, KY: Westminster John Knox, 1993), 299.

23 Blumenthal, *Facing*, 211–225. See also, for example, Jonathan Brumberg-Kraus, 'Contemporary Jewish Theologies: An Essay Review', *The Reconstructionist* (1994): 86–94; Isabel Wollaston, 'The Possibility and Plausibility of Divine Abusiveness or Sadism as the Premise for a Religious Response to the Holocaust', *Journal of Religion and Society* 2 (2000): 1–15.

24 For a recent survey of Jewish theodical and anti-theodical responses see David Tollerton, 'Reconfiguring the Theodicy-Antitheodicy Boundary between Responses to the Holocaust', *Journal of Jewish Thought and Philosophy* 26 (2018): 278–292.

25 Quoting Psalm 94.22, or possibly 18.2, or 61.3, or Proverbs 18.10. For a recent Trinitarian theology of a God unable to prevent traumatising evil see Jennifer Baldwin, *Trauma-Sensitive Theology: Thinking Theologically in the Era of Trauma* (Eugene, OR: Cascade Books, 2018).

26 Such as Richard Swinburne, *Providence and the Problem of Evil* (Oxford: Oxford University Press, 1998); Alvin Plantinga, *God, Freedom and Evil* (Grand Rapids, MI: Eerdmans, 1977).

such theodicies have been corrosively analysed by Terrence Tilley and D.Z. Phillips[27] and also by Kenneth Surin, with his emphasis that we must allow the narratives of victims to interrupt the narratives we tell, and John Swinton, with his sense that the proper response to suffering, is found not in theory but in lament, forgiveness, thoughtfulness, hospitality, and friendship.[28]

Is there then an approach that retains the personal character of God, *contra* Wildman, without seeking either to exonerate God as per White or yet to characterise God as 'abuser' as per Blumenthal?

That God might be the author of suffering is familiar ground in the Hebrew Bible, and Christians need, I believe, to take with more seriousness texts such as Deuteronomy's 'See now that I, even I, am he; there is no god besides me. I kill and I make alive; I wound and I heal; and no one can deliver from my hand' (Dt 32:39). 'The Lord kills and brings to life; he brings down to Sheol and raises up' (1 Sm 2:6) and Deutero-Isaiah's description of God as the author of 'weal and woe alike' (Is 45:7).[29]

It is an interesting question, far beyond the scope of this chapter, why Christianity has largely parted company with these insights into the mystery of God. But two reasons may at least be glimpsed: first, that a sense of the fallenness of the world, deriving especially from Augustine's reading of Paul's reading of Genesis 3, made it possible for centuries of Christian thinkers to 'park' the disvalues of God's creation at the door of some agency other than God[30] and, second, because of a sense in so much Christian thought that Christ's self-giving on the Cross is somehow the ultimate answer to all questions about suffering in the world.[31]

But I wonder whether these moves, so embedded in much Christian imagination, do not need further honest reflection on their completeness. After all, Christianity shares with Judaism the foundational story of the deliverance of the people of God from slavery, a release involving God's use of the

27 Terrence Tilley, *The Evils of Theodicy* (Georgetown, VA: Georgetown University, 1991); Dewi Zephaniah Phillips, *The Problem of Evil and the Problem of God* (London: SCM, 2004).

28 Kenneth Surin, *Theology and the Problem of Evil* (Oxford: Basil Blackwell, 1986), 161–162; John Swinton, *Raging with Compassion: Pastoral Responses to the Problem of Evil* (Grand Rapids, MI/Cambridge: Eerdmans, 2007).

29 See M. Daniel Carroll R. and J. Blair Wilgus, eds., *Wrestling with the Violence of God: Soundings in the Old Testament* (Winona Lake, IN: Eisenbrauns, 2015) for recent engagement with these and other problematic texts.

30 We see this approach persist, in different ways, in the work of Messer, Deane-Drummond and Hoggard Creegan cited earlier and in Michael Lloyd, 'The Fallenness of Nature: Three Nonhuman Suspects', in *Finding Ourselves After Darwin*, ed. Stanley P. Rosenberg et al. (Grand Rapids, MI: Baker Academic, 2018), 262–279.

31 So in the powerful and important work of Jürgen Moltmann on the Cross, *The Crucified God: The Cross of Christ as the Foundation and Criticism of Christian Theology*, trans. R.A. Wilson and J. Bowden (London: SCM, 1974), 276, he writes that 'He [God] humbles himself and takes upon himself the eternal death of the godless and the godforsaken, so that all the godless and the godforsaken can experience communion with him.'

powers of the natural world. And much Christian eschatology insists that in the Christ event, the cosmos has already been reconciled with God its creator (Col 1:20). *And yet* there seems a deficit of explanation as to why when the assumption of order that humans need to live by is shattered,[32] there is not a stronger response, among Christians traumatised by natural disaster, that the God who created everything out of nothing, who is also confessed as the God of deliverance, has failed them.[33]

The extraordinary power of Blumenthal's paragraph quoted earlier lies in that willingness to accord blame to God and yet to continue 'In spite of all this . . .'. It is reminiscent of Samuel Terrien's formulation of Israel's relationship with her Lord, written in the context of the story of the near sacrifice of Isaac: 'The sign of purity of faith was love at any cost for a God who conceals his Godhead in appearance of hostility'. Israel's religion, for Terrien, is

> based on the courage to face the abyss of being, even the abyss of the being of God, and to affirm . . . the will to gamble away not only one's own ego but even one's hope in the future of mankind.[34]

This conclusion about the God of the Hebrew Bible theophanies is too much tidied up in too many Christian preachers' accounts of God's ways with the world. Karkkainen again: 'Much of Evangelical spirituality and theology, especially in its popular, devotional form, is a misguided effort in whitewashing the walls of our world with sentimental talk about God's love'.[35]

I suggest that recognising God's responsibility for natural evil counts as a helpful story in Hauerwas and Burrell's terms because (1) it releases us from destructive alternatives, whether they be that humans are so utterly corrupt that even a newborn baby deserves destruction, or that blame must be assigned to human groups judged especially immoral[36] (and so also keeps us from having to resort to violence); (2) it provides us with ways of seeing through current distortions, such as the sentimental whitewashing just referred to, and finally (3) it enhances and attunes our sense of the

32 Cf. Ronnie Janoff-Bullman, *Shattered Assumptions: Towards a New Psychology of Trauma* (New York: Free Press, 1992).

33 For a sociological study of the acceptability of anger against God in a North American context see Julie J. Exline, Kalman J. Kaplan, and Joshua B. Grubbs, 'Anger, Exit and Assertion: Do People See Protest Toward God as Morally Acceptable?' *Psychology and Religion and Spirituality* 4, no. 4 (2012): 264–277.

34 Samuel Terrien, *The Elusive Presence: Toward a New Biblical Theology* (Eugene, OR: Wipf and Stock, 2005), 83–84.

35 Karkkainen, 'Evil', 231.

36 As in the extraordinary assertion in a flyer from an American Baptist Church that the 2004 tsunami had done a good, in resulting in the deaths of many Swedish people in Thailand, because of the extent of homosexuality in Sweden. 'Tsunami: where was God?' (documentary, director Mark Dowd, broadcast by Channel 4 and available on YouTube).

tragic – neither humanity nor even God seems to have the power to realise certain sorts of goods except through suffering.

So Christians, I suggest, must be honest, banishing sentimentality and the temptation to whitewash in acknowledging God's responsibility for the violent and harmful character of the natural world. For both Frances Young and myself, the Incarnation of Jesus, God's astonishingly intensified commitment to the world, culminating in the Cross, is God's taking responsibility for the suffering-filled world.[37] Perhaps this is for Christians the beginning of the framing of an 'In spite of all this' that is the sequel to the chronicle of God's complex relationship with the people of God in the Hebrew Bible.

I want to consider how a Christian community that had undergone terrible suffering might rewrite the second half of Blumenthal's remarkable paragraph. This is not in any way to seek to detract from the horror of the Holocaust (and the particular horror for Christians that it was perpetrated by a nation with a strong Christian tradition), or yet to seek to detract from the force, authenticity or importance of Jewish formulations of relationship with God. But it is possible to imagine Christian communities too feeling let down, abandoned, and neglected, if not positively abused by, sufferings from natural disaster, sufferings for which God seems principally responsible, and by God's seeming failure to respond to the extremity of their situation. The God of such situations seems at once devastatingly powerful and yet powerless.

It is, of course, possible to frame theodicies of natural evil, and I have been part of extensive conversations about these.[38] Sitting in a university study, it is easy to pronounce, for example, that a world of tectonic activity, a world therefore of earthquakes, volcanoes, and tsunamis, is a world in which many processes that enhance living organisms are made possible. But in the face of the *experience* of disaster such long-distance, on-balance reflections look out of place, if not positively offensive.[39]

Three-lensed seeing

In more recent work, I have considered God's involvement in natural evil from the standpoint of the contemplation of divine glory.[40] There, I propose that God's glory is typically best understood as a visible sign of the deep reality of God. In the natural world the massive power of physical forces,[41] the

37 Frances Young, *God's Presence: A Contemporary Recapitulation of Early Christianity* (Cambridge: Cambridge University Press, 2013), 247; Southgate, *Groaning*, 83.

38 See, for example, Southgate, *Groaning*; Southgate, 'Free-Process'; Christopher Southgate, 'Cosmic Evolution and Evil', in *The Cambridge Companion to the Problem of Evil*, ed. C. Meister and P.K. Moser (Cambridge: Cambridge University Press, 2017), 147–164.

39 On the offence of theodicy, see, for example, Tilley, *Evils*.

40 Christopher Southgate, *Theology in a Suffering World: Glory and Longing* (Cambridge: Cambridge University Press, 2018).

41 The tectonic slippage that caused the Indian Ocean tsunami is estimated to have had 23,000 times the energy of the atomic bomb dropped on Hiroshima.

skill of predators and even the ingenuity of parasites can all be considered signs of the creative work of God.[42] As we have just been discussing, the signs of God's creative activity in the natural world include forces of great violence and capacity to cause harm and also ingenious pathogenic strategies that can likewise occasion great suffering. Hints here of what for Luther is the *opus alienum Dei*?

But that is not the whole story of God with the world. I argue that a full contemplation of events in the natural world, with all their violence and ambiguity, involves what I term 'three-lensed seeing'.[43] By this I mean the need to consider every event in relation to *Gloria mundi*, signs in the creation of the creative activity of God; *Gloria crucis*, signs associated with God's self-giving in the Passion and death of Christ; and *Gloria in excelsis*, God's bringing of all of creation to consummation.

Such seeing will involve attending carefully to the experience of the sufferers of natural evil, as Surin urges,[44] and allowing that experience to interact with convictions about God's taking responsibility for all suffering at the Cross of Christ. It will involve protest and lament, as Swinton suggests.[45] It will involve seeing the extraordinary gift in creation that is human life and holding on also to the belief that God holds out a future for God's creatures, including those that have died in terrible suffering.[46]

Blumenthal himself advocates a strategy of 'tacking'.[47] By this he means advancing not wholly directly into the challenges of life, now prioritising reason, now spiritual practice, now the insights of the arts. 'One tack in our lives is to confront what we would rather avoid, with as much courage as we can muster'.[48] Given the content of the rest of his book, this must include facing up to the blameworthiness of God, and finding the language for that, as well as for praise and hope. Three-lensed seeing endeavours to be more 'synoptic' than a strategy involving tacking between blame, lament, and praise. That perhaps makes it more theologically acceptable than Blumenthal's characterisation of the 'abusing' God, although at the risk of taking the edge off the radical character of the protest at God that is so important in the Jewish tradition, especially deriving from the Psalms and the Book of Job.

Three-lensed seeing and the Eucharist

This three-lensed seeing, this bringing of the whole story of God's ways with the world into every event, however shocking and full of harm, finds

42 Southgate, *Theology*, Ch. 3.
43 Southgate, *Theology*, 14–15.
44 Surin, *Theology*, Ch. 5.
45 Swinton, *Raging*.
46 Southgate, *Groaning*, Ch. 5.
47 Blumenthal, *Facing*, Ch. 5.
48 Blumenthal, *Facing*, 54.

for Christians (or should find) its outward expression in the actions of the Eucharist. There everything that has happened to the participants and the context of which they are a part is brought to God and interacts with the threefold narrative structure of creation, Cross and eschaton. Stephen Garrett writes that

> *our performance of the Eucharist serves to triangulate our actions in the present as we live in the presence of the risen Christ in the Spirit with reference to redemptive history yet in light of his eschatological glory*. A robust imagination is necessary to integrate our remembering and envisaging – what *was* with what *is* and *is to come*, bringing a sense of meaning and understanding to the present so we can participate fittingly and creatively in the dramatic movements of God's triune life.[49]

That (for Christians from sacramental traditions) the Eucharist can be intensely meaningful in traumatising contexts is confirmed by the recent experience of Alan Everett, parish priest at St Clements near Grenfell Tower.[50] O'Donnell writes of the Eucharist's underlying movement as one that gathers the people into a place of safety and forgiveness, constructs a narrative that makes sense of their experience, and reconnects them with society.[51] But is there a danger that some Eucharistic practice may seem to some people all much too neat? Is there a risk that the tripartite story there enacted, of creation, reconciliation through the Passion, and eschatological hope may too readily tidy up the rawness and agony of human suffering in time of disaster? Does the Eucharist as usually practised, with its emphasis on the redemption of human sin, provide sufficient opportunity to struggle to forgive God, to 'pray angry' at God's involvement in suffering?[52]

Robert Orsi writes this of 'Frank', a Catholic priest who had suffered sexual abuse at the hands of priests:

> Frank's theodicy of praying angry directly addresses this reality. "What more can God do to you?" he says. To have seen God at God's worst is to be liberated from the old relationship with an omnipotent God, and this opens a way for a new relationship. Survivors are free not only to express their doubts, their sense of betrayal, and their anger with God, but also to consider the articulation of these feelings as prayer. There is a hard edge to Frank's theodicy of prayer. Survivors have got God's number; they meet God without illusions about God. But this does not

49 Stephen L. Garrett, *God's Beauty-in-Act: Participation in God's Suffering Glory* (Eugene, OR: Pickwick, 2013), 192 (emphasis in the original).

50 Alan Everett, *After the Fire: Finding words for Grenfell* (Norwich: Canterbury, 2018).

51 O'Donnell, *Broken Bodies*, 179–180.

52 Robert Orsi, 'Praying Angry', http://forums.ssrc.org/ndsp/2013/08/27/praying-angry, accessed July 20, 2018.

> drive them away from God, or it need not do so in Frank's theology. Rather, it permits them to pray fearlessly and freely, to pray as they really are as persons, to open their inner lives in all their turmoil and anger to God who must take them as they are . . .
>
> So Frank invites survivors not to resolve their problems with "prayer," but instead to see what is unresolvable as prayer itself. This refusal of closure restores the tension . . . between persons praying and the divine other. Praying angry is the medium of this new relationship with God, its ground, and its safeguard.[53]

While sexual abuse poses very particular challenges in terms of prayer and liturgy, explored by Carla A. Grosch-Miller in this volume, some of these reactions could well apply to communities devastated by natural disaster. They, too, may have the feeling that they 'have seen God at God's worst'. They, too, need to be able to 'pray angry' and not to accept premature closure.

One might imagine a Eucharist in such a community lasting many hours and containing a long vigil and time of lament. Such Eucharistic practice would find room not only for Jesus's words over bread and wine at the Last Supper – words not necessarily uttered in calm certainty but, rather, torn from him as the beginning of his agony – but also for his prayer in Gethsemane, his own 'In spite of all this . . .' acceptance of the future mapped out for him by God. Such Eucharists might also provide a way in which the dynamic of Good Friday leading not directly to Easter Sunday but first to Holy Saturday, identified both by Shelly Rambo and by Jennifer Baldwin as the moment in the Christian year most in tune with the experience of survivors of trauma, might find expression.[54]

The vigil and lament, times of silence and praying angry, might be followed by music inspired by Christ's Passion and, in turn, by a Eucharistic prayer that included a sense of God's taking responsibility for the suffering-filled world God has made. The invitation to communion would recognise that it might take a long time for someone to be ready to accept God's gift of Christ's body and blood and that, for others, it might on that occasion be impossible to accept the 'staged reconciliation' with God that taking communion would symbolise. To return to Garrett's helpful formulation quoted earlier, the integration of 'remembering and envisaging' may come at different rates for different people, not because some possess more 'robust imagination' than others, but because the histories of trauma that we each bear as humans interact differently with present sufferings and future hopes. It would be important that those who could not receive were still held by the community as full members.

53 Orsi, 'Praying Angry'.

54 Shelly Rambo, *Spirit and Trauma: A Theology of Remaining* (Louisville, KY: Westminster John Knox, 2010); Baldwin, *Trauma-Sensitive Theology*.

The theme of Eucharist in relation to trauma is further explored in the work of O'Donnell in her chapter in this volume. What I advocate here is that the use of the Eucharist in traumatised congregations, especially those where the 'perpetrator' is God in Godself, is not rendered too tidy but that its full possibilities for holding a space of pain and anger are explored.

In spite of all this . . .

I began the second half of this chapter from that remarkable (and to some extent notorious) paragraph of Blumenthal's at the end of *Facing the Abusing God*. I posed the question as to how a Christian community, devastated by a natural disaster, might frame the second part of that paragraph, the 'In spite of all this . . .'.

Perhaps such a community's prayer might run something like this, rewriting Blumenthal:

> You God, made the great forces that have destroyed our homes, our livelihoods, and taken from us those we held dear. You did not warn us of disaster; you did not have regard to all our prayers and worship. We know of your loving-kindness from both Testaments of our Scriptures, but we have not felt it. Though we sought to bless you, our lives are broken.
>
> In spite of all this, we will pray for Your comfort and mercy. We will use the life, Passion and Resurrection of Jesus as our clue to what life with You might ultimately be. We will believe in You because of Him, we will place our hope in You because of Him. Though His care could show partiality,[55] and His teaching an almost unbearable sternness,[56] yet we believe he shared to the uttermost in our Godforsakenness. Because of His life and His Passion we will yearn for Him, groaning prayerfully within the greater groans of the Holy Spirit (Rom 8:23–27). We will wait for the Christ's return, and we will anticipate the time when we will see You in His risen glory. We will love one another and seek even to love the enemy. We will seek to build Your Kingdom as He described it.

This is a radical formulation, and most Christian experience will, I suggest, lie between this and the all-too-common whitewashing of experience found in so much worship and preaching. But I suggest that this paradoxical prayer has wider application than only to communities shocked by sudden natural disaster. Every Christian community contains those subject to sudden tragedy, unexpected or long dreaded, explicable through understood causes or

55 As at the story of the Syrophoenician woman at Mk 7:24–30.

56 As, for example, in the teaching on faith dividing families at Matthew 10:35–36.

simply mysterious.[57] Perhaps it is time that some Christian liturgies were constructed more along these lines, and Christian hymnody diversified to inhabit more of the territory so importantly marked out by the Psalms.

Conclusion

In this chapter I have considered God's involvement in horrific events, both those caused by moral evils – either malicious or arising out of negligence – and those natural evils in which God is the principal cause of the harms and suffering. I drew on resources from both the Christian tradition and contemporary Jewish theology to imagine what responses might be made by Christian communities faced with such natural disasters, both in terms of prayer and liturgy. My conclusion is that reflection on the impact of traumatising events, and honest, unsentimental reflection on God's ways with the world, should lead not only to a richer vein of Christian contemplation but also to radical and paradoxical answers to the question as to what should be prayed in time of disaster.

Select references

Blumenthal, David R. *Facing the Abusing God: A Theology of Protest*. Louisville, KY: Westminster John Knox, 1993.

Southgate, Christopher. *The Groaning of Creation: God, Evolution and the Problem of Evil*. Louisville, KY: Westminster John Knox, 2008.

Southgate, Christopher. 'Cosmic Evolution and Evil'. In *The Cambridge Companion to the Problem of Evil*, ed. C. Meister and P.K. Moser. Cambridge: Cambridge University Press, 2017, 147–164.

Southgate, Christopher. *Theology in a Suffering World: Glory and Longing*. Cambridge: Cambridge University Press, 2018.

Surin, Kenneth. *Theology and the Problem of Evil*. Oxford: Basil Blackwell, 1986.

Swinton, John. *Raging with Compassion: Pastoral Responses to the Problem of Evil*. Grand Rapids, MI/Cambridge: Eerdmans, 2007.

57 See Christian Wiman, *My Bright Abyss: Meditations of a Modern Believer* (New York: Farrer, Strauss and Giroux, 2013), for whom the sense of Godforsakenness in Christ's cry of dereliction at Mk 15:34 is what held him within Christian faith despite being diagnosed with a rare and agonising cancer at the age of 39.

8 Trauma and the narrative life of congregations

Christopher Southgate

This chapter explores the narrative life of congregations and their vulnerability to trauma. It also suggests ways in which congregations might be helped to become more resilient in the face of the shock events to which all communities will tend to be exposed. The chapter takes as its point of departure the innovative work on congregational narrative produced by James Hopewell in his book *Congregation: Stories and Structures.*[1] I extrapolate here from Hopewell's account, drawing on my own experience of ministry and the training of ministers. I acknowledge that I write very much from my own context in a very affluent society, that of the England of the second decade of the 21st century and, within that, in the region of the south-west, which has many problems but lacks others associated with more urbanised and post-industrial areas.

It is appropriate, given the methodology outlined in the first section of this book, which emphasises the primacy of experience, that we begin from Hopewell's account of the last phase of his life. The story of how, from his hospital bed, with a terminal diagnosis, he inferred the narrative genres that were being used to counsel him on his experience of cancer, and extended this to the life of congregations, is a remarkable one. Hopewell noticed that four narratives of health and illness lay behind his visitors' approaches.[2]

Some hospital chaplains and seminarians pointed to cases where the threat of cancer evoked stresses that proved unnecessary. A deeper knowing, 'getting with' the cancer, 'can unite self and body and interrupt the malignant relationship'.[3] In contrast, some charismatic seminarians urged an adventurous approach, 'venturing into the unknown, battling the evil, finding the good, and in the end gaining the prize, which, in my case, would be the release from my cancer as well as an experience of God's intimate

1 James F. Hopewell, *Congregation: Stories and Structures*, ed. Barbara G. Wheeler (Philadelphia: Fortress, 1987).

2 For a different theological use of four stories of advanced cancer see Deanna A. Thompson, *Glimpsing Resurrection: Cancer, Trauma and Ministry* (Louisville, KY: Westminster John Knox, 2018).

3 Hopewell, *Congregation*, 59.

presence.'[4] Family members and fellow ministers offered Hopewell their conviction that he must be reconciled to his life and lot 'and even more to my God, bending my remaining time to God's will'.[5] Therein lay his path to salvation. Whereas his fellow faculty members 'recognized the absurdity of my situation and did not predict my cure'.[6] Working from the literary analysis of Northrop Frye,[7] Hopewell characterised these approaches as exhibiting comic, romantic, tragic and ironic genres, respectively.[8] I develop the description of these genres further below.

To discern this range of narratives from within the experience of incurable cancer was striking enough, but Hopewell's further proposal that these narrative genres characterise congregational life is a further and much underused insight.[9] Arguably less helpful is Hopewell's theological translation of Frye's literary genres, in which comic, romantic, tragic and ironic genres are parsed as gnostic, charismatic, canonic and empiric, respectively.[10] So this chapter uses the literary terms. The other essential caveat to introduce at this stage is that a genre description of congregational story is not any sort of complete account, nor would one expect congregational narratives to fall neatly into one genre. As Hopewell himself puts it,

> [r]emember that the congregation is idiomatic; it constitutes itself by a very distinctive language whose indicative aspect identifies a world in some ways allied with the metaphors widely employed in the culture but in other ways peculiar to that group alone. The world view categories [genres of internal narrative] may help organise the interpretation of idiom elements, but they do not describe the full richness of parish settings.[11]

4 Hopewell, *Congregation*, 59–60.
5 Hopewell, *Congregation*, 60.
6 Hopewell, *Congregation*, 61.
7 Northrop Frye, *The Anatomy of Criticism* (Princeton, NJ: Princeton University Press, 1957).
8 For a recent re-appropriation of Frye's work on genre in the context of the Fourth Gospel see Brian Larsen, *Archetypes in the Fourth Gospel: Literature and Theology in Conversation* (London: T&T Clark, 2018).
9 Works of practical theology often acknowledge Hopewell without pursuing his methodology. For an example of efforts to use insights into narrative genre, and narrative therapy, in congregational development and healing, see the project at the Alban Institute directed by Larry Goleman; for example, Larry A. Goleman, ed., *Finding Our Story: Narrative Leadership and Congregational Change* (Lanham, MD: Rowman and Littlefield, 2010). See also Vaughan S. Roberts and David Sims, *Leading by Story: Rethinking Church Leadership* (London: SCM Press, 2017). Roberts and Sims helpfully elaborate Hopewell's scheme by distinguishing between interpretive, identity, and improvised stories, but in doing so they seem to lose sight of Hopewell's key insight into genre.
10 I also find Hopewell's effort in the later part of his book to establish the (literary) myth of congregations to be trickier and more tenuous territory, so this chapter uses only his insights into genre.
11 Hopewell, *Congregation*, 87.

This type of genre analysis should be seen as a heuristic tool rather than an overarching or self-contained metanarrative. But Hopewell's point, again derived from Frye, that some pairs of genres cannot be combined – the comic with the tragic, the romantic with the ironic – continues to be important.[12] And his overall proposal forms a useful diagnostic tool as to the interior life of a congregation.

The four genres illustrated

I now give a brief account of the four genres of narrative and illustrate each of them by means of a literary example, a scriptural narrative and a hymn that would tend to be popular within this internal narrative.

Comic stories unfold from problem (often more apparent than real) to solution, often expressed in terms of unions such as marriages. Those Shakespeare comedies that rely on mistaken identity are classic of this genre, but so is Dante's great mystical journey in *The Divine Comedy* in which the disoriented protagonist is guided through great difficulty to a paradisal union with the divine. Jesus also told comic stories, of which that of the Lost Son (Lk 15:11–32) is a striking instance. The lost son faces an apparently insuperable difficulty in regaining the esteem of his father, but the father runs to embrace him and restore his status in full. More generally, it could be said that the Gospels (with the important exception of the shorter ending of Mark) tell a comic narrative, in which the apparently devastating disaster of the Master's arrest and execution is triumphantly reversed by resurrection appearances that show Christ's reunion both with his followers and his Father.[13]

Hymn preferences form a useful diagnostic of a congregation's dominant internal narrative. In the singing of what type of hymn is a congregation's expression of its narrative life most characteristically expressed? Readers will be familiar with churches where only triumphant, Resurrection hymns can be sung, and this may be indicative of a strongly comic narrative, in which it is always Easter and never Good Friday. A slightly more subtle form of this genre might be found in churches who love Sydney Carter's 'Lord of the Dance', where the Good Friday observation 'It's hard to dance / with the devil on your back' is followed by the coda beginning 'They cut me down / and I leapt up high / I am the life / that'll never never die'.[14]

12 Hopewell, *Congregation*, 61.

13 The difficulty for some individuals and groups of continuing to operate in this narrative genre in the face of their own experiences of suffering is what leads Shelly Rambo, *Spirit and Trauma: a theology of remaining* (Louisville, KY: Westminster John Knox, 2010), to her analysis of the importance of Holy Saturday, the time before the fact of the Resurrection has given final shape to the narrative of the Gospel.

14 Sydney Carter, 'Lord of the Dance', *BBC Songs of Praise, Music Edition* (Oxford: Oxford University Press, 1997), 142–143.

Romantic narratives are often characterised by the pursuit of a quest. As Hopewell puts it: 'The hero or heroine leaves familiar surroundings and embarks on a dangerous journey in which strange things happen but a priceless reward is gained'.[15] The contemporary taste for quest narratives is shown by the enormous popularity of the films of *The Lord of the Rings*. Biblically, the narrative of the Passover and Exodus from Egypt shows many of the characteristics of a romance. Hopewell quotes Frye: 'The hero of romance moves in a world in which the ordinary laws of nature are . . . suspended: prodigies of courage and endurance unnatural to us are natural to him'.[16] Of course, the great adventure of the Exodus moves later into other types of genre, an example of the literary insight that the point at which a story is ended has a profound effect on the genre in to which it falls. Hopewell identifies this congregational story as 'the charismatic negotiation',[17] often, although not exclusively, associated with churches with a charismatic spirituality. Many hymns and songs of the charismatic movement fall into this narrative genre of the romantic; of more traditional fare Bunyan's 'To Be a Pilgrim' is an example of such a genre.

In a tragic narrative, 'the hero is shaped by the pattern of the Other and is obedient to it unto death'.[18] Hopewell quotes Frye: 'tragic heroes are wrapped in the mystery of their communion with that something beyond which we can only see through them, and which is the source of their strength and their fate alike'.[19] Most famously, Hamlet epitomises this genre of hero. Some of the Israelite kings may be seen in this light, but most strikingly the Christian Church inhabits this genre on Good Friday, when the story is halted at the tragedy of the Lord Jesus pitted unavailingly against the oppressive powers of the world.[20] That magnificent Passiontide hymn 'When I Survey the Wondrous Cross' belongs to this genre. Although as Hopewell insists, '[d]enominations do not determine world view',[21] it may be that many conservative Protestant churches will incline to this genre of narrative, because of their theological anthropology and soteriology.

Finally, I consider Frye's fourth genre, that of the ironic, brilliantly evoked in the 20th century by such authors as Beckett and Kafka. As Hopewell characterises this genre, '[m]iracles do not happen; patterns lose their design; life is unjust, not justified by transcendent forces'.[22] Godot never comes; no system of justice ever emerges in *The Trial*. This genre is adept at accommodating

15 Hopewell, *Congregation*, 59.
16 Hopewell, *Congregation*, 59, quoting Frye, *Anatomy*, 33.
17 Hopewell, *Congregation*, 75–79.
18 Hopewell, *Congregation*, 60.
19 Hopewell, *Congregation*, 61, quoting Frye, *Anatomy*, 208.
20 On the tragic view of the atonement see Frederick W. Dillistone, *The Christian Understanding of Atonement* (Welwyn, UK: Nisbet, 1968), 115–160.
21 Hopewell, *Congregation*, 96.
22 Hopewell, *Congregation*, 61.

paradox, as in Beckett's famous 'I can't go on. I'll go on'.[23] Interestingly the wisdom literature of the Bible knows this genre well. Irony lurks on the edge of the Book of Job (and is only whisked away in a most unsatisfactory fashion by the self-satiric-seeming ending). But it is the Book of Ecclesiastes, with its hypnotic refrain that all is 'vanity' and that there is no escape from the rhythms of the natural world, that most completely epitomises this genre. It is a challenge to find a hymn in this genre, although 'Brother, Sister, Let Me Serve You' has been proposed. Indeed, that song has a sense that authenticity of friendship may be all we have, and it evokes that 'time to laugh, time to weep' of Ecclesiastes, but it cannot resist the eschatological promise of the penultimate verse, beginning 'When we sing to God in heaven',[24] a signal of unironic movement towards a hoped-for destination.

I now proceed to apply these insights of Hopewell's, using my own experience of working with generations of ordinands on the stories of their churches. It is my observation that congregations' internal narratives are indeed deeply held, although often not articulated. Furthermore, they have often been shaped by a defining event that is construed in narrative terms within one (or a combination of two) of the four genres. Thus, for example, the breaking down of an old rivalry through an unforeseen event – for instance, a fire in a church building that forces a new intimacy of worship in an improvised setting, and a creative re-appraisal of the part music plays in liturgy – might predispose to a comic congregational narrative. A form of resurrection has been experienced and continues to shape communal life. The unexpected healing of the minister (or other key figure) after a campaign of prayer might predispose to a romantic narrative in which supernatural deliverance is continually expected and sought. (This might have happened in Hopewell's case but in practice did not.) A tragic narrative may be inhabited if a church benefits from a pair of churchwardens who serve it diligently into old age and then die at the same time. Their joint funeral, and the sense that they have left a pattern of service that would take decades for others to grow into, might deeply mark a small church. Whereas if the 'trophy' young couple in such a church take on the Sunday School and the family service and are then implicated in multiple cases of child abuse, that would predispose to an ironic internal narrative.

Note that I am proposing that actual events of only local significance can decisively shape congregational narrative. I acknowledge also that larger events may be hugely important. For the generation born between the wars, which ran so many churches until very recently, the impact of war and post-war rationing on internal narrative should not be underestimated. Indeed, the intergenerational difference of experience between that group and baby-boomers may explain the congregational dynamics of many churches where

23 Quoted in Thompson, *Cancer*, 14.

24 Richard Gillard, 'Brother, Let Me Be Your Servant', in *BBC Songs of Praise, Music Edition* (Oxford: Oxford University Press, 1997), 708.

the internal narrative life of the community has been split. Also of profound importance is the theological tradition of the church, as expressed in its doctrinal statements, preaching, and use of the Bible. However, I note Hopewell's point that response to credal assertions (as an indicator of theological tradition) is not as big a predictor of congregational dynamic as might have been expected.[25]

The four genres and the impact of traumatic events on the internal narratives of congregations

Hopewell's work is mentioned, often in passing, in many texts on the nature of congregations.[26] Often, however, Hopewell's insights are only cited as a preliminary to a more general ethnographic treatment of congregations in their normal functioning. I have not encountered any previous attempt to discern how trauma affects congregations' internal narratives, understood in the genre terms to which Hopewell points us. Hopewell himself, working in a less trauma-sensitive era, gives this relatively little attention, but in his guided interviews of congregants, he does steer them towards consideration of the death of friend or relative and other situations when life seemed out of control. Hopewell thus realises that it is consideration of huge events that tends to show what internal story congregants are truly carrying, as opposed to what they think they ought to believe.[27]

In this next section I consider how different genres of congregational narrative may be affected by a shock event or disclosure. Comic, romantic and tragic narratives all contain, in their different ways, trust, hope, and a sense of the meaningfulness of reality. It is the comic genre, in which narratives have surprising positive resolutions, that is perhaps most characterised by *trust* in the fabric of reality. The romantic genre, in which the community is on a shared quest, reliant on the supernatural intervention of the forces of good against the powers of evil, is most typified by a reliance on *hope*. The tragic genre of narrative may be deeply pessimistic about the nature of unredeemed humanity but strongly affirms the underlying *meaningfulness* of the world.

As we discussed in the opening section of this book, the prime characteristic of trauma is the overwhelming of resources. At an individual level this begins as a whole-body physiological response, characterised by fight–flight impulses and an initial suppression of higher intellectual functions. We are

25 Hopewell, *Congregation*, 84.

26 For a survey see Linda Woodhead, Mathew Guest, and Karen Tusting, 'Congregational Studies: Taking Stock', in *Congregational studies in the UK: Christianity in a post-Christian context*, ed. Mathew Guest, Karen Tusting and Linda Woodhead (Aldershot: Ashgate, 2004), 1–23.

27 Hopewell, *Congregation*, 91. He does also incorporate the death of a pastor's baby into one of his mythologisations of congregational story (p. 125).

concerned here rather with how a community processes an experience that has overwhelmed the resources of some or all of its members. Here the internal narrative of the community becomes very important, and I hypothesise that those communities with internal narratives that fall into some genres will tend to experience trauma more profoundly and collectively than those principally informed by other genres. In what follows, I consider mainly local traumatising events rather than huge disasters, such as a major fire, flood or terrorism, where all resources are in the first instance overwhelmed.

A diagnostic of what type of narrative has been damaged in the case of a congregation is – which of its favourite hymns can be sung when the community first re-gathers after the traumatising event? I was very moved by my conversations with clergy of the Diocese of Christchurch, New Zealand, as they reflected on the aftermath of the earthquake that destroyed their cathedral (and continued through its aftershocks to threaten church life in the Diocese for another two years). 'It was hard to choose hymns' was an understated but profound comment. Hymnody (as opposed to psalmody) tends always to express trust and hope in ways that may be hard indeed for communities to express. But to attend to *which* particular hymns seem no longer remotely appropriate might help in the discernment of how a congregational narrative has been damaged.

The Virgin train on which I first drafted this chapter had a witty announcement in the toilet asking that a whole series of things not be flushed away, including sanitary towels, extra sweaters, etc. The list ended, 'hopes, dreams and goldfish'. Particularly devastating to communities with a strongly hopeful internal narrative are events that metaphorically do just that to hopes and dreams. The resources provided by that narrative in terms of worship, prayer, hymnody and mutual support will be especially vulnerable to being overwhelmed by an event that severely erodes a sense of hope. An example would be if a new young minister, who seemed to offer a fresh direction and sense of exploration to a church, were suddenly to be signed off on indefinite sick leave with an entirely unforeseen illness (physical or mental).

Betrayals of trust will also tend strongly to exacerbate collective trauma. This is most familiar in cases of sexual or financial abuse by those in positions of responsibility. As we shall go on to discuss in Part V of this book, it is a characteristic of such scandals, particularly when they have a sexual basis, so that the evidence concerned is intimate and disputable, that the church community tends to split, some siding with the perpetrator and some against him or her. In such a case, trust is broken not merely between the perpetrator and the church but between church members, each faction unable to credit the judgement of the other in a sensitive matter. Interior narratives based on a comic genre, where union is emphasised, will be hit particularly hard by such rifts.

All the preceding reflections might seem to commend a congregational narrative in the ironic mode, from which hopefulness, trust in persons and institutions, and a sense of the meaningfulness of the underlying structures of reality are all absent. Hopewell in his description of 'the empiric negotiation' draws on the work of Wade Clark Roof. A certain sort of religion in this genre 'affirms: a) the centrality of ethical principles in their meaning systems; b) a parsimony of beliefs, few attributions of numinosity; c) breadth of perspective; d) piety defined as a personal search for meaning; and e) license to doubt'.[28] There can be a sense in this genre of internal narrative that everything has been tried and nothing made any real difference, that individuals who were a focus of hope invariably disappointed and that even if there has been no scandal the denomination, as underlying locus of trust, has offered less and less by way of inspiration and resource. Indeed, I suspect there are many more churches, particularly of the communal, as opposed to the gathered, variety, operating in this genre than might be recognised by their denominations.

Indeed, the strength of this genre is that whatever shock event happens is recognised for itself. Little effort will be made by the community to recast the story of the traumatising event in illusory and overly hopeful or overly trusting terms. Little is believed, and still less is believed corporately, so the corporate shock is less than it might be. If there is heroism in the response, little may be made of it beyond the matter-of-factness of action. 'We just got on with it' may be a typical congregational reflection.

I suspect, however, that the loss of trust, hope and a sense of meaning to reality is too great a concession for a Christian church to make.[29] The Gospel cannot meaningfully be proclaimed on a sustained basis within the thought-world of Qoheleth, where all is 'vanity'. Nevertheless, that genre of narrative may find its place in the 'disillusionment' phase of a community's life after a traumatising event.

Indeed, it seems possible that for many churches that operate within an ironic mode, not believing that anything much can change, or that sustained growth or transformation can take place, the underlying reason for this internal narrative is unprocessed past trauma. A community can be trapped in the disillusionment phase of trauma response[30] if what has happened and its effects cannot be articulated and witnessed to. This can happen if betrayals of trust are covered up, or if communities cannot express, and grieve over, a loss of hope. More generally, churches can be locked into an extreme form of a particular genre of internal narrative if those responsible for guiding its life lack the awareness to explore the effect of what has happened.

28 Hopewell, *Congregation*, 82.

29 Though see William L. Randall, 'The Importance of Being Ironic: Narrative Openness and Personal Resilience in Later Life', *The Gerontologist* 53 (2013): 9–16, for advocacy of the health of this genre of internal narrative.

30 Laurie Kraus, David Holyan and Bruce Wisner, *Recovering from Un-natural Disasters: A Guide for Pastors and Congregations After Violence and Trauma* (Louisville, KY: Westminster John Knox, 2017), xiv–xvi.

The interior narrative of congregations and good ministerial practice

I now turn, therefore, to consider what good ministerial practice might look like in relation to the internal narrative of congregations. First I note one of the key inferences that may be drawn from Hopewell's work – that if a minister's (narrative) worldview differs markedly from that of the congregation, much energy will be expended in mutual misunderstanding.[31] A minister determined to lead his or her congregation on a supernaturally inspired quest will struggle to communicate with a church that has the sense that everything has been tried and nothing much is possible. Conversely, a church that feels itself to have experienced resurrection will feel frustrated in its efforts to communicate with a minister whose spirituality is rooted in meditation on the sinfulness of individuals and their need for salvation through penance.

This, in turn, points to the importance of a new minister taking a great deal of trouble to understand the idiom of the congregation as a whole – as well as making all the individual visits with which a ministry might well begin.[32] One way of approaching this is to set up a meeting to go through a timeline of the church's history.[33] The response to such a proposal will itself be diagnostic. How far do people suggest going back in the history? What are taken to constitute foundational events? What are taken to be the successes within that history, and who is given credit for them (the Holy Spirit, a minister, the congregation as a whole?). Especially noteworthy would be a widespread resistance to undertaking the exercise – that would be, in itself, diagnostic of an ironic narrative, one not given shape by achievement or rescue or yet tragedy. In the context of the present study, events that are registered in a church's history as having been traumatic, at least for some, to have overwhelmed expectations and comfort zones, will be especially significant. Are those events registered as able to have been learned from? Are they still contested histories, suggesting that further work may be necessary to reflect on their importance? How have those events affected the church's interior narrative?

Earlier I suggested that a narrative that can be called Christian must rest on convictions about trust, hope and meaning that prevent a congregation from lapsing into a purely ironic mode of internal life. In turn, that imposes on the leadership great responsibilities in terms of the maintenance of trust and the management of hopes and expectations. But there is another

31 Hopewell, *Congregation*, 98.

32 For some suggestions on how to conduct this form of exploration positively, as 'appreciative inquiry', see Susan Beaumont, 'Giants and Grasshoppers: Stories that Frame Congregational Anxiety', in Larry A. Goleman (ed.), *Finding Our Story: Narrative Leadership and Congregational Change* (Lanham, MD: Rowman and Littlefield, 2010), 91–104.

33 The 'historical' element of 'identity narratives' in Roberts and Sims, *Leading*, Ch. 7.

dimension to the way ministers work with the interior narrative of congregations that I consider of particular importance in respect of trauma. That concerns how the Bible is used in worship and preaching. In my summaries of the character of the different narrative genres, I made clear that all these genres can be found in the Scriptures. But preachers and churches not making consistent use of the Lectionary so often default to a particular micro-canon. For years I sat and listened to a particular preacher who only ever spoke about the Gospel stories of Jesus's life. No other aspect of the New Testament, let alone the Old Testament, received any coverage. Other churches expound a narrow canvas of Pauline themes. Readers may want to consider when they last heard a sermon on a psalm or yet on Ecclesiastes or Lamentations.

My proposal is that the gift of the breadth of the Scriptures is a vital gift for ministering in a world full of traumatising events. In her essays, Megan Warner notes the traumatic context of the origin of many of these texts, and how the Psalms provide a particular resource in times of pain and lament. Indeed, the Psalter, with its constant shifts of mood, and its willingness to rail at God and to make the turn to praise, seems to me to be an important antidote to an overly ironic worldview. But equally, aspects of the Wisdom literature, especially Ecclesiastes, guard against an overly naïve celebration of the charismatic victory of the good over demonic opposition. I referred earlier to the risks of inhabiting only Easter Sunday or only Good Friday. The Lectionary and the liturgical year, though not without their flaws (the addition of the Season of Creation is an overdue corrective to some of the latter) are a very important resource in practising the inhabiting of a range of narrative genres.

That is not to say that congregations will not retain their characteristic genre of interior narrative, but a church that genuinely inhabits the range of biblical texts offered by the Lectionary will have an imaginative suppleness that will stand it in good stead in the face of sudden shocks. To say this is not to understate the difficulty of many biblical texts – their patriarchality, sexism, racism and xenophobia – but again, these factors are not to be ducked but engaged with.

It may be, too, that a shock event makes a particular text very difficult. The project team have been profoundly moved by our contact with the Revd Nick Bundock, who had to minister after the suicide of a teenage girl who was a member of his congregation at St James and Emmanuel, Didsbury.[34] The Gospel reading for the Sunday after her death was the story of the raising of the little girl (*Talitha cum*) in Mk 5. But Bundock's preaching was exemplary. He did not change the text; he did not duck the text. He spoke honestly about the church's inability to pronounce that beautiful Aramaic

34 Carla A. Grosch-Miller tells the story at greater length in Chapter 2 in this volume, although there neither the parish nor the minister is identified.

bidding. The little girl in everyone's thoughts could not be raised up by the community's faith because of the choice she had made. I recall another service following a suicide of a young woman when the many friends of hers gathered, unfamiliarly for them in a church, to remember her. The wave of relief that flooded through that church when it became clear that there would be honesty about what had happened is something I shall never forget. The beginning of a response to a tragic event includes the recognition that what has happened has happened. Although humankind, in T.S. Eliot's memorable phrase, 'cannot bear very much reality',[35] the reality of shock events must be borne if healing is to ensue.

Preachers and liturgists, then, must be honest and fearless performers of our sacred canon, not editing that performance out of fear or avoidance or theological partiality. But neither should ministers suppose that they can by force of their own conviction and preaching transform the interior narrative of a congregation. Neither can they determine the character of the response to trauma. The dynamic by which disillusionment must follow heroism and be succeeded only eventually by a new wisdom cannot be subverted.[36] Ministerial wisdom must consist rather of discerning the dynamics of a church's response and making the right spaces at the right junctures for reflection on that response. It is the contention of this chapter that a deep understanding of the interior narrative (or narratives) carried by a congregation is a vital aid to considering the extent and the character of the wounds that have been suffered and hence being able to journey creatively through the process of disillusionment that may ensue.

Last, I return to that same tragic event at St James and Emmanuel, Didsbury mentioned earlier. The church grieved for the young suicide. But the inquest then revealed that her concerns about the church's possible reaction to her sexuality played a part in her decision to end her life. The church now found itself (unconsciously) in the role of 'perpetrator'. It was challenged to 'recast' its self-understanding in the light of what had happened.

Admittedly, this is a relatively unusual aspect of the response to trauma. Very many events do not have causes in which churches are implicated as communities (even if it becomes known that a particular individual has breached the bounds of trust). But Bundock's experience is important because many communities can benefit from the quality of interior reflection to which his church members found themselves so tragically and distressingly called. And although few churches will suddenly find themselves in the position of perpetrator, many will find themselves responding to a tragedy with some measure of regret and yearning, an 'if only'. Again, a minister may be able to discern why a particular interior narrative leads to a particularly strong 'if only'.

35 T.S. Eliot, *Complete Poems and Plays* (London: Faber and Faber, 1969), 271.
36 See Kraus et al., *Re-covering*.

Conclusion

This brief exploration has emphasised the claim, deriving from the work of Hopewell, that congregations carry strong internal narratives and that those narratives tend to fall into one (or, at most, a mixture of two) classic types of genre. I went on to suggest that understanding of the genre of congregational narrative might be particularly important in understanding the damage done to a community by a shock event and that inhabiting all four genres of story in the performance of Scripture might be important to congregational health and resilience.

Select references

Frye, Northrop. *The Anatomy of Criticism*. Princeton, NJ: Princeton University Press, 1957.

Goleman, Larry A., ed. *Finding Our Story: Narrative Leadership and Congregational Change*. Lanham, MD: Rowman and Littlefield, 2010.

Hopewell, James F. *Congregation: Stories and Structures*, ed. Barbara G. Wheeler. Philadelphia: Fortress, 1987.

Kraus, Laurie, David Holyan and Bruce Wisner, eds. *Recovering From Un-natural Disasters: A Guide for Pastors and Congregations After Violence and Trauma*. Louisville, KY: Westminster John Knox, 2017.

Roberts, Vaughan S. and David Sims. *Leading by Story: Rethinking Church Leadership*. London: SCM, 2017.

Woodhead, Linda, Mathew Guest and Karen Tusting. 'Congregational Studies: Taking Stock'. In *Congregational Studies in the UK: Christianity in a Post-Christian Context*, ed. Mathew Guest, Karen Tusting and Linda Woodhead. Aldershot: Ashgate, 2004, 1–23.

9 Responding to disaster in an Afro-Caribbean congregation

Deanne Gardner

The voices of non-white congregations are often missing from UK Christian literature. Afro-Caribbean congregations form an important part of multi-cultural communities, in which the church is often considered a place of support and solace when individuals and communities are confronted with personal and national tragedies. The pastor and, if married, his or her spouse are pivotal in supporting both the church and community at such times. This chapter discusses the collective congregational response to disasters and how faith and historical experiences inform those responses. The author draws on her experience as the wife of a pastor within a Pentecostal church.

> Tragedies are commonplace.
> All kinds of diseases, people are slipping away.
> The economy's down; people can't get enough pay.
> As for me, all I can say is, thank you Lord for all you've done for me.
> (Walter Hawkins)[1]

Afro-Caribbean congregations

Afro-Caribbean congregations, sometimes referred to as 'black-led churches', have been present in the United Kingdom since the 1940s.[2] Their emergence and establishment came predominantly, although not exclusively, out of the Windrush era, with an influx of Black people migrating to the United Kingdom from the West Indies. Many individuals who came to the United Kingdom were Christians or had been regular churchgoers in the Caribbean. Stories are told that upon arriving in the United Kingdom, many Afro-Caribbean people searched for a place of worship akin to what they had left in the West Indies. Individuals reported experiencing a cool reception from members

1 Walter Hawkins, 'Thank You', *Love Alive IV*, 1990.

2 Israel Olonfinjana, 'The History of Black Majority Churches in London (ND)', www.open.ac.uk/arts/research/religion-in-london/sites/www.open.ac.uk.arts.research.religion-in-london/files/files/ecms/arts-rl-pr/web-content/Black-Majority-Churches-in-London.pdf.

of mainstream majority-white churches.[3] The experience of rejection and a different style of worship led individuals, some who had held positions of leadership within the Caribbean churches, to start churches or small groups in living rooms and community centres. Some individuals who had held pastoral positions within churches in the Caribbean came to the United Kingdom and started a branch of the church they had left in their home island.

Afro-Caribbean people sought others with whom they could identify, who shared a similar culture and faith background. Today, Afro-Caribbean congregations tend to be found within the Pentecostal tradition. The migration of people from the West Indies, including Antigua, Barbados, Jamaica, St Lucia, Nevis, St Kitts, Trinidad, Martinique and St Martin, has made up many Afro-Caribbean congregations. While this was the majority group within such congregations for some time, Afro-Caribbean congregations have experienced changes in terms of cultural mix; with new waves of migrants coming to the United Kingdom from the continent of Africa and many European Union countries, churches have become visibly diverse.

Shared points of identity

The historical context and social background of Afro-Caribbeans are important elements to explore in order to gain some understanding of how Afro-Caribbean congregations respond to disasters. Within Afro-Caribbean congregations, there is a feeling of togetherness, validation and shared identity that allows for growth and a sense of acceptance. This approach to life originates from the collectivist position from which Afro-Caribbean communities are considered to come and in which the individual is considered as 'we' rather than 'I'.[4] An understanding of corporate identity that recognises the whole as 'one body and the sum of many parts' fits with Paul's teaching about being part of one body with each part having value (1 Cor 12:12) and has similarities with the Aristotelean school of thought to the effect that 'the whole is greater than the sum of its parts'. Biblical images and principles are adopted and interpreted in ways that underpin this collectivist understanding; 'I am my brother's keeper' and 'doing unto others as you would have them do unto you' are biblical ideas that guide behaviour and relationships with others. The underlying ethos is of a shared responsibility for the well-being of others. Communities hold the image of Jesus being in relationship and contact with others, thus showing the significance of connection and togetherness and informing the Afro-Caribbean congregation of the importance of maintaining the collectivist stance. With this collectivism comes a collective voice, responsibility and celebration of achievements.

3 Mike Phillips and Trevor Phillips, *Windrush: The Irresistible Rise of Multi-Racial Britain* (London: Harper Collins, 1998).

4 Colin Lago, *Race, Culture and Counselling* (2nd Ed.; Berkshire: Open University Press, 2006).

However, the collective stance also brings collective shame and shared impact of trauma. Therefore, cautiousness may be observed in groups maintaining a collectivist stance. There may be a concern about a possible risk of harm to individuals who are isolated, so an attitude of 'strength in numbers' is perpetuated. This idea may have evolved from a duality of experiences, both past and present. It is known that individuals can be at risk of attack for being different, and within our society, skin colour has caused many tragic experiences for the Afro-Caribbean individual. Alongside this, the history of slavery continues to have undercurrents.

The need to stick together and support one another for survival developed as a result of the threat to life. People from the Caribbean are not strangers to experiences of tragedy and resulting trauma, and it is important to hold this in mind when considering the shared historical context of a large group of people. Historical slavery, colonisation and the Windrush era of migration led to displacement and multiple layers of loss of identity, family, property and future for countless thousands of people over many generations. Migration saw groups of people leaving their homelands to move to various countries, including the United Kingdom. Individuals from the Commonwealth, including the Caribbean, were invited to come to the United Kingdom to share their skills and help the mother country; some individuals came in the hope of a better future. While the purpose of the move was to a great degree accomplished, it usually came at an emotional cost, which may in itself be considered as a personal and collective tragedy. The collective result of experiences, such as racism, rejection and being viewed with suspicion, initiated the formation of various groups, including church congregations which now include first, second and third generations born to parents of Afro-Caribbean descent. It might be asked whether the impact of first-generation trauma continues to ripple through to future generations several decades after the initial disaster or tragedy has been experienced.

Interpretations of disaster

> Folks without homes, living out in the streets
> And the drug habits some say, they just can't beat
> Muggers and robbers, no place seems to be safe
> But You'll be my protection every step of the way
> And I want to say, thank you Lord for all you've done for me.
>
> (Walter Hawkins)

The national news reports yet another stabbing within the local community; rival gangs of youths, some who until recently attended Sunday school at one of the local black-led churches, have been caught up in the conflict.

National and local news reports often remind ethnic minority groups that they are part of a community, and that, although living within a dominant culture, they are different and not always accepted. Their journeys and experiences are akin to those of the children of Israel within the Old Testament. Afro-Caribbean congregations can sometimes feel like a minority within a minority. By that I mean that being black and part of a faith group can have an impact on internal responses whenever the black and minority ethnic (BME) community is highlighted by negative news. Although Afro-Caribbean congregations are not devoid of disasters or trauma, the word *disaster* is rarely used within such congregations.

According to the *New Oxford Dictionary of English*,[5] *disaster* is 'a sudden accident or a natural catastrophe that causes great damage or loss of life' or 'an event or fact that has unfortunate consequences'. *Tragedy*, meanwhile, is defined as 'an event causing great suffering, destruction, and distress, such as a serious accident, crime, or natural disaster'.[6] The historical and ongoing experiences of people within Afro-Caribbean congregations and communities suggest that the life stories of many, if not all, fit disconcertingly well with these dictionary definitions. This may cause outsiders to question levels of personal and congregational awareness about experiences of personal and national tragedies and their effects on survivors. It may also lead to questions about whether coping mechanisms within Afro-Caribbean congregations are understood and accepted by those from more individualistic communities. If traumatic experiences are and have been an integral part of life for a collective group, might this cause outsiders to believe that congregants from this setting lack self-awareness or display avoidant behaviour? Might personal experience of tragedy indeed inform the response to disasters? In order to answer to this, we need to consider the following: the role that the individual's relationship with God plays in traversing difficulties, teachings within specific church settings and expectations with regard to coping with difficulties and the place and importance that the Holy Spirit plays in the lives of Afro-Caribbean congregations.

The direction, guidance and comfort of the Holy Spirit is sought in the lives of individual members of Afro-Caribbean congregations who, taking the Bible as divinely inspired and often translating it literally, base their faith and belief systems on God's constant guidance and purpose. Seeking to develop a personal relationship with God, they endeavour to live their lives in accordance to the direction given in the Bible and believe that there is a reason or divine purpose for events that take place. A personal relationship with God is understood to assist the individual to navigate their way through their thought processes, and the difficulties and traumas experienced in life. Storytelling and sharing one's experiences through narrative have always been media used within the black community as a way of unburdening oneself of the weight of personal troubles and worries. While speaking of the facts of an event is not new, exploring the impact of such experiences has

5 Judy Pearsall, ed., *The New Oxford Dictionary of English* (Oxford/New York: Oxford University Press, 1998), 524.

6 Pearsall, *New Oxford*, 1965.

been a new approach, fostered by the introduction of dedicated counselling services within churches.

The opening lines of the song 'Thank You', by American gospel singer Walter Hawkins (reproduced earlier), reflect both the acceptance of life's problems and the reliance on God that many Afro-Caribbeans adopt, as well as an aptitude for looking at things from an alternative perspective, becoming thankful for the blessings that have been given rather than focusing on the tragedy that has happened. The standpoint that 'things could be far worse' is often adopted, particularly by senior congregants, in spite of whether an individual is pessimistic or optimistic by nature. As a result, the age difference in Afro-Caribbean congregations and correlation with patterns of personal responses to disasters and subsequent trauma may be worthy of further deliberation. A further standpoint adopted by individuals, noting that the Scriptures speak of attacks from the enemy of our souls, is that 'nothing bad happens without a reason'. This standpoint may lead individuals to apportion to the enemy blame for tragedies experienced by the self or other people. Living 'by the word' means that difficulties and tragedies that are encountered or experienced can be 'spiritualised'. This is not a derogatory standpoint; in line with the Scriptures, many turn to the Bible to find an identifying point and an experience that relates to their situation. There are no set Church teachings with regard to how disasters are to be managed and dealt with, but the Scriptures are the main source of guidance. The Scriptures and spoken word are sought for solace, with Psalms being a particular favourite.

Taking time to reflect on the meaning of disaster and tragedy, when considering the manner in which various cultures respond to tragedies, we need to think about how faith informs responses to adversities within Afro-Caribbean settings. Certain personal events that may be deemed to be a disaster in non-faith-based settings are sometimes interpreted by individuals as trials and tests within the Church. Often, the difficulties faced in everyday life are considered as preparation for some greater difficulty or a means to develop one's character (this thought is based again on the Bible's text – Rom 5:4). Natural events, such as hurricanes and earthquakes affecting many lives simultaneously, while terrible and catastrophic, may be viewed philosophically as a reminder that God has total control. Alongside this, there may be an observable difference with regard to how different age groups within such congregations respond to such adversities. Seniors may take a pragmatic approach, while younger members may adopt an idealistic attitude.

Becoming visible and audible

> Social workers have secured a high court order to remove two young children from the home of their mother and grandmother. The children were said to have been neglected and beaten by their mother, who struggled with

> mental health issues and said that voices had told her that her children were possessed by bad spirits. The grandmother was said to be a member of the local church.

It might be assumed that a collectivist group brings with it the strength of presence, an audible voice and visual prominence. However, whilst this might be so for African American congregations, with the voices of black people and people of faith being heard within the United States via preachers and social advocates, there is evidence that this public boldness and togetherness has yet to transpose itself onto UK soil in a way that makes a significant mark, particularly when responding to disasters. There is a sparseness of literature sharing the history of Afro-Caribbean congregations, and the importance that such churches have on the communities within which they are set, and yet it is known that the Church is sought by individuals within BME communities as the first place of support and help for spiritual or emotional needs.[7] At times of national disasters and international tragedies, Afro-Caribbean churches are adversely affected, and this is particularly so when events have involved ethnic minorities and especially when there is a religious or spiritual element involved. Depending on the event and by the harm done, and by whom, there is a collective internalised shame that has a historical context. From a collectivist viewpoint, there is the notion of 'what affects you affects me' and results in an eternal wail from our women and a difficult silence from our men. Pain is felt as though it were our own, and our own experience of pain is a touchstone, used to inform us of the pain of others. Within such congregations a deep level of empathy is evident, but the impact of tragedy and trauma is internalised, and as mentioned earlier, while the details of an event are shared, the inner experiencing of the tragedy is rarely articulated. It might be said that tragedies are dealt with silently, and there is an unhealthy internalisation process. Perhaps decades of having to internalise the effects due to being a minority within a dominant society has reinforced this behaviour.

It is important to state that within Afro-Caribbean communities, as with other collective cultures, mental health and spirituality are often interlinked, and one is viewed as having an impact on the other. Individuals will often seek help from the church first when struggling with emotional health, rather than seeking the help of general practitioners or the community mental health team. The church responds to such individuals by offering whatever support it might, although often the persons providing the help may not be professionally trained.

7 T. Scott Bledsoe, Kimberly Setterlund, Christopher J. Adams, Alice Fok-Trela and Melissa Connolly, 'Addressing Pastoral Knowledge and Attitudes About Clergy/Mental Health Practitioner Collaboration', *Social Work & Christianity* 40, no. 1 (2013): 23–45.

Being heard is affirming, gives one identity and a louder voice and places one within the setting in which one lives. It might be questioned why do we not hear more from Afro-Caribbean congregations regarding life in the United Kingdom, including how we share personal and collective responses to disasters. Is there a mind-set that 'we don't share our business' caused by a fear of how it might be perceived by the dominant context within which we live? The fear of judgement and the assumed preconceptions of black people and people of faith may be one answer to this question. Have congregations inculcated the way of being within the dominant society in which they live, or is there fear regarding the reactions of others in how we deal with 'our stuff'? Might it be that the use of language within BME communities and Afro-Caribbean congregations, and ways in which experiences are shared by way of stories, metaphors and parables, is questioned and therefore devalued by others and interpreted as lacking coherence and acceptable articulation?

The richness of Afro-Caribbean congregations

It could have been me (thank you)
Outdoors (thank you)
With no food (thank you)
And no clothes (thank you)
Or left alone (thank you)
Without a friend (thank you)
Or just another number (thank you)
With a tragic end (thank you)
But you didn't see fit to let none of these things be (thank you)
'Cause everyday by Your power (thank you)
You keep on, you keep on keeping me, I wanna say
(Thank you Lord for all You've done for me).
(Walter Hawkins)

> A young lady comes to the UK fleeing the awful experiences of her own country. She has lost everything that she had, she has no family and knows no-one within her new community. She seeks a place to be free of fear, a place to find and be herself, and be accepted.

What does the Afro-Caribbean congregation have that provides us with the ingredients for responding to disasters and draws individuals through the doors of our churches as the first port of seeking help and support for some trauma that has been experienced? The answer may be the following: warmth, a sense of belonging, identity, community, ownership, shared labour (we are in this together). These elements draw and invite the weary and wounded from within the congregation and community to be fed and restored.

Within their structures/walls Afro-Caribbean congregations are not silent. The basic needs of every human being, food, shelter and companionship are offered to the fellow traveller. Along with this, four components are presented as practices that are valued and helpful: prayer, congregational worship, sharing God's word through preaching and, last, practical support. The worship style is often energetic, vibrant and inclusive and invites participation from everyone. The interactive service is experienced as cheering and comforting; it is a valuable medium and a reminder of God's continued care and presence. It may also help to alleviate some of the physical elements of trauma experienced through some tragedy. Prayer, considered the stable diet within the majority of such congregations, is often sought first when those in need make contact. The preached word is accepted as spiritual and emotional food, particularly when navigating through difficulties and personal or national crisis.

As little is written from the context of the United Kingdom on the subject being discussed, it has been useful to consider some literature from the United States in terms of black congregations. Sandra L. Barnes discusses the importance of what she terms 'the church toolkit' in enhancing the social action and community coherence, both of which are deemed important when responding to personal and national tragedies.[8] The toolkit includes prayer and music by way of Gospel songs and preaching. Her study explores the experiences or influences of such tools within black churches based in the United States. As to whether these tools assist coping with disasters or seek to avert such experiences is not evident. Prayer is said to be significant, and here in the United Kingdom, it is equally significant in black congregations, with a petitionary style being adopted, in order to claim God's promises. The drive for social justice and fairness, while not spoken of as loudly and powerfully as by our counterparts in the United States, nonetheless has some bearing on our behaviour towards those within our communities.

One way of responding to disasters, then, can be reflected in the worship style and the coming together as a congregation. This may be viewed as simplistic, but many people place great importance on the constancy of the church service when life has become unpredictable. Regular church attendance may not be practised by all individuals from the Afro-Caribbean community. However, turning to the church is regularly seen when an individual is experiencing some kind of difficulty or disaster. The Church/God is sought in order to make sense of what is happening, for solace or for an impending difficulty to be diverted. Critics of this type of responding may argue that responding is internalised (takes place within the church building) rather than externalised (the church going into the community).

8 Sandra L. Barnes, 'Black Church Culture and Community Action', *Social Forces* 84, no. 2 (2005): 267–994.

The song quoted at the beginning of this chapter testifies to the fact that within such congregations a song can be heard for every experience. Similarly, the Bible is used as a road map. Having a deep faith and sense of God often transcends the here and now (experiencing the problem) to the there and then (difficulties and their effects are no longer experienced). Afro-Caribbeans, whose roots more often than not can be traced back to the continent of Africa, turn and hold tightly to their faith and spirituality in times of disasters. Having something bigger than themselves to believe in in the face of adversity was, and still is, key to survival. Historical events, leading to displacement, the annihilation of self-identity, loss of family, belongings and language, run through the veins of the Afro-Caribbean people. When one has faced his or her worst fears or experienced an existential angst, spirituality plays an important role in giving some form of an anchor – knowledge of how to integrate and process difficult and traumatic experiences based on the word of God. The Church is often sought as a place of comfort and solace by both the congregants and individuals within the community setting. The diversity and inclusiveness of such settings invite and offer support to those who are experiencing difficulties or personal struggles. Within such congregations, the pastor is often called on to pray with an individual or to give a word of encouragement.

Leadership

> A murder has taken place, and the police contact the Church Pastor informing him that a member of his congregation has lost their life and a suspect is being held who is known to several members of the church.

What does it mean for a pastor and his or her spouse (if married) that the Church can be the first port of call when faced with some dilemma? There is an expectancy that the Church will provide an answer that would not necessarily be forthcoming from the regular community networks. It is felt that individuals will be heard, understood and not judged and will not need to explain themselves in terms of their language and ways of communication. As the wife of a pastor, I have observed that within Afro-Caribbean churches, the clergy/pastor plays a pivotal part in how the congregation responds to tragedies within the church and the community. As the leader, the pastor may provide a template that is followed by the congregation. Within Afro-Caribbean communities, the church congregation has certain expectations of their leader and, to some extent, the leadership couple. The leader, and if married his or her spouse, is given a great responsibility, and the manner in which situations are responded to has an impact on the overall health of Afro-Caribbean congregations.

The pastor and spouse may be approached for guidance, counselling, information, spiritual support and practical help, to name but a few expectancies.

It is to the minister that both congregants and the local community turn when there is some problem with which help is needed. Akin to the head of a family, the pastor's response, and that of his or her spouse, can facilitate the congregation's individual and collective response to tragedies and the impact of traumatic events. It also allows individuals to explore how they might process their own traumatic experiences within the Christian faith, such as thoughts regarding mental health, loss, relationship breakdowns and natural disasters.

We have observed African American churches in which the minister is regularly both visible and audible on issues of injustice, events that have had an impact on the community and church, and the need for social action. The response of the leader appears to some extent to give members of the congregation a voice and permission to speak out about their experience of experiences. Barnes discusses the African American church's place within the community and use of mediums already mentioned, such as prayers, songs and preaching, to spur congregations into social action and community activities.[9] Sadly, while such mediums are used within the church services in Afro-Caribbean services in the United Kingdom and are very much a source of comfort, encouragement and inner strength, the voices of black ministers from Afro-Caribbean congregations are infrequently heard within the local and national media in the United Kingdom. Social issues and tragedies such as the recent Windrush experience is one such example. While community leaders from the Afro-Caribbean community and elsewhere became audible, this was not equalled by our church leaders on the public stage. An image might be held of the quiet father who, confronted with the risks of speaking out and being attacked and of harm to himself and the congregation, remains silent and safe.

Harris speaks of the purpose of Christianity and religion within the lives of black Americans and how these nurture social action in the form of engagement with politics and poverty, in ways that respond to difficulties and tragedies.[10] Black-led churches have become the centre of life at some point or other for many Afro-Caribbean people and African Americans post-slavery, and it appears that leaders are striving at getting an appropriate balance between social action and meeting spiritual needs. Considering the continuation of community cohesiveness, immigration and shared experiences, leaders within black American churches have been seen to become a voice in the community for others when tragedy strikes. It is evident that there is a noticeable silence within the United Kingdom. Fighting for rights is not a shared experience, and similar to children emulating the behaviour of a parent, might it be that congregants might emulate the behaviour of the

9 Barnes, 'Black Church Culture', 967.

10 Frederick C. Harris, 'Black Churches and Civic Traditions: Outreach, Activism, and the Politics of Public Funding of Faith-Based Ministries', www.trincoll.edu/depts/csrpl/Charitable%20Choice%20book/Harris.pdf, accessed July 2018.

pastor with regard to remaining silent regarding the experiences and impact of tragedy and trauma?

Taking into consideration the question of silence, Kay suggests that the personality of the Pentecostal minister in the United Kingdom tends to be extroverted and posits that this may have an impact on evangelistic activities.[11] Moving this thought further, the personality of the minister may then inform how the congregation responds to tragedies. The importance of what the pastor preaches in motivating the congregation into taking social action and supporting the community appears pivotal. Is it that there may be a lack of confidence in taking a stand and putting one's head above the parapet? It could be that historical experiences may influence the pastor in taking a stand, albeit subconsciously. The biblical principle of being a peacemaker, and how this may be interpreted into everyday action, comes to mind. Writers of American literature have discussed the value of the church in social action involvement and stressed the importance of the church leadership in guiding the congregation. There is, however, little discussion in the United Kingdom, as a collective, with regard to the impact of disasters and response, and unlike some UK counterparts, such as the Church of England, Afro-Caribbean congregations do not have a prescribed toolkit for responding to disasters or tragedies, either nationally or individually. However, this does not mean that there is no involvement or response. Although pastors may not be as vocal as their counterparts in other places in the world, they nonetheless encourage congregants to offer food, shelter, monetary help and a listening ear to those who require it.

Conclusion

It is hoped that this chapter has helped give an understanding of the frame of reference for the interpretation of and responses to disasters within the Afro-Caribbean community. It does not speak for all black-led churches, which have different cultural backgrounds. Echoing the words of the songwriter Walter Hawkins, tragedies are a common event in life, and within the Afro-Caribbean community and congregation, difficulties are considered a continuation of our history and ongoing experience. Working through the experiences of traumatic events on a public platform is still very new. The question, 'How does that make you feel?' – in response to the onslaught of news in the media – is rarely asked within Afro-Caribbean churches or communities. Tragedies that affect people locally, nationally and internationally have a ripple effect throughout black communities. Fellow humans are embraced in line with the Bible as a neighbour and one of our own. It could be argued that from an emotional context, there is the risk within Afro-Caribbean congregations of minimising the impact of experiences of tragic

11 William K. Kay, *Pentecostals in Britain* (Carlisle: Paternoster, 2000), 265–297.

events. However, as a counterargument, it could be said that our response to disasters is informed by past experiences and the need for survival of self and others. This is our history, and so we carry on and get on with life, normalising the experiences to regulate emotions. What might be the consequences? Being overlooked and not having a voice, with society thinking that we are OK?

Within our communities, more diverse than ever, it is possible to observe a search for likeness. Family systems are important, and the Church is considered a family (as well as a body), with the local community and the world seen as an extended family. The importance of the leader as an interactive and involved person is paramount. The pastor may be seen as the father of the congregation, just as some pastors' wives may, in some congregations, be viewed as the mother of the church, and be expected to represent our saviour in his role of shepherd.

Although not visible or represented in many mainstream settings, and possibly becoming a smaller group compared to the growing number of African congregational churches in the United Kingdom, Afro-Caribbean congregations are important in terms of the support they provide within the community, particularly in times in distress. What has become clear from this reflection is that while we are competent at responding to the individual who has encountered tragedies and turns to the Church for sanctuary, things seemed to be a little less structured and blurrier when it comes to responding to disasters outside of the walls of the church building. There may be many reasons for this, some of which have been explored through this chapter, but which constellate around the need to have the courage to take a stand and the silence of the dominant community.

This chapter has explored how Afro-Caribbean communities respond to disasters. While reflecting on current practices, it has highlighted the need for further reflection, particularly in light of increasing demands for support from the Church at a time when many seek help, not only financial but also in their search for the meaning to life and ease from dis-ease.

Select references

Barnes, Sandra L. 'Black Church Culture and Community Action'. *Social Forces* 84, no. 2 (2005): 267–994.

Bledsoe, T. Scott, Kimberly Setterlund, Christopher J. Adams, Alice Fok-Trela and Melissa Connolly. 'Addressing Pastoral Knowledge and Attitudes About Clergy/Mental Health Practitioner Collaboration'. *Social Work & Christianity* 40, no. 1 (2013): 23–45.

Kay, William K. *Pentecostals in Britain*. Carlisle: Paternoster, 2000.

Lago, Colin. *Race, Culture and Counselling*, 2nd ed. Berkshire: Open University Press, 2006.

Phillips, Mike and Trevor Phillips. *Windrush: The Irresistible Rise of Multi-Racial Britain*. London: Harper Collins, 1998.

Part IV

Liturgical responses

Introduction to Part IV

This part opens with an essay addressing a range of liturgical responses to traumatising events. Carla A. Grosch-Miller, writing with Megan Warner and Hilary Ison, addresses two questions: First, how should trauma-aware liturgists address the challenges inherent in facilitating acts of worship, rhythms of worship, and other uses of sacred space in the phases that follow a shock event? Second, what can be learned from the way ministers have faced the types of extraordinary challenge posed by such events as a terrorist attack or a life-destroying fire?

Woven together in this chapter is theological reflection about what should be done and why, as a community responds to a shock, together with commentary on remarkable examples of ministers crafting liturgical acts (some of which are set out in full in the Appendices). The authors consider the opportunities and challenges created by the liminal role that liturgy can play in the journey communities must make towards a new wisdom, how liturgies can offer words into experiences that baffle or silence those most affected and how liturgies can bind communities together. All these considerations have to be combined with a sensitivity not only to the phase of trauma response that the community is in but also with an understanding of context. The latter is particularly important in multicultural settings, exemplified very particularly by the challenge of crafting the service six months after the Grenfell Tower fire (see Appendix 6).

These liturgical acts often involve settings outside 'sacred space' and people not familiar with traditional liturgical wordings. So the issue of choice of language is also hugely important, as is a choice of symbol. And after the immediate aftermath comes the question of anniversaries – how, and for how long, should these events be commemorated?

Two especially important dimensions of Christian liturgy are explored in the other chapters in this section. The first is arguably the most neglected inheritance from Christianity's Jewish roots, the practice of lament, the outpouring of pain and anger in the face of suffering in which God seems either complicit or passive. Megan Warner examines how the psalms of lament function and how their composition contributes to their effectiveness. She argues that these psalms supply canonical and authorised words in situations of confusion – words of solidarity and of witness.

Warner goes on to ask about the controversial turn toward praise, hope and trust, that many psalms of lament make, and how that movement relates to our understanding of trauma. Finally, she considers the use of laments in contemporary Christian practice.

The last chapter is Karen O'Donnell's study of the eucharist. In contrast to the practice of lamenting, this is a practice central to very many Christian churches. O'Donnell reiterates the fundamentally embodied nature of trauma (introduced in Part II), rupture of bodily integrity, of normal timelines and of cognition. The Eucharist is, on one hand, a profoundly material and body-making practice, but O'Donnell also notes that it can be problematic – overly hierarchical, discriminatory and colluding with oppression.

Nevertheless, she develops her argument by exploring the importance of the eucharist in post-traumatic remaking, with its repair of what has been so damaged in the traumatising experience. This includes the location of the survivor within a profound narrative of healing, both in individuals and in the community.

10 Enabling the work of the people

Liturgy in the aftermath of trauma

Carla A. Grosch-Miller, with Megan Warner and Hilary Ison

Christian worship is at the heart of the community of faith. Regular and extraordinary services for specific purposes affirm being, create belonging and enable becoming. They are particular expressions of the human phenomenon of ritual, present in cultures around the world. Rituals structure and facilitate the most central and basic dilemmas of human existence: birth and death, continuity and change, mortality and transcendence.[1] Aidan Kavanagh describes ritualisation as essential to human development.[2]

The importance of ritual in human life is reflected in the etymology of the word *liturgy*, from the Greek *leitourgia* (*leitos* from *laos*: people + *ergō*: to work). Liturgy, then, is the (religious) work of the people. In the aftermath of trauma, facilitating the work of the people – to gather, to lament and to traverse the valley of the shadow of death – is a key task for ministers.

This chapter explores the conceptual understandings and practical considerations that go into shaping meaningful liturgy that fosters healing in individuals and communities whose lives have been shattered by tragedy. It is rooted in a series of interviews that members of the team have conducted with UK ministers and can be read partly as an introduction and guide to the Appendices. The contents of the Appendices relate to liturgies that have been performed in the United Kingdom following traumatic events that have had an impact on congregations, which we have graciously been permitted to share more widely. The chapter explores the functions and movements of liturgy generally before focusing on the role of liturgy in the aftermath of a disaster. It explores liturgical responses suitable to all stages of trauma response, beginning with the days immediately following a disaster, the first Sunday after the disaster, the weeks and months following the disaster, and, finally, extraordinary liturgical responses that might be appropriate at a range of stages after the traumatic event. Throughout the chapter, there are extensive quotations from ministers who have been interviewed for the 'Tragedy and Congregations' project and extracts from the liturgies they have prepared and performed.

1 Fiona Bowie, *The Anthropology of Religion: An Introduction* (Oxford: Blackwell, 2006), 168.
2 Aidan Kavanagh, 'The Role of Ritual in Personal Development', in *The Roots of Ritual*, ed. James Shaughnessy (Grand Rapids, MI: William B. Eerdmans, 1973), 145–160.

Liminality, language and love

Anthropologist Arnold van Gennep presents the structure of a rite of passage as a threefold journey that incorporates separation from daily life, transition and incorporation or re-entry into daily life.[3] In the aftermath of trauma, rites that negotiate passage through trauma begin by creating occasions for gathering in a safe place (separation), continue through the structuring of liminal communal and individual activities (transition)[4] and conclude with a sending out of the gathered people (re-entry).[5] Of course, no one ritual or liturgy will accomplish the full journey. Rather, different ritual acts ease the passage through the complex and lengthy process of post-traumatic remaking.[6]

Victor Turner, developing van Gennep's work, identified the second stage as the central liminal 'betwixt and between' phase. Likening liminality 'to death, to being in the womb, to invisibility, to darkness, . . . to the wilderness',[7] Turner conceptualised the liminal phase of a ritual as a place of possibility that can hold chaos and non-sense.[8] As trauma gives rise to disorder and shatters meaning, liminal spaces and practices have the capacity to hold the people as they grieve and mourn and prepare to pick up the pieces and adjust to a new normal that contains great loss. Well-crafted liturgy is a container for the bedlam, strong emotion and imaginative possibility that will fuel movement through the threshold towards re-entry into the world.

Liturgy also offers a language of suffering when trauma silences, shutting down the Broca's area in the brain and leaving the traumatised without words or means to express what is happening to them.[9] Megan Warner writes about the traumatic origins of core Christian texts, and about liturgical (and non-liturgical) uses of the lament psalms in trauma contexts in her chapters 'Bible through the Lens of Trauma' and 'Teach to your Daughters a Dirge' elsewhere in this volume. While words have power in liturgy, so, too, do silence and ritual actions that embody the movement through the

3 Arnold van Gennep, *The Rites of Passage*, trans. Monika B. Vizedom and Gabrielle L. Caffe (Chicago: University of Chicago, 1960).

4 From the Latin *limen*, meaning 'threshold', liminality is the central concept in the working of a ritual.

5 See, further, Karen O'Donnell's essay in this section.

6 'Post-traumatic remaking' more accurately describes what happens in the aftermath of trauma than the term *recovery*. See Karen O'Donnell's essay in this section, crediting Hilary Scarsella for the term.

7 Victor Turner, *The Ritual Process: Structure and Anti-Structure* (New York/London: Aldine Transaction, 2008), 95.

8 Frank C. Senn, *Christian Liturgy: Catholic and Evangelical* (Minneapolis, MN: Fortress, 1997), 11.

9 This area in the human brain is strongly associated with language. See Bessel A. van der Kolk, *The Body Keeps the Score: Brain, Mind and Body in the Healing of Trauma* (New York: Penguin, 2014), 43–45.

threshold, and Karen O'Donnell's chapter in this part explores this latter phenomenon. The power and provisionality of both words and actions will be taken up later.

Finally, the work of ritual and liturgy is premised on the understanding that human beings are made by and for relationship. Rituals take place in communities (Turner emphasises the role of *communitas*).[10] In the immediate aftermath of a traumatising event, people need to be together. Where trauma isolates, gathering consoles. The human nervous system operates optimally when it is in harmonious relationship with another human nervous system. 'Resonant caring', as described in the essays by Hilary Ison and Kate Wiebe in this volume, is the single most effective healing response in trauma. We are, indeed, made for love, and it is love that liturgy channels to embrace suffering in the aftermath of trauma.

In the early hours

The work of the people in the immediate aftermath of a traumatising event is to gather and to acknowledge the horror of what has happened. In crafting any liturgical response, knowing and engaging with the context is foundational. An authentic religious response comes out of the embodied practices that the church has engaged in over time and involvement with what people are thinking and feeling. The Reverend Prebendary Alan Everett, in his memoir and theological reflection on the 2017 Grenfell Tower fire in London, tells how, as the tower was consumed by fire, he opened nearby St Clement's Church, turned on the lights and lit candles on the altar as a sign of God's presence and as an invitation to prayer.[11] He reflects that opening the church and turning on the lights were the most significant things he had ever done as a priest, encapsulating not only his own ministry of presence but also trying to create light and open doors for more than 30 years.

Opening the safe and sacred space of a church, to whoever might be seeking solace or companionship in the face of disaster, is an act of humane hospitality that counters the inhumanity of violence and destruction, and that constructs a counternarrative of goodness in the face of malevolence or indifference. Churches have significant resources that are readily marshalled in the event of a crisis: physical premises, tea-making facilities, volunteers who can listen and, most important, an ethos of servanthood. Putting these resources to work for the good of the community activates two of the three essential responses traumatised people need: calming (safety) and caring (resonance as warm and precise listening).[12] Churchwarden of St Ann's

10 Turner emphasises the 'essential and generic human bond, without which there could be *no* society', *Ritual Process*, 97, see also 126–129.

11 Alan Everett, *After the Fire* (Norwich: Canterbury, 2018), 4.

12 The third thing that people need (the third 'C') is the communication of clear information.

Church, Manchester Liz Agbetto wrote in *CRUX*, the diocesan magazine, shortly after the Manchester Arena attack,

> St Ann's Church became a focal point for many people who needed to pray, to talk and to seek solace. In the immediate aftermath of the blast, our priority was to comfort the throngs of visitors pouring through our doors. We laid aside our own feelings of grief and disbelief in order to support others.[13]

Thinking more liturgically, what liminal practices might be offered in an initial gathering? Candle lighting is an act of defiance against encroaching darkness; memorial books or notes place the names and pleas of the people before the community and God; shared silence weaves a bond of unity whilst making room for a diverse experience; singing regulates breath and calms racing pulses. All these activities are containers for strong emotions, enabling some catharsis and countering disorder and despair.

A particularly effective liminal practice in the immediate aftermath of disaster is lamentation: the outcry of pain and injustice meant to sear the heart of God. As Megan Warner observes in the next chapter of this volume, individual and communal psalms of lament make up the largest single genre group in the Book of Psalms.[14] Yet, as she also notes, the Revised Common Lectionary often omits or edits out those most uncomfortable of offerings. What is lost when a congregation sings only the joyful songs of the Lord is the capacity and ability to stand naked and raw before the Holy and, if necessary, to hurl invectives over the pain and injustice of one's condition . . . setting it within the ambit of God. Such a direct address is an act of faith, and lays the foundation for the traumatic remaking that, it is hoped, will occur in the months that follow.

As trauma isolates and fragments, the best responses bring together and unify. Collaboration with other faith groups and local agencies sends the silent message of human goodness and mutuality. Against the devastation wreaked by individuals or an unruly earth (flood, earthquake), a cooperative human response consoles the sorrowful and fuels hope.

The first Sunday

In the aftermath of a traumatising event, it is important to continue with 'normal' events unless it is clear that is not appropriate. The normal church diary can help structure people's time and stabilise their expectations. However,

13 See Appendix 2 for an extended extract.

14 That lamentation has been important in human life throughout the ages is reflected in the fact that there are three kinds of songs in every culture: lullabies, wedding songs and laments (including dirges for the dead: Nancy C. Lee, *Lyrics of Lament: From Tragedy to Transformation* (Minneapolis, MN: Fortress, 2010), 7.

life is no longer normal. And the loss of normality must be reflected in some way on that first Sunday. In general, the first Sunday's liturgy should neither avoid nor totally dwell on the tragedy. The liturgy can be trusted to bring people into God's presence, hold the pain and confusion people are feeling, give a language to the suffering and create the space where over time post-traumatic remaking will occur. You can see each of these elements reflected in the sermon preached by the Dean of Southwark, Andrew Nunn, in Southwark Cathedral on the first morning that it was able to open its doors after the Borough Market attack.[15]

Sometimes the Lectionary offers a surprising and unsettling gift. Christopher Southgate, in his essay 'Trauma and the Narrative Life of Congregations' in this volume, tells the story of how a priest preaching on the first Sunday after the suicide of a female teenager was faced with the lectionary story of a 12-year-old girl whom Jesus raises to life with the words *talitha cum*. His honest admission from the pulpit that 'there will be no *talitha cum*' for *their* child released a torrent of grief, enabling people to begin to accept what had happened and sparking a turn towards greater honesty and depth in the congregation.[16] On the first Sunday after Cockermouth in Cumbria was flooded, a minister stumbled over the set Psalm 93, 'the floods have lifted up their voice; the floods lift up their roaring. More majestic than the thunders of mighty water . . . is the Lord!' The recitation of this psalm, incredibly appointed for the day, provoked strong emotion and theological reflection.[17]

Alan Everett describes the power of silence and sacraments on St Clement's first Sunday after the Grenfell Tower fire:

> The Mass itself was intensely moving. Approximately 150 people were packed into the small church. The atmosphere was subdued, attentive. From the moment we stood for the opening hymn and prayers, there was a palpable sense of unity. The sermon, preached by Robert Thompson, part-time priest and a Labour councillor in Dalgarno Ward, spoke of an inherent brutality in our social system, with its disregard for the poor, and quoted Pope Francis:
>
> > The Gospel tells us constantly to risk a face-to-face encounter with others, with their physical presence which challenges us, with their pain and their pleas, with their joy which infects us in our close and continuous interaction. True faith in the incarnate Son of God is inseparable from self-giving, from membership in the community, from service, from reconciliation with others.
>
> The sermon may have provoked strong feelings among some members of the congregation, but whatever anger they felt, it was contained.

15 See Appendix One.

16 The Revd Nick Bundock, Interview with the Tragedy and Congregations Project, March 28, 2017.

17 The Revd Alistair Smeaton, Interview with the Tragedy and Congregations Project, March 9, 2017.

> There was then an emotional transition. We stood for two minutes' silent prayer. Immediately afterwards, virtually everyone came forward to light a candle in sand trays positioned around the church. There was a deep sense of release as, for some, this was the first time they were able to weep. The mutual support in those few minutes was transformative.
>
> The structure of the liturgy enabled us to feel that the chaos of the situation – the turmoil of our feelings, the overwhelming sense of grief and loss – was in some small way being expressed in a safe place before God.[18]

After the first Sunday

After the first Sunday, as weeks and months go by, the regular worship diet of the congregation will resource people to heal and make sense of what has happened. Elements of the liturgy mirror elements required for post-traumatic remaking. People can only begin that journey in safety; it is to be hoped that the church is as safe a place as possible. Broken relationships are addressed through confession and reconciliation. Scripture and sermons fund the task of the construction of a coherent narrative that includes and makes sense of the tragedy. The 'robust' character of the biblical narratives,[19] and their genesis in traumatic experiences, fits them to support the congregation as it painstakingly pieces together a new story. Finally, through the prayers of intercession and the sending out, people are reconnected to the world around them.

In the most difficult phase of the journey through the valley (the disillusionment phase),[20] people will need support to grapple with the pain and confusion of what has happened. Lamentation may be a feature of worship for some time during this period. Preaching may need to be more directive, particularly to address unhelpful pressures to simply 'forgive and forget' or to blame victims (especially common in clergy sexual abuse cases), for example. Both comfort and challenge have a place in worship during this phase. It is not a time to duck issues or sugar-coat. Trauma strips away illusions and unmasks assumptions; it has the capacity both to annihilate and to reshape faith. The pulpit is a powerful permission giver for honest emotion and deep wrestling, resourcing and supporting a nascent story of faith in the face of adversity. Kraus *et al.* observe that 'a balance of lament, compassionate comfort, and emergent hope will shape a pastoral approach to preaching during this time'.[21]

18 Everett, *After the Fire*, 24–25, quoting from *Evangelii Gaudium*, 88.

19 See Megan Warner's essay, 'Bible Through the Lens of Trauma', in this volume.

20 A helpful chart of the phases of trauma response can be found on the website of the Institute for Congregational Trauma and Growth, at www.ictg.org/phases-of-disaster-response.html.

21 Laurie Kraus, David Holyan and Bruce Wismer, *Recovering From Un-natural Disasters: A Guide for Pastors and Congregations after Violence and Trauma* (Louisville, KY: Westminster John Knox, 2017), 74.

The Grenfell Tower National Memorial Service, held at St Paul's Cathedral in London on the six-month anniversary of the fire and discussed at greater length later, is a paradigmatic example of a worship event that enabled movement through the valley of the shadow of death. The welcome included these words:

> In this service we come together as people of different faiths and none, as we remember with love before God those whose lives were lost, and pray for them to be at peace; as we are alongside brothers and sisters who have lost their homes and their community and those they love; as we commit ourselves to care for each other and to be united in the face of suffering and sorrow; as we seek each other's help and resolve to build on our hopes for a future in which the tragedy that struck the peoples of Grenfell Tower will never happen again. So now, together, we remember and reflect.[22]

The service followed on with an anthem of consolation, the reading of the Beatitudes, a sound montage of voices from Grenfell introduced by the haunting sound of an oud, a song by the Al-Sadiq and Al-Zahra Girls Choir and other elements of worship including the commemoration of the dead, prayers, hymns, music from a steel band, a poem by Rumi and an Act of Commitment.

When originally consulted, local religious leaders had thought it was too soon for such a service. The community leaders, however, were clear that it was absolutely the right time. The service, which was televised by the BBC, made the event heard, seen and known and expressed the grief of the nation. The Bishop of Kensington's sermon spoke of a determination to get to the heart of how such a tragedy happened, acknowledging the grief and anger that were still palpable in the community. After the service, the local religious leaders reflected that it had happened at the right time and was a real moment of transition for the community.[23]

As a congregation begins to emerge from despair and is able to accept what has happened and that there is also good in life (moving into the rebuilding and restoration phases), lamentation will no longer seem necessary or appropriate. Sermons become less directive, opening a space for 'appreciative wondering'.[24] The congregation is still being re-formed and remade,

22 St Paul's Cathedral, *Grenfell Tower National Memorial Service*, London, December 14, 2017. See Appendix 7.

23 Conversation with the Reverend Prebendary Alan Everett (St Clement & St James, North Kensington), the Revd Mike Long (Notting Hill Methodist Church) and Fahim Mazhary (Inter-faith Adviser, Al-Manaar Cultural Centre and Mosque), in preparation for the 8 March Bishop's Study Morning *Pastoral Ministry in Times of Tragedy: Grenfell Tower and After*, at Birmingham Cathedral, Birmingham, March 7, 2018.

24 Kraus et al., *Recovering from Un-natural Disasters*, 95.

and there will be dips in mood and difficult moments, but the direction will be towards a future with hope. Liturgy that contains space and silence into which the unspoken can be brought will enable people to be real and present to the movement of the Holy. There may be a need for special services: the rededication of ruined or violated sacred space, blessing services for children, anniversary services. It is to services like these and other extraordinary services that our attention now turns.

Extraordinary services

Wherever the congregation finds itself on the journey towards remaking, extraordinary services may aid its movement forward.

The Appendices contain a range of liturgical resources, most of which relate to 'extraordinary services'. Readers will find much in them to prompt reflection or to assist in thinking through the preparation of their own liturgies in the aftermath of traumatic events. Designing special services for particular purposes offers scope for the imagination and requires prayerful consideration of many factors, some of them highly sensitive. Following a brief introduction to these resources in the Appendices, most of which take the form of actual liturgies held in the wake of the disasters that hit the United Kingdom in the summer of 2017 (arranged in roughly chronological order, in terms of the stages of disaster response), the remainder of this chapter explores some of the more challenging factors that demand the attention of liturgists in crafting extraordinary liturgies that respond to traumatic events. It includes extracts of interviews in which members of the team spoke with ministers who have written and/or conducted extraordinary liturgies in the wake of disasters, including the liturgies reproduced in the Appendices.

Appendices 1 and 2 have already been referred to here and, strictly speaking, do not fit the category of extraordinary services. Appendix 1, as noted earlier, contains the sermon preached by the Dean of Southwark on the first Sunday on which it was possible to conduct services in Southwark Cathedral after the London Bridge and Borough Market attack. Appendix 2 contains extracts from *CRUX*, the magazine of the Diocese of Manchester, published on July 2017, shortly after the Manchester Arena attack. The extracts contain, variously, an episcopal message and the reflections of clergy and people of St Ann's Church, located near the Manchester Arena, on the impact of the disaster on the congregation and on the interfaith response.

Appendices 3 and 4 contain liturgies for extraordinary services that are 'public' and 'outdoor' and so, to some degree, informal. Of the two, the Appendix 3 liturgy is briefer and less formal. It was designed to facilitate and honour the removal of flowers, teddy bears, sticky notes and other offerings from the makeshift memorial that sprang up on London Bridge after the attack there and in Borough Market, and, like each of the resources in the Appendices, is discussed in more detail later. Appendix 4 contains a reclaiming liturgy, held at the Maltings in Salisbury, following the Novichok nerve-agent attack there in early 2018 and designed to 'reclaim' the place for the people of Salisbury.

Appendix 5 contains a reflection by a London-based minister on a liturgy she conducted with the particular goal of traumatic remaking within the congregation amongst whom she ministers. The liturgy itself was not reduced to writing. In reflecting further about this, the minister wrote,

> I had used occasional written liturgies in this church before and they largely fell flat. This was odd as it is a liturgical church. They just didn't like anything different from what was in the Common Worship Booklets. What worked on this occasion is that the liturgy and the ritual action came seamlessly out of the sermon and it was preached from the heart and mostly without notes. What the congregation encountered was an immediacy and authenticity from their priest that spoke into their experience of the church. In such a wounded church this was very important. If they had pieces of paper in their hands with responses it would have diluted the effect.[25]

The liturgy in Appendix 6, conversely, is extensive and formal. The Grenfell Tower National Memorial Service was held at St Paul's Cathedral six months after the fire and, as the name suggests, was envisaged, at least in part, as an opportunity for memorial, memory and looking forward for the whole nation. It was also, of course, very much envisaged as being for the survivors and bereaved and their local communities as well, but it presented a unique opportunity for those groups of people to know themselves to be held in the imagination and care of the nation as a whole.

Factors to be addressed in designing extraordinary liturgies in the wake of traumatic events

Context, purpose and timing

The first and primary consideration is the context, purpose and timing of the service. Who are the intended beneficiaries of the service? What do they need? What will work? Finding answers to these questions may require extensive consultation.

Shortly after the Grenfell Tower fire, the Dean of St Paul's approached the Bishop of Kensington to offer anything that St Paul's could do to help the local community. Three months later, the Bishop – after discussions with survivor and bereaved family groups – passed on the message that they thought it would be helpful for the Cathedral to do something. The Grenfell people

25 Personal communication.

decided that they would like something on 14 December 2017, the six-month anniversary of the fire. A team from the Cathedral then began a prolonged period of consultation with the Bishop, the Al Manaar Mosque and people from Grenfell, where bodies were still being discovered. Emotions were often raw. The Dean calls the process 'deep listening': 'simply hearing what people felt and then going away to put something together which we thought would meet the needs that people had'.[26] The listening was a necessary preparation. It was also

> very much pastoral in the sense of being there to listen and not to do things to people. The Church was seeking to model a healthy way of relating to people who felt they were having things done to them by others, as of course the whole Grenfell disaster was something that was done to a group of vulnerable people. So how do you not do things to them or patronise? How do you help them articulate where they are, what their needs are and how they want those needs to be met? Also bring to bear the realities of what will or won't work. One of the roles that we have is to be witnesses to the lives of others and to say, 'What happens to you matters because you matter in the sight of God, and I'm living that out with you'.[27]

Supporting the agency of people who have been traumatised is a healing act. It can, however, take a minister to an uncomfortable place, as the Grenfell service planners discovered. The discussion of another important consideration for extraordinary services, whom to invite, proved particularly difficult. Should people who had oversight of the Tower (the Council), the cladding of which appeared to be the cause of the rapid spread and destruction of the fire which claimed 72 lives, be present? Survivor groups were adamant and angry and did not want them present; the Dean was torn ('as Christians you want to work for reconciliation'). In the end the Council decided not to send Council representatives in an official capacity, out of respect and solidarity with the families and community.

Collaboration is another approach, like consultation, that aids decisions about context, purpose and timing. Several of the ministers interviewed for this project observed that the relationships they had built *before* tragedy struck made possible strong pastoral and liturgical collaboration. The Dean of Southwark had nurtured strong relationships with the Borough Council, Borough Market residents and businesses based at Borough Market. Then the London Bridge and Borough Market terrorists struck on 3 June 2017. The Dean reflected later that 'you don't realise why you're doing it till a

26 The Very Revd David Ison, Dean of St Paul's, Interview with the Tragedy and Congregations Project, London, July 27, 2018.

27 David Ison, Dean of St Paul's, Interview with the Tragedy and Congregations Project, London, July 27, 2018.

moment like this comes along'.[28] Because of the trust that had been built, the Borough Council chose to rely heavily on the Cathedral and its clergy to articulate what was going on and what people were feeling, and this spawned meaningful liturgical opportunities.

Similarly, a United Reformed Church minister in West Cumbria observed that long-established ecumenical relationships and a functional ministers' group helped to promote quick and coordinated responses when floods inundated the area in 2009.[29] Worship spaces were shared as some churches were flooded out for months and Churches Together in Cockermouth and in Keswick and Workington found themselves at the forefront of relief work in the community.

Collaboration in multifaith areas brings additional challenges and opportunities. Southwark Cathedral is located in an area with a large Muslim population. Before the attack, cathedral staff had planned to host an Iftar – a traditional breaking of the Ramadan fast evening meal.[30] Deciding to go ahead with it, they hosted the 'Grand Iftar' on the first anniversary of the attack. It featured a rehearsal of the story, thereby incorporating the story of the tragedy within the larger story of the shared community.[31] The booklet guide for the Grand Iftar begins with this message from the Bishop of Southwark and the Chair of the Bankside's Residents' Forum:

> We are delighted to welcome you to this Grand Iftar at Southwark Cathedral, marking the first anniversary of the London Bridge attack.
>
> Over the last year Bankside Residents' Forum, in partnership with Southwark Cathedral, has gained a reputation in its efforts towards community cohesion and collaboration with all age groups, genders, ethnicities, faiths including those of no particular faith and the LGBT community.
>
> We remember the mindless violence which took place on the evening of 3rd June 2017. We remember the courage and solidarity of the community in the immediate aftermath of the London Bridge attacks and the unity which has shone through that day and every day since.
>
> From out of the bad came good, and a determination to rebuild. Together, we have reclaimed our community. That which was broken is now refined and more beautiful than ever.
>
> We are glad you could join us in this act of Peace, Hope and Unity. Let us carry the spirit of love into the days, weeks and months to come.

28 The Very Revd Andrew Nunn, Dean of Southwark, Interview with the Tragedy and Congregations Project, London, November 8, 2017.

29 Alistair Smeaton, United Reformed Church minister, serving West Cumbrian Network, Interview with Tragedy and Congregations Project, Cockermouth, March 9, 2017.

30 Andrew Nunn, Dean of Southwark, Interview with Tragedy and Congregations Project, London, May 14, 2018.

31 *Testimony*, a community memory project, was performed at the Grand Iftar held Sunday, June 3, 2018.

> Let us act to make our world, whether near or far, a better place. This means working together for the common good, playing our part whether small or big by giving something of ourselves to others.
>
> We wish you all a wonderful and peaceful Ramadan.
>
> Ramadan Kareem.[32]

The Iftar began with the Borough Market Choir singing Bill Withers's 'Lean on Me' and included addresses by the Secretary General of the Muslim Council of Britain, the Bishop of Southwark and the Chair of the Bankside Residents' Forum. At the heart of the event was the performance of *Testimony*, a community memory project that recorded the stories of many people caught up in or affected by the 3 June attack. *Testimony* maps the horror and the pathos of the attack and the unexpected, costly gifts that came thereafter. It ends with a stylised 'conversation' between the Bishop of Southwark, the Chair of the Bankside Residents' Forum and representatives of the residents. In the conversation, the Bishop remembers the courage the community showed on the night of the attack and during the weeks and months afterwards. The Bankside Residents' Forum expresses gratitude for the kindness and understanding shown to Muslims in the wake of the attack. The residents – a man and a woman – express confidence that violence and hatred will not affect their lives and values – that 'Love will win', that healing comes from acknowledging, rather than hiding from pain, and that in ten years' time what will be remembered will not be the attacks but the way in which the community withstood them and even flourished. Finally, the Bankside Residents' Forum Chair pronounces that 'Light will always defeat Darkness . . .'.

As St Paul's Cathedral crafted the Grenfell Tower National Memorial Service, its clergy worked to incorporate elements that would speak to the significant Muslim population affected by the fire.[33] After much discussion about how to relate to Islam within a service in a Christian context, they settled on having an oud (an Arabic stringed instrument) player perform meditative music before and after the three-minute media piece of voices from Grenfell, and on having a Muslim Girls' Choir. The Grenfell banner that processed in for the beginning of the service and out at the end was carried jointly by a local Roman Catholic priest and a support worker from the local mosque. A steel band also played during the service to resonate with the Afro-Caribbean population of Grenfell.

Language

Language is a powerful element in liturgy, and each of the ministers interviewed by the team reflected on the care they had taken in choosing words for the liturgies they'd constructed.

32 The Grand Iftar booklet, June 3, 2018, reproduced with the kind permission of the Dean of Southwark, the Very Revd Andrew Nunn.

33 David Ison, Dean of St Paul's, Interview with the Tragedy and Congregations Project, London, July 27, 2018.

Particular issues around language arise if the liturgy is to be held outside of the church's walls. The Dean of Southwark reflected that finding the right words and the right register 'comes out of being in conversation because when you're in conversation with people of course you hear their vocabulary about the event'.[34] He concluded that 'trying to draw back from what everybody knows are the fundamentals of our faith does not serve the whole process of inter-faith at all well. So I was unashamedly Christian but not insensitively Christian'.

An especially difficult question can be whether (and, if so, how) to include deceased perpetrators in the prayers and how generally to speak of them. Here, again, like the question of whom to invite, sensitivity to the intended beneficiaries of the service may dictate the answer. Shared silence can provide a meaningful container for diverse emotion, thought and reflection, as can instrumental music. Finally, what matters most can be *how* things are said rather than *what* is said. An authentic and warm, resonant delivery communicates care beyond what words can say.[35]

Symbolic actions and congregational movement and activity

Silence and delivery are but two tools of nonverbal communication. Symbolic actions and congregational movement and activity bring human bodies and the gathered body into liminal space. The Grenfell service made use of numerous symbolic actions. For example, white roses were placed on the seats reserved for the survivors and the bereaved, the bereaved were invited to bring photographs of their deceased loved ones, a banner was processed in at the start of worship and led the congregation out at the end, and small green hearts were scattered by schoolchildren to represent those who had lost their lives in the fire.

After the London Bridge and Borough Market terrorist attack, people began leaving flowers and sticky note messages near the huge spike at the end of the bridge near Southwark Cathedral. Two weeks later, the flowers were beginning to rot. The Borough asked the Cathedral to design a sensitive way to move them. The plan was for the Dean to say a simple prayer[36] and for the Mayor, followed by a few clergy and members of the Muslim community, to pick up a few bunches and move them towards the van where workers would load them. What happened next was surprising and very moving:

> We thought that that would be the symbolic thing and then we'd stand back and the council workers would move everything, but it didn't

34 Andrew Nunn, Dean of Southwark, Interview with Tragedy and Congregations Project, London, May 14, 2018.

35 R. Ruard Ganzevoort, Conversation with Tragedy and Congregations Project Advisory Board, London, November 12, 2018.

36 The entire prewritten liturgy, which consists, essentially, of the simple prayer, is reproduced in Appendix 3.

> happen like that. Everybody there suddenly silently got into this procession and picked up flowers and moved them without any fuss, without any kind of organisation onto the vans. And it became quickly very clear that what the community wanted to do was to clear it themselves . . . it became a people's liturgy.[37]

This event underscores the importance of planning, flexibility and trusting that people know what they need. The flowers were taken to be composted, and the sticky notes were archived by the Borough. At the anniversary Grand Iftar, some of the composted flowers were in the pot holding a mature olive 'Tree of Healing'. Inscribed on the pot is *And the leaves of the tree are for the healing of the nations*. The tree lives in the Cathedral churchyard, the church holding the community memory of the events.

In further public liturgy at Southwark that included movement and symbolic action the Bishop, Dean, Precentor and other cathedral clergy walked through the Borough Market, stopping at key places where violence had occurred to pray, sprinkle with holy water and cense those places. On another occasion, the Dean led a blessing of the Black and Blue restaurant, where a number of people had sought safety during the attack. By means of these informal, public rituals, the cathedral clergy symbolically 'reclaimed' the area for renewed use by local residents, stall-holders and businesses. There have been a number of such 'reclaiming' liturgies performed around the United Kingdom in recent years and in a variety of contexts. The liturgy for a reclaiming service performed partly in a parish church and partly near the site of the Novichok nerve-agent attack in Salisbury, in which that place, too, was ritually 'reclaimed' for public use through prayer, censing and sprinkling with water is reproduced in Appendix 4. In other examples, the Cockermouth United Reformed Church building in Cumbria was rededicated once flood damage had been repaired,[38] as was the churchyard of a Somerset church where a man had killed himself after murdering another.[39]

Anniversaries

Anniversary services are commonplace. In the first year they can be particularly meaningful and helpful to survivors and bereaved people and communities. Thereafter, questions arise if and how to remember tragic events in years to come. Kraus *et al* tell the story of the one-year anniversary liturgy marking the murder of the sexton and a parishioner in the sanctuary of a church. In an act of prayer, members of the congregation wrote down their

37 Andrew Nunn, Dean of Southwark, Interview with Tragedy and Congregations Project, London, May 14, 2018.

38 The Revd Alistair Smeaton, *Cockermouth United Reformed Church Rededication Service*, June 27, 2010.

39 The Revd Paula Hollingsworth, *St Lawrence's Churchyard and Church, Saturday 16th April 2011, Service of Remembrance and Hope*, Westbury sub Mendip, 2011.

hopes and fears, which were then ritually burned.[40] The liturgy was repeated on the second and third anniversaries, but the focus of the symbolic action in the third year shifted away from the double murder to the general hopes and fears of parishioners. There was no request from the congregation or the lay leadership to repeat it on the fourth anniversary. There comes a time when the tragic event stops being a defining moment in the congregation's life. The Dean of St Paul's says the question is, 'What new thing will bring life into this situation now?'[41]

On 7 July 2007, a bomb exploded in a London tube carriage resulting in the death of eight people and the injury of many more near the Aldgate tube station. St Botolph's, the church next to the station, became a focus as the churchyard was filled with flowers and a service for the emergency responders was held.[42] On the first and tenth anniversary of the bombing, St Paul's Cathedral held large public services. But annually, there has been an intimate anniversary commemoration around the plaque in Aldgate station.[43] Bereaved family members, a few tube drivers and the priest of St Botolph's gather at the plaque for a simple liturgy that has remained unchanged. People appreciate the consistency and particularly want the names of those killed read out each year. Asked how long she will continue to run this service, the priest replied,

> As long as they [the families] want to have it.
> I feel quite strongly about that, because it is a clear need . . . this idea that I'm praying these prayers for them because they're not able to is really strong.
> For me, turning up at 9:30 and having the tea and coffee is as important as doing the liturgy, to demonstrate to them that they are important. We haven't forgotten them, that they're somehow held.[44]

In Hyde Park, at noon on the same day, survivors from the bomb blast have gathered for a secular event that has featured a Gospel choir. Survivors have not tended to attend the Aldgate station service; the priest wonders if it is difficult for survivors to be in the same place as those who have lost somebody. The Grenfell planners also observed the differences between the two groups – survivors and bereaved. Sensitivity to the needs of each can help shape appropriate liturgical responses.

40 Kraus et al., *Recovering*, 95–98.

41 David Ison, Dean of St Paul's, Interview with the Tragedy and Congregations Project, London, July 27, 2018.

42 The Revd Laura Jorgenson, Interview with Tragedy and Congregations Project, London, March 16, 2017.

43 Laura Jorgenson, *Aldgate liturgy*, 2018, personal communication.

44 Laura Jorgenson, Interview with Congregational Tragedy Project, London, May 15, 2018.

Commemorative objects

Connected with the issue of anniversaries is the question of commemorative objects. The considerations that shape liturgy (e.g., context, consultation) also help determine what might be a helpful and appropriate commemorative object and the capacity of churches to maintain memorials that would not be welcomed in other places. Southwark Cathedral, as already noted, has become the site of the Tree of Healing – the market stall-holders did not want the terror attack to be a defining moment that would scare off trade. A church can hold the community memory of tragedy more comfortably, as it is a repository for community history and memory in many places. During the Borough Market attack, the police believed the perpetrators had entered the Cathedral, and in their pursuit of the perpetrators, the police battered the sacristy doors. Cathedral clergy decided to make the doors secure but not to fill in or replace the wood that was damaged, letting the building bear the marks for future generations:

> Reflecting around the resurrection appearances and what Paul says – we bear in our bodies the marks of Jesus – and how the church needs to have the confidence to bear the marks and not do what we like to do and airbrush out the evidence.[45]

Care must be always be taken, as commemorative items created by a church or local agency without consulting the people most affected by the tragedy may not be welcomed or serve their intended needs.

The long aftermath

Liturgy may serve to heal hearts and enable movement along the journey of post-traumatic remaking long after tragic events have struck. It may, for example, be an important and effective tool in helping a congregation to 'reframe' its story. In one church that had been beset by a series of traumas – a building loss, conflict over whether women should be permitted to be priests, the closure of a sister church and others – a priest used the regular service on the first Sunday of Advent as an opportunity to encourage the congregation's reframing of the story of the church. The Lectionary's appointed Gospel reading for the day was the parable of the fig tree, so the priest used that story as a framework. Naming the traumas one by one and lighting a candle for each, she talked about the congregation's responses of denial, anger and depression and used, as a repeated refrain, the phrase 'and yet we are faithful and prayerful'.[46] She reported that the Parochial Church

45 Andrew Nunn, Dean of Southwark, Interview with the Tragedy and Congregations Project, London, November 8, 2017.

46 The full text of the report of this 'remaking' exercise is included in Appendix 5.

Council (PCC) meeting the following day was lighter and more positive in tone than previous PCC meetings.

Conclusion

Churches are in a privileged position when it comes to responding to disasters:[47] with recognised sacred spaces, a treasure trove of trauma-tested texts, a language for suffering and for new life coming from death, and an understanding of the power and promise of ritual, church leaders can create liturgies that help to heal traumatised brains and broken hearts, restore relationships and spark imaginations to write new stories of God and God's people in the aftermath of tragedy. The journey of post-traumatic remaking is a long and arduous one. Liturgy is a tool that helps the lame to walk and those blinded by pain and fear to come to a new vision.

This chapter has highlighted positive examples of liturgy that have helped people and communities in the aftermath of trauma. There also abound scores of examples of missed opportunities, liturgies that miss the mark, commemorations that offend and other *faux pas* that could be cited . . . all of them opportunities for learning. It is only too easy to misstep in this fraught territory.

Finally, liturgy is an instrument of power. Not only is it impactful in the moment, but it also transmits a view of the human being before God. One of the challenges for liturgists in times of trauma is that, although key biblical stories are steeped in trauma, standard liturgies focus on sin. The result is that the experiences and needs of the sinner are addressed at greater length than those of the wounded.[48] The creativity invited in special gatherings to lament, memorialise and bless may help to redress this deficit, providing balm to hearts, minds and bodies that have been shattered by tragedy.

This chapter closes with a final offering, a litany in the wake of trauma from the pen of Christopher Southgate:

Creator of a cosmos of mourning and wonder

Have mercy upon us and hear our prayer

Word made flesh, traumatised as our servant

Have mercy upon us and hear our prayer

47 Hence, the very particular challenges for liturgy, and ministry in general, when the church in question is unusable either because it is a crime scene (as was the case for Southwark Cathedral following the London Bridge/Borough Market attack) or has been rendered unsafe by, for example, an earthquake (as was the case for the Cathedral and other city churches following the 2011 earthquake in Christchurch, New Zealand and during the extended aftershock period). The sermon preached by the Dean of Southwark on the first Sunday it was possible to conduct worship in the Cathedral after the attack is contained in Appendix 1.

48 R. Ruard Ganzevoort, Conversation with the Tragedy and Congregations Project Advisory Board, London, November 12, 2018.

Spirit, companion of lives that carry death within them

Come close in time of pain.

Empower us to bear reality

What has happened to us has happened.

Help us to see even disaster

As part of the fabric of God's creation

Help us to bring even the rawest tragedy

To the foot of Christ's Cross.

Help us to be authentic bearers of the hope

That one day there will be no more crying, for God will be all in all.

Enfold us in love that is strong as death.
Enfold us in the grace that sin can never exhaust.
Enfold us in the fellowship that will never let us go.

And the Grace of our Lord Jesus Christ, the love of God and the fellowship of the Holy Spirit be with us, now and for evermore. Amen.[49]

Select references

Everett, Alan. *After the Fire*. Norwich: Canterbury, 2018.

Kavanagh, Aidan. 'The Role of Ritual in Personal Development'. In *The Roots of Ritual*, ed. James Shaughnessy. Grand Rapids, MI: William B. Eerdmans, 1973, 145–160.

Kraus, Laurie, David Holyan and Bruce Wismer. *Recovering From Un-natural Disasters: A Guide for Pastors and Congregations After Violence and Trauma*. Louisville, KY: Westminster John Knox, 2017.

Senn, Frank C. *Christian Liturgy: Catholic and Evangelical*. Minneapolis: Fortress Press, 1997.

Swinton, John. *Raging With Compassion: Pastoral Responses to the Problem of Evil*. Grand Rapids, MI/Cambridge, UK: William B. Eerdmans, 2007.

Turner, Victor. *The Ritual Process: Structure and Anti-Structure*. New York/London: Aldine Transactions, 2008.

49 Christopher Southgate, January 2019, personal communication.

11 Teach to your daughters a dirge[1]

Revisiting the practice of lament in the light of trauma theory

Megan Warner

John Swinton opens his study of the practice of lament with the story of a disconnect.[2] He describes attending worship at his local church the day after the Omagh Bombing in 1998 and encountering a liturgy of unrelieved praise and thankfulness. By not a single word or gesture was the carnage of the day before acknowledged, let alone confronted. This experience, he writes, led him to new insights about the worship practice of his congregation:

> I suddenly understood clearly that there was no room in our liturgy and worship for sadness, brokenness, and questioning. We had much space for love, joy, praise, and supplication, but it seemed that we viewed the acknowledgement of sadness and the tragic brokenness of our world as almost tantamount to faithlessness.[3]

Swinton is by no means alone in having experienced, and reflected on, a disconnect of this kind. Don E. Saliers writes of what he terms 'lament denial' as follows:

> At the same time, individual and family grief and bereavement continue to affect persons in every congregation. These, too, are brought to Christian liturgical assemblies. Yet a disconnect between the sorrowing, the grieving, and the poetry of the biblical Psalms occurs too frequently. Even funeral liturgies often fail to invite a shared anger and lament over loss, to sing, in Brian Wren's language, 'an honest aching song'.[4]

Kathleen Norris's sense of disconnect between her childhood experiences in the world (and in the world of her faith) and in her church, where she perceived a relationship with God as being somehow caught up in the need to

1 The title comes from Jer 9:20, which continues, 'and each to her neighbour a lament'.
2 John Swinton, *Raging With Compassion: Pastoral Responses to the Problem of Evil* (Grand Rapids, MI: Eerdmans, 2007), 90–129.
3 Swinton, *Raging*, 92–93.
4 Don E. Saliers, 'Psalms in Our Lamentable World', *Yale Journal of Music and Religion* 1, no. 1, Art. 7, 104, https://doi.org/10.17132/2377-231X.1013.

be 'dressed up', both outwardly and inwardly, finds expression in her brief poem:

> They pounded nails into his hands
> After that, well, after that
> Everyone wore hats . . .[5]

She further writes that what went wrong for her in her Christian upbringing was bound up with 'the insidious notion that I need to be a firm and even cheerful believer'.[6]

Swinton, Saliers and Norris each go on to discuss the psalms of lament of the Old Testament (OT) as an answer, if not *the* answer, to the disconnect they identify. Similarly, Denise Ackermann (whom Swinton cites in his essay) writes in an open letter to her daughters that she has 'found' and 'discovered' the ancient tradition of lament and that it offers a 'language that can lead us out of' a situation of lack.[7] Indeed, it seems that almost every writer on the subject of lament psalms is inclined to identify a gaping gap in Christian practice to which the lament psalms are the antidote, so this essay might very well have begun, 'It is a truth universally acknowledged that the Church lacks a practice of the expression of grief, shock and anger and the lament psalms are the answer'.[8]

This is not supposed to sound flippant but, rather, to reflect something of the extent and force of the consensus, both academic and popular, that the psalms of lament have a great deal to offer Christian practice and that this truth has somehow been overlooked, obscured or forgotten in most non-monastic Christian traditions.

In this chapter, I propose, after setting out some of the reasons why the consensus is held so ardently, to tease out some questions about the understanding of lament psalms and their use in the aftermath of traumatic events which arise when biblical scholarship and trauma theory are brought together with considerations of practical and pastoral theology. I round out the discussion with an exploration of practical issues around the liturgical and non-liturgical use of lament psalms.

5 Kathleen Norris, *The Cloister Walk* (New York: Riverhead, 1996), 107.

6 Norris, *Cloister Walk*, 107.

7 Denise M. Ackermann, *After the Locusts: Letters from a Landscape of Faith* (Grand Rapids, MI: Eerdmans, 2003), 108.

8 With apologies to Jane Austen. For a helpful survey of the 'loss' and the 'recovery' of the lament tradition in Christianity see Kathleen D. Billman and Daniel L. Migliore, *Rachel's Cry: Prayer of Lament and Rebirth of Hope* (Eugene, OR: Wipf & Stock, 1999). Billman and Migliore's work draws heavily on the work of Walter Brueggemann, who could be considered the grandfather of Christianity's renewed interest in the lament tradition. See Walter Brueggemann, *The Message of the Psalms* (Minneapolis, MN: Augsberg, 1984) and Patrick D. Miller, ed., *The Psalms and the Life of Faith: Walter Brueggemann* (Minneapolis, MN: Fortress, 1995).

What is it about the lament psalms?

It is possible to identify two elements in the disconnect described by Swinton, Saliers and Norris to which psalms of lament respond. The first element is the observation that the church lacks a language for the expression of 'negative' emotions, such as grief, shock and anger.[9] The second element is a fear that such a language, even if the church possessed it, could express only faithlessness. What is remarkable about the lament psalms is that they address both these elements strongly and definitively. As regards the first, the psalms contain within them expressions of just about every kind of emotion there is. Many are edifying, while others, like those expressing a desire for vengeance,[10] tend to be less comfortable for 21st-century churchgoers. This sense of discomfort is arguably exacerbated by the lectionary practice of omitting the more violent and vengeful portions of psalms and other biblical readings, thus shielding congregations from the full range of emotions expressed biblically while limiting and sanitising their understanding of the breadth of worship that is possible.[11]

The Psalms offer not only language but also authorised literature for the expression of a full range of emotions.[12] For those finding it challenging to get in touch with, identify or express their emotions (a category of people into which most of those affected by trauma will fall), the Psalms offer a collection of authorised texts, each one having been used by countless suffering people and peoples. In these prayers, individuals and congregations have a library of ready-made vehicles for the expression of complaint and suffering that also draws them together with countless generations of lamenters before them. Furthermore, the fact that the psalms address these emotions

9 Norris's verse points out that this is so despite the violent beginnings of the Christian faith itself.

10 The classic example of the expression of a desire for vengeance is found in Psalm 137:8–9:

> O daughter Babylon, you devastator!
>
> Happy shall they be who pay you back
> what you have done to us!
>
> Happy shall they be who take your little ones
>
> and dash them against the rock!

11 Billman and Migliore, *Rachel's Cry*, 25, write that '[t]he Temptation to hear the joyful voices and dismiss the anguished voices among the biblical witnesses tempts us again and again. When the church succumbs to this temptation, the result is always the impoverishment of Christian life and ministry.'

12 John Goldingay has reportedly, and rather wonderfully, quipped that the psalms are 'one hundred and fifty things God doesn't mind having said to him'. The fact that Goldingay himself does not recall having used this phrase does not stop significant numbers of his students attributing it to him.

to God directly means that they express not faithlessness but precisely the opposite.[13] Implicit in the psalms is a conviction that God is in control and, even if not entirely responsible for the situation in which the lamenter finds him- or herself, holds the key to its resolution.

As noted earlier, many writers have reflected on what it is about the lament psalms that mean that they offer us so much in terms of response to tragedy, violence and hurt. Swinton writes, for example,

> Lament gives a voice to suffering and releases rage in a context of faith and compassion. In so doing, it opens up the possibility of life and liveliness in the face of those forms of evil that would seek to destroy both. Engagement in such a practice of lamentation is a pastoral practice that enables one to hang onto one's humanity in the midst of apparent dehumanization and to emerge from the silence that is forced upon us through our encounters with evil.[14]

Ackermann, writing an imagined theological letter to her daughters, says,

> The integrity of the psalms grips me. When the psalmists lament, they shape our experience of despair. Could Jesus have felt the same when he cried out on the cross: 'My God, my God, why have you forsaken me? (Ps. 22:1) . . . The psalms say it all – God absent, God present, God mysterious, God known, God of wrath, and God of love and mercy.[15]

Earlier in the letter, Ackerman tells her daughters that she has found a language 'that can lead us out of the temptation to apathy, muteness and anger, and that does not resort to atheism'.[16] Lament does indeed offer a 'language' in contexts in which one is needed, and the lament psalms offer a set of ready scripts for conversation with God that is impassioned, real, unapologetic, therapeutic and faithful.

The impact of trauma

Trauma theory suggests that the gift of lament psalms to traumatised people may be even greater than already suggested. One of the markers of trauma is that it leaves its victims feeling overwhelmed, helpless and mute. Quite literally, a traumatised person may find themselves physically unable to speak. When a person has become 'stuck' in the fight or flight response, the parts of

13 So, for example, Howard Neil Wallace, *Words to God, Word from God: The Psalms in the Prayer and Preaching in the Church* (Aldershot, UK/Burlington, VT: Ashgate, 2005), 80, writes, 'It suggests that an expression of protest is not to be equated with a lack of hope, or for that matter, a lack of faith itself. In fact, since it is a protest *to God* it embodies a level of trust and expectation.' (emphasis in the original)

14 Swinton, *Raging with Compassion*, 105–106.

15 Ackermann, *After the Locusts*, 115–116.

16 Ackermann, *After the Locusts*, 108.

the brain that regulate speech will be 'shut down' to some degree as the body mobilises its capacity to run, do battle or hibernate.[17] This physical barrier to speech is compounded by further effects of trauma that limit the ability of a traumatised person to tell a coherent story. In normal memory processes, experiences are stored as memories that can be retrieved and recounted. The overwhelming nature of trauma, however, means that the brain's capacity to store the experience as memory is compromised – literally overwhelmed. In fact, as outlined in some of the other chapters in this volume, because the event is never really 'experienced', no memories are formed. Instead, the body retains isolated and jagged impressions of the event, which become stored not in the brain but in the body more generally.[18] These may come into consciousness unexpectedly and painfully (as flashbacks) but not with sufficient detail or coherence to support a construction of the story of the event. Thus, once a traumatised person recovers the physical gift of speech, she may nevertheless find telling the story of the trauma to be beyond her.

The painful irony here is that the received wisdom has tended to be that traumatised people will recover from the effects of their trauma only once they have been able to 'tell the story' of the traumatic event. Judith Herman, one of the pioneers of trauma theory, for example, writes, 'Remembering and telling the truth about terrible events are prerequisites both for the restoration of the social order and for the healing of individual victims'.[19] More recent scholarship has revisited this view, and cautions that compelling a traumatised person who does not wish to tell his story, or cannot, is unhelpful and may lead to re-traumatisation. Instead, academics and practitioners are exploring different approaches to trauma recovery that focus on the body and on physical movement that have the capacity to release painful shards of stored traumatic experience. EMDR (Eye Movement Desensitising and Reprocessing) is possibly the best known of these, but the field is growing.[20] Encouragement to 'tell the story' remains a central therapeutic approach, but it is today supported by a number of alternatives.

Fortunately, *any* speech about the traumatic event and expression of the emotion connected to it, even without an accurate and full narration of the story itself, may be therapeutic, and significantly so.[21] Extraordinarily,

17 See, for example, Bessel van der Kolk, *The Body Keeps the Score: Brain, Mind and Body in the Healing of Trauma* (London: Viking, 2014), 43–45; David G. Garber, Jr. 'Trauma Theory', in *The Oxford Encyclopaedia of Biblical Interpretation*, ed. Steven L. McKenzie (Oxford: Oxford University Press, 2013), 421–428.

18 Thus the title of Van der Kolk's, *The Body Keeps the Score*.

19 Judith Herman, *Trauma and Recovery* (New York: Basic, 1992), 1.

20 See the latter chapters of Van der Kolk, *Body Keeps the Score*; Peter Levine, *Waking the Tiger: Healing Trauma* (Berkeley, CA: North Atlantic, 1997).

21 Brent Strawn, 'Trauma, Psalmic Disclosure, and Authentic Happiness', in Elizabeth Boase and Christopher Frechette, *Bible Through the Lens of Trauma* (Atlanta: SBL, 2016), 143–160, 144–149, argues strongly that disclosure (of whatever kind) of traumatic experience acts to counterbalance and redress the negative health impacts of non-verbalisation or inhibition of traumatic experience.

research into the health benefits of confronting and expressing the impact of traumatic events has suggested that expression and non-expression of the emotions connected to traumatic experiences are more predictive of health outcomes than even the nature and scale of the traumatic events themselves.[22] This is where the real gift of lament psalms to traumatised people becomes apparent. These Psalms express the full range of emotions about traumatic events. Brent Strawn writes, 'The psalmists have experienced events that are properly called traumatic – to greater and lesser degrees and in a wide variety of circumstances'.[23] Strawn also notes that the lament psalms themselves are often elusive, hazy and riddled with gaps when it comes to describing the traumatic events themselves. While the emotions expressed can be raw, details of the petitioner's complaint are often limited. This, together with the fact that lament psalms are *authorised* (in the sense that they comprise part of the canon of the Scriptures, and so can be prayed with confidence), can make them ideal vehicles for the expression of strong, violent, unspeakable emotions connected with traumatic events in the lives of people today.[24]

One further dimension of lamenting is important here. Recovery from trauma is connected not only with the expression of emotions but also with the witness of such expression. Gabor Maté, for example, writes that '[t]rauma is not what happens to us, but what we hold inside in the absence of an empathetic witness'.[25] Shelley Rambo also writes movingly about the therapeutic importance of the witnesses to the expression of trauma-related emotions.[26] For example, in the discussion of the power of the 'healing circle', she writes, 'It is not just that one's "hurt" recognizes the hurt in another, but that the collective attunement to pain forges routes of healing that did not previously exist'.[27] The lament psalms address the need for witnessing. Although it is quite possible to pray the lament psalms while alone, the Psalms are in their essence *liturgical*; that is, they presuppose performance in company. A congregation, or a smaller group, become witnesses to the performance and therefore to the pray-er's expression of emotion. Communal lament psalms, in particular, have the capacity to respond to the sense of isolation that is

22 See James W. Pennebaker, *Opening Up: The Healing Power of Expressing Emotions* (New York: Guilford, 1997) and discussion of Pennebaker's findings in Strawn, 'Trauma, Psalmic Disclosure, and Authentic Happiness'. Strawn notes (at 149) Pennebaker's observation that prayer is a form of 'disclosure' or expression for these purposes.

23 Strawn, 'Psalmic Disclosure', 152.

24 Hugh G.M. Williamson, for example, writes, 'the language is such that it is capable of serving to articulate an almost infinite number of such experiences, and this no doubt accounts for the enduring value that is set upon them'; see Williamson, 'Reading the Lament Psalms Backwards', in *A God So Near: Essays on Old Testament Theology in Honor of Patrick D. Miller*, ed. Brent A. Strawn and Nancy R. Bowen (Winona Lake, IN: Eisenbrauns, 2003), 3–16, 4.

25 Gabor Maté, 'Foreword', in Peter Levine, *In an Unspoken Voice: How the Body Releases Trauma and Restores Goodness* (Berkeley, CA: North Atlantic, 2010), xii.

26 Shelly Rambo, *Spirit and Trauma: A Theology of Remaining* (Louisville, KY: Westminster John Knox, 2010) and *Resurrecting Wounds: Living in the Afterlife of Trauma* (Waco, TX: Baylor University Press, 2017).

27 Rambo, *Resurrecting Wounds*, 130.

one of the features of traumatisation. Performance of communal psalms of lament by victims of trauma guarantees witnesses for expression,[28] but also has the potential to re-unite those who have undergone a common traumatic experience but whose traumatisation has led to feelings of isolation.[29]

The structure and function of psalms of lament

The Psalter contains two distinct types of psalms of lament – individual and collective – and together, they account for approximately a third of the psalms.[30] The two forms of lament psalms, individual and corporate, share many common features, and indeed their essential structural elements are more or less the same:

1 an address to God;
2 a statement of the lament, which may include a description of the problem; and
3 a request, or petition, for God's intervention.[31]

These 'essential structural elements' may be, and typically are, supplemented by further additional elements. Individual lament psalms lament a variety of experiences of individual people; they may include, additionally, a confession of innocence, a confession of confidence, a vow of praise and an expression of an assurance of being heard. Communal laments lament losses that impact the entire community. They may include additionally, therefore, a recital of Israel's history of salvation (which stands in contrast to the current experience of loss, devastation or abandonment),[32] an appeal to God's name or honour, a confession of sin or declaration of innocence and a vow of praise or statement of assurance of being heard by God.

These additional structural elements should not be thought of as marginal or unusual. Many scholars of the Psalms, including the most prominent scholars of the last 50 to 100 years, consider some or all of them essential or universal. Walter Brueggemann, for example, considers that a typical lament psalm could be expected to contain address to God, complaint, petition,

28 It is not essential that witnesses have shared in experience of the traumatic events. See, for example, Rambo's discussion (*Resurrecting Wounds*, 114–130) of the ministry of (non-veteran) 'Warrior's Journey Home' members to returned veterans suffering with PTSD.

29 This is of particular relevance in cases of major public traumas, such as terrorist attacks or natural disasters, but may also apply within congregations where multiple members are affected.

30 Assignment of psalms to *genre* is not an exact science, but the number may be somewhere between 47 and 52. Jan Christian Gertz et al., *T&T Clark Handbook of the Old Testament: An Introduction to the Literature, Religion and History of the Old Testament* (London/New York: T&T Clark, 2012), 527–549, esp. 537–541 offers a helpful introduction.

31 Gertz et al., *Handbook of the Old Testament*, 538–539.

32 For a discussion of the recitation of Israel's history in Psalm 78 through the lens of trauma, see Rebecca W. Poe Hays, 'Trauma, Remembrance and Healing: The Meeting of Wisdom and History in Psalm 78', *JSOT* 41 (2016): 183–284.

motivations (for God to act), imprecation (curse), assurance, payment of vows and, finally, doxology and praise.[33] In particular, many scholars consider a final expression of praise of God and/or hope that God will answer the petition to be an essential, or universal, element of psalms of lament (both individual and corporate). Brueggemann, again, takes the view that lament *always* turns to praise.[34] Swinton shares this view: 'Lament provides us with a language of outrage that speaks against the way things are, but always in the hope that the way things are just now is not the way they will always be. Lament is thus profoundly hopeful.'[35] He goes on to assert that '[s]uch a return to God in faith and hope is really the only resolution that Scripture gives to the problem of evil.'[36]

As Swinton's comments would suggest, the most common place for expressions of hope or praise in the lament psalms is at the end, so that the mood of the psalm travels from desolation towards hopefulness. The movement is not always smooth; in fact, the transition from one mood to the other is often sudden or abrupt. Psalm 13, which Swinton reproduces in his study of the lament psalms, is a good example. The psalm begins with the desolate cry 'How long, O LORD? Will you forget me forever?' and verses 1 to 4 continue the psalmist's complaint. Suddenly, in verse 5, the psalmist speaks of trust and rejoicing, and it appears that the LORD has already granted the petition and that the petitioner's suffering is in the past. This abrupt shift of mood and related questions about its function and the possible reasons for it have been the single most pressing issue for modern biblical scholarship on the lament psalms.

A range of reasons has been suggested for this abrupt shift in the lament psalms from desolation/complaint to hope/praise. Prominent explanations have been liturgical and editorial.[37] Increasingly, the most persuasive explanations for an abrupt change of mood in the lament psalms have been *psychological*. These suggest that the experience of expressing the lament directly to God is effective in changing the mood of the petitioner so that by the time the petitioner reaches the end of the psalm, she is ready to express trust, hope and praise.[38] In the case of a psalm as brief as Psalm 13, this is not an easy argument to maintain(!), but nevertheless, psychological explanations have been influential, at least in persuading scholars that reciting the

33 Walter Brueggemann, *The Message of the Psalms: A Theological Commentary* (Minneapolis, MN: Fortress, 1985), 54–56.

34 See a critical assessment of Brueggemann's views in Frederico G. Villanueva, *The Uncertainty of a Hearing: A Study of the Sudden Change of Mood in the Psalms of Lament* (VTSupp 121; Leiden: Brill, 2008), 18.

35 Swinton, *Raging with Compassion*, 105.

36 Swinton, *Raging with Compassion*, 112.

37 As to the former, see for example, Joachim Begrich, 'Das priesterliche Heilsorakel', ZAW 52 (1934): 81–92, as to the latter, Gertz et al., *Handbook of the Old Testament*, 539.

38 See, for example, Erhard S. Gerstenberger, *Der bittende Mensch* (WMANT 51; Neukirchen-Vluyn: Neukirchener, 1980), 163–169.

psalms is effective in *beginning* a movement in the petitioner from lament to trust, hope and praise.

One explanation for the shift in mood that stands as out as being radically different is that of Hugh Williamson. In an essay titled 'Reading the Lament Psalms Backwards', Williamson has suggested that the lament psalms are not, in fact, laments at all, but psalms of praise written *after* God has intervened to answer prayer or to resolve some situation of disaster.[39] The lament elements, on this argument, function to heighten the drama of the psalm and to contextualise and heighten the offered praise. If Williamson is right, then the lament psalms are not and *should not be* effective liturgical and pastoral resources for those experiencing tragedy, loss and trauma.

There is, however, a problem with all this discussion, and Williamson's argument serves to highlight it. The problem is that *it is simply not the case that all lament psalms move from lament to praise*. There are several patterns of mood shift in the lament psalms. Some begin with a mood of praise and introduce lament later. Others shift backwards and forwards between lament and praise, some concluding with praise and some not.[40] At least one lament psalm, Psalm 88, includes no element of hope or praise at all. Williamson acknowledges the 'pure' lament psalms (offering Psalm 88 as an example, as well as Psalms 25, 70, 141 and 143), but he does not explicitly address the issue of psalms that begin with praise elements and move toward lament.[41] This variation in the form of lament psalms is explored by Frederico Villanueva in *The Uncertainty of a Hearing*, in which Villanueva adopts and challenges the paradigm of lament psalms that sees them move uniformly from lament to praise.[42]

There are, of course, significant pastoral implications of a paradigm of lament psalms in which lament, complaint and request give way to expressions of trust, hope and praise. Such a paradigm suggests that in addition to providing both a language and a literature for the faithful expression of 'unspeakable' emotions and experiences, lament psalms offer a vehicle for the passage of inner states from desolation to hopefulness, so that a modern

39 Williamson, 'Reading the Lament Psalms Backwards', 13 and *passim*.

40 Trauma theory notes the potential for movement between a range of psychological states. For example, an initial period of exaltation can give way to a sense of disillusion, and joy and despair can continue to rub shoulders. Something similar was proposed early by Friederich Heiler, *Das Gebet: Eine Religionsgeschichtliche und Religionspsychologische Untersuchung* (München: Ernst Reinhardt, 1921), 380: 'The petitioner carries on an internal conflict between doubt and certainty, hesitation and assurance, until finally faith and trust break through with victorious power'.

41 Although Williamson refers in his title to reading psalms backwards (i.e., from praise back to lament), his primary argument is that it should not be assumed that the situation of the psalmist at the *beginning* of the psalm is the situation of the psalmist at the time of writing the psalm. Williamson argues that logic points to the time of writing being a time *after* the resolution of the psalmist's complaint.

42 Villanueva, *The Uncertainty of a Hearing, passim.*

'pray-er' may, by praying the lament psalms, expect to experience movement from his original emotional state to a new, more hopeful one. The observation that the lament psalms do not as a collective group show evidence of a single pattern of movement from lament to praise but that the overall picture of the form of lament psalms is more varied and complex complicates the pastoral implications of the paradigm as currently understood.

Movement from lament to hope in liturgical practice with traumatised people

If a movement from lament to praise is not universal in the lament psalms, how clear is it that hope and praise are appropriate elements in practice of lament with traumatised people? Nearly all those who address the pastoral value of the lament psalms foreground the movement to praise within lament psalms and present it as one of the most valuable features of lament psalms in terms of their pastoral use. Swinton, for example, adopts Brueggemann's observations about the *formful* character of suffering to argue that the psalms of lament *form* human pain and suffering; lament psalms offer a means of 'reframing' suffering 'in the light of the hope and promises of God', and this reframing 'enables, or at least initiates, movement from hurt and brokenness to joy and praise'.[43] It would be wrong to say that Swinton sees this as the only or even principal function of the lament psalms; he also, for example, highlights the subversive character of lamentation as an act of resistance.[44] Nevertheless, in his instructions for writing one's own lament psalm, borrowed from Ann Weems and set out at the end of the chapter, he includes both an expression of surety and a vow of praise as essential elements.[45]

How are hope and praise best addressed with victims of trauma? Laurie Kraus, David Holyan and Bruce Wismer, writing about working with congregations in the immediate aftermath of major trauma events, including 9/11 and the Boston Marathon bombing, caution against the temptation to avoid suffering by too hasty a movement toward hope:

> Pastors may unintentionally enable such avoidance by moving too quickly toward words of comfort, hope, forgiveness, and reconciliation. In so doing, they ignore what needs to be faced: the pain and hurt, the rip in the fabric of life, the taste of tears shed in disbelief and anger. . . . The time will come when hope, peace, and love emerge in celebratory ways. But it may take years for the energy of a traumatic event to dissipate fully. In the early stages lament and compassionate presence are appropriate congregational responses.[46]

43 Swinton, *Raging with Compassion*, 108–109.
44 Swinton, *Raging with Compassion*, 111.
45 Swinton, *Raging with Compassion*, 126–128.
46 Laurie Kraus, David Holyan and Bruce Widmer, 'Post-Traumatic Ministry: Pastoral Responses in the Aftermath of Violence', *Christian Century* March 29 (2017): 22–25, 23.

Kraus, Holyan and Wismer suggest Psalm 23's image of the Valley of the Shadow of Death as helpful in this context as a direction for movement. Rather than hopefulness, they suggest, it is likely to be most pastorally helpful to encourage the need to walk through the valley – potentially for a long period.

> Walking through the valley involves a slow deliberate journey through the very places that cause the most fear. God may provide reassuring presence along this journey, but God does not save people from having to make the trek. It's impossible to go back and undo a disaster. And it's unhealthy to avoid the pain that violence imprints upon a communal landscape . . . .
>
> A worship service in the time of lament might be thought of as a walk through the valley of the shadow of death in three movements:
>
> *Letting go* (releasing what was and seeking sanctuary in the presence of God)
> *Letting be* (being present to God and to one another in the midst of distress)
> *Letting begin* (beginning to walk and work in the valley of the shadow)[47]

This model incorporates the sense of movement and progress that is at the centre of the paradigm of movement from lament to praise but without risk of avoidance of the pain and work that is itself essential to any real and lasting recovery and healing. Kathleen Norris senses something similar about the relationship between pain and praise:

> There's a fine line between idealizing or idolizing pain, and confronting it with hope. But I believe that both writers [Emily Dickinson and Walter Brueggemann] are speaking the truth about the psalms. The value of this great songbook of the Bible lies not in the fact that singing praise can alleviate pain, but that the painful images we find there are essential for praise, that without them, praise is meaningless. It becomes the 'dreadful cheer' that Minnesota author Carol Bly has complained of in generic American Christianity, which blinds itself to pain, and thereby makes a falsehood of its praise.[48]

All the literature on trauma points to recovery being a long process and supports these observations that the pain of trauma cannot be avoided but must

---

And see, more generally, Laurie Kraus, David Holyan and Bruce Widmer, *Recovering From Un-natural Disasters: A Guide for Pastors and Congregations After Violence and Trauma* (Louisville, KY: Westminster John Knox, 2017).

47 Kraus, Holyan and Widmer, 'Post-Traumatic Ministry', 23.

48 Norris, *Cloister Walk*, 112–113.

be engaged directly and worked through before healing can be possible. It is also clear that lament psalms offer a language and a body of literature than can aid and progress that engagement and work. How helpful is a 'movement' from lament to praise in that context? Is there a danger that praise and hope might be introduced too quickly if these (non-universal) aspects of the psalms are too strongly emphasised? Is there at least a case for delaying (perhaps for significant periods) such emphasis in use of the lament psalms with traumatised people?

This chapter opened with a discussion of Swinton's identification of a disconnect between the real experiences of the world and his experiences of Christian worship. Joyful worship songs functioned in the context of the service he attended on the day after the Omagh bombing to facilitate avoidance of the pain of that shocking event. Swinton and others rightly look to the psalms of lament as an antidote to this inclination to avoidance of what is painful. Tendencies on the parts of academics working on the lament psalms to focus on the movement to hope, and on the part of pastors working with traumatised people to move them toward hope too fast, may be part and parcel of the same inclination.

Nevertheless, it important not to discount entirely or to hamper the impulse of the movement towards hopefulness that is found in the majority of lament psalms, where it is discerned that that impulse feels authentic to a traumatised person. The lament psalms perform a significant liturgical and theological role in holding together expressions of despair and pain with joy and hopefulness. One of the most painful aspects of traumatic injury can be the sense that the traumatic experience is incompatible with a continuing faith in God's goodness and care. The psalms of lament, like the passage from David Blumenthal's book *Facing the Abusing God* that inspired the title of Christopher Southgate's essay 'In Spite of All This, We Will Yearn for You' in this volume, hold together in uneasy, but powerful tension anguished cries of betrayal with statements of faith and hope in the very God accused as betrayer.

Liturgical use of lament psalms: when and how?

Clearly, it would benefit the Church to recover its tradition of lamentation. How should the lament psalms be used? For example, should use, or 'performance', be liturgical or non-liturgical, or both? Should there be any distinction drawn between individual and communal lament psalms in this regard? And to what degree, if any, should the 'performers' be encouraged to express the emotions suggested by the words? Should performance be 'embodied', for example?[49]

49 The likely benefits of embodied performance are suggested by the tendency of trauma to be held in the body, discussed earlier, and see Van der Kolk, *Body Keeps the Score*.

Swinton promotes engagement with the lament psalms in small groups[50] and notes that Denise Ackermann also nominates the small group as the ideal locus for lament psalm practice.[51] He writes, 'Such groups hold the potential to become places for honest rage and compassionate listening, places where an individual's pain and hurt can be "heard into speech" in the presence of God and within the fellowship of God's people'.[52] Small-group practice suggests a context that is non-liturgical and in which alternatives to ritual are available.

Practising lament in small groups need not, however, mean that ritual and liturgical expression must be foregone. Swinton notes that the Eucharist 'has the potential to provide a significant dimension of this process', and he connects the role of the Eucharist with the movement from despair to hope already discussed.[53] Similarly, Ackermann sees a vital role for the Eucharist: 'I imagine small, vital groups of people who, after lamenting together, give thanks for memories of God's loving power in the past and thereby affirm this power in the present'.[54] A Eucharistic practice must mean either, of course, that the small group contains a priest or other duly authorised minister amongst its members or that it must introduce such a person to the group for the proposes of the Eucharistic liturgy. This latter possibility may or may not challenge the dynamic of the group, depending on the nature of the relationships that have been developed and the sensitivities of the minister.

Kraus, Holyan and Widmer's work points to another locus for lamentation practice entirely. They envisage lament practice on the part of an entire congregation in the context of its usual weekly worship.[55] They do not offer practical suggestions about how the lament may be 'enacted' in this context. One could well imagine a coordinated approach in which reflection in the context of a sermon, homily or talk could offer some introduction to communal 'performance' of lament psalms during a period of intercession.[56] There might, additionally, be some added degree of performance in which

50 Swinton, *Raging With Compassion*, 121–128.

51 Swinton, *Raging With Compassion*, esp. 122–125, and with particular reference to Denise M. Ackermann, '"A Voice Was Heard in Ramah": A Feminist Theology of Praxis for Healing in South Africa', in *Liberating Faith Practices: Feminist Practical Theologies in Context*, ed. Denise M. Ackermann and M. Bons-Storm (Leuven: Peeters, 1998).

52 Swinton, *Raging With Compassion*, 122.

53 Swinton, *Raging With Compassion*, 124–125, and see the essay by Karen O'Donnell in this volume.

54 Ackermann, 'A Voice Was Heard in Ramah', 99 (cited also by Swinton).

55 Kraus, Holyan and Widmer, 'Post-Traumatic Ministry'. They do not stipulate either Eucharistic or non-Eucharistic worship, simply that what is envisaged is the ordinarily weekly worship gathering of the congregation.

56 Saliers, 'Psalms in Our Lamentable World', 110, writes, 'Each Sunday most Christian communities offer prayers of intercession. The psalms of lament both within and outside the discipline of the Lectionary's appointed psalms, provide a biblical and theological resource for deepening the assembly as a community of intercession in the face of the world's injustice and suffering.'

an individual or group 'performs' psalms (perhaps in quite a dramatic sense) with the congregation in the role of witness. A congregation might, additionally, be encouraged to meet as a whole outside regular worship times for lamentation practice which, while still incorporating ritual, is not necessarily liturgical.

Such a 'congregational' approach does not offer the *same* kind of benefits as the small group approach. A congregational approach will not offer the same opportunities for deep reciprocal sharing. In general, too, it may limit the opportunity for the overtly emotional performance of lament psalms, at least in certain cultures, unless the option of co-opting an individual or group to lament dramatically on behalf of and in the presence of the congregation is adopted. A congregational approach may also tend to inhibit the full expression of trauma experienced by members or by the group as a whole, as appropriate sensitivity is applied to what may and not be expressed publicly - for reasons such as an ongoing dispute between congregation members, confidentiality, a legal process or the potential for retraumatisation.[57]

In situations in which the congregation *as a community* has suffered trauma, however, congregational lamenting may be highly effective in facilitating the communal expression of a shared trauma and in rebuilding a sense of the congregational identity. For a congregation which has been physically close to traumatic events, and perhaps also closely involved in related recovery operations (for example the congregations of the churches/cathedrals closest to the Westminster and London Bridge attacks and to Grenfell Tower) this may be especially important. In such circumstances, a careful choice of communal psalms of lament will be appropriate.

The potential for building shared understanding and identity that is found in congregational performance of lamentation may perhaps, in addition, in some senses, substitute for, the *physical, embodied experience* of lamenting of the individual, whether alone or in smaller groups. A congregation is not embodied in the same manner as an individual, but the congregation is itself a body and the act of expression, through the use of lament psalms, of a common trauma may help to reconstitute that body.

Conclusion

We have seen a high degree of consensus, both scholarly and popular, that the practice of lamentation, and in particular through performance of the psalms of lament, is a resource of the church that has in some sense been 'lost' and that potentially offers a great deal both to individual Christians and to Christian communities. This is particularly so in cases in which there has been an experience of trauma. The preceding discussion has suggested,

57 Kraus, Holyan and Widmer, 'Post-Traumatic Ministry', 24.

however, that bringing together practical and pastoral theology with biblical scholarship and trauma theory points to a number of areas in which both creative imagination and fruitful caution will be called for in the Church's reclaiming of this valuable resource.

Select references

Ackermann, Denise M. *After the Locusts: Letters From a Landscape of Faith*. Grand Rapids: Eerdmans, 2003.

Brueggemann, Walter. *The Message of the Psalms: A Theological Commentary*. Minneapolis: Fortress, 1985.

Kraus, Laurie, David Holyan and Bruce Widmer. 'Post-Traumatic Ministry: Pastoral Responses in the Aftermath of Violence'. *Christian Century* (2017): 22–25.

Norris, Kathleen. *The Cloister Walk*. New York: Riverhead, 1996.

Strawn, Brent. 'Trauma, Psalmic Disclosure, and Authentic Happiness'. In *Bible Through the Lens of Trauma*, ed. Elizabeth Boase and Christopher Frechette. Atlanta: SBL, 2016.

Swinton, John. *Raging With Compassion: Pastoral Responses to the Problem of Evil*. Grand Rapids: Eerdmans, 2007.

12 Eucharist and trauma

Healing in the B/body

Karen O'Donnell

Trauma is a notoriously difficult thing to define. It took the best part of a century, from Freud and his psychoanalysis, through the so-called hysteria of late 19th-century women, the First and Second World Wars, to the return of soldiers from the Vietnam War and the rise of the women's movement,[1] to acknowledge post-traumatic stress disorder (PTSD) in the diagnostic handbook of the American Psychiatric Association.[2] This is, in part, due to the slippery nature of trauma. It is notoriously individual, hidden; it follows no set patterns of onset or development; and its causes are difficult to pinpoint. Two people might experience the exact same event and only one of them find it traumatic.

But for all its trickiness and nebulous nature, trauma is real and is on the rise.[3] Most groups of people, congregations included, are likely to include someone who has experienced trauma, whether or not they have a pathological diagnosis of PTSD. It might be the veteran who served in the armed forces decades ago, the young wife hiding abuse, the couple devastated by the loss of a child, or the individual who was raped or abused.

Many of these hidden trauma survivors will join in, or be present for, the celebration of the Eucharist. Most gatherings of Christians for worship will include some sharing of bread and wine in memory of the Last Supper and death of Jesus. Whilst, of course, different Christians understand this ritual in a multitude of ways, nonetheless, it is a corporeal practice that forms the

1 Judith Herman, *Trauma and Recovery: The Aftermath of Violence – From Domestic Abuse to Political Terror* (2nd Ed.; New York: Basic, 1997), 9–32, 33: 'Psychological trauma is an affliction of the powerless. At the moment of trauma, the victim is rendered helpless by overwhelming force. When the force is that of nature, we speak of disasters. When the force is that of other human beings, we speak of atrocities. Traumatic events overwhelm the ordinary systems of care that give people a sense of control, connection, and meaning.'

2 American Psychiatric Association, *Diagnostic and Statistical Manual of Psychiatric Disorders (DSM-III)*, Vol. 3 (Washington, DC: American Psychiatric Association, 1980), 236.

3 Ben Farmer, 'Cases of PTSD on the Rise as More Veterans Seek Help for Mental Health Problems', *The Telegraph*, September 9, 2016, www.telegraph.co.uk/news/2016/09/09/cases-of-ptsd-on-the-rise-as-more-veterans-seek-help-for-mental/.

core of much of Christians' worship around the world and has done so for centuries.

In this chapter, I outline the ways in which trauma must be understood as a corporeal experience before considering the ways in which participation in the Eucharist has the potential to retraumatise trauma survivors and to draw congregations into unjust practices. But hope is not lost because, as I demonstrate, the Eucharist is redolent with the scent of post-traumatic remaking and, when carefully curated by the celebrant and the gathered congregation, can model the process of post-traumatic remaking and provide a space for witnessing to the experience of trauma.

Trauma is corporeal

Trauma is not a condition unique to the modern world, although it is in the modern context that trauma has been named and known and it is in this contemporary world that trauma has moved from the uncommon to the common. Trauma, or at least the risk of trauma, is an ancient experience. The most ancient of Western literature, Homer's epics *The Iliad* and *The Odyssey*, are, amongst other things, accounts of the experience of trauma and PTSD.[4] Sadly, soldiers have always been sent off to fight wars; women have always been raped – trauma has always happened, and it is a relatively common experience today.

It is in the 20th century that trauma made the shift from uncommon to common experience. Judith Herman, whose life's work has been dedicated to understanding trauma, notes,

> It was once believed that such [traumatic] events were uncommon. In 1980, when post-traumatic stress disorder was first included in the diagnostic manual, the American Psychiatric Association described traumatic events as "outside the range of usual human experience." Sadly, this definition has proved to be inaccurate. Rape, battery, and other forms of sexual and domestic violence are so common a part of women's lives that they can hardly be described as outside the range of ordinary experience. And in view of the number of people killed in war over the past century, military trauma, too, must be considered a common part of human experience; only the fortunate find it unusual.[5]

Trauma is a thing of the body; it is corporeal. Whilst neuroimaging clearly demonstrates the ways in which trauma impacts on the brain, the memory of trauma crouches inside the body like a wounded animal, deaf to talking

4 See Jonathan Shay, *Achilles in Vietnam: Combat Trauma and the Undoing of Character* (New York: Simon and Schuster, 2010); Jonathan Shay, *Odysseus in America: Combat Trauma and the Trials of Homecoming* (New York: Scribner, 2002).

5 Herman, *Trauma and Recovery*, 33.

therapies, teeth bared and eyes wide, ready to strike; it is in the tense body, the elevated heart rate, the arm poised to strike, the recoil from oncoming onslaught. The memories of a traumatic event are not located in the same place other memories. The memory of a rape, of warfare, of abuse does not sit alongside memories of happy birthdays and jolly summer holidays. These happier memories sit in the verbal, reasoning, rational part of the brain. In contrast, the memory of trauma sits in the deeper regions – the amygdala, the hippocampus, the hypothalamus, the brain stem – all regions of the brain that are only marginally affected by thinking and cognition. The core of trauma lies in somatic memory, not in semantic memory.[6] Bodies are central to understanding the experience, impact, and afterlife of trauma.

If bodies are key to understanding the experience of trauma, they are equally critical to post-traumatic remaking.[7] Whilst talking therapies are useful in some cases, they are frequently insufficient on their own as a tool for the post-traumatic remaking of a trauma survivor. Similarly, post-traumatic remaking can rarely begin with the abstract thought, but rather, finding a bodily practice that puts the traumatised person in touch with their body is a far more successful starting place.[8] Trauma expert and psychiatrist Bessel van der Kolk notes,

> The body keeps the score. If the memory of trauma is encoded in the viscera, in heartbreaking and gut-wrenching emotions, in autoimmune disorders and skeletal/muscular problems, and if mind/brain/visceral communication is the royal road to emotion regulation, this demands a radical shift in our therapeutic assumptions.[9]

Whilst there have been a number of attempts to categorise the experience of trauma, to put the experience and the impact it has into neat boxes that can then be 'fixed', the reality is that the experience of trauma is an individual one, even when it affects whole communities. Sitting in the individual body, trauma feels different for everyone. And a corporate body that is constituted of individually traumatised bodies can be a very volatile and unpredictable body. Bearing this individuality and volatility in mind, it is possible to outline three impacts that trauma usually has on those who experience it is

6 Bessel van der Kolk, 'The Body Keeps the Score: Memory and the Evolving Psychobiology of Post Traumatic Stress', *Harvard Review of Psychiatry* 1, no. 5 (1994): 253–265.

7 I consciously use the term *post-traumatic remaking* instead of *trauma recovery* as it more accurately names the process a trauma survivor will go through in the aftermath of trauma. I am grateful to Hilary Scarsella for her use of this term.

8 In her account of her own trauma recovery, Serene Jones notes the significance of practices like yoga and acupuncture (corporeal practices) in her recovery, alongside prayer and sacraments: Serene Jones, *Trauma and Grace: Theology in a Ruptured World* (Louisville, KY: Westminster John Knox, 2009), 157–161.

9 Bessel van der Kolk, *The Body Keeps the Score: Mind, Brain and Body in the Transformation of Trauma* (London: Penguin, 2015), 86.

possible. These three impacts are best characterised as ruptures. One might consider trauma to be an earthquake that shakes through a person – opening fissures, destroying structures, uprooting firmly held ideals – leaving behind it destruction, an unrecognisable landscape, and a deep sense of instability.

The first of these three ruptures caused by trauma is a rupture of bodily integrity. In many experiences of trauma, the body is unwillingly violated by another. This might be with the manipulation of the mind in the case of psychological abuse and torture; the insertion of the penis, fingers, or other object into the body; or the causing of an injury with intent to harm or kill. The body is no longer a safe place: '[B]eing frightened [as a trauma survivor] means that you live in a body that is always on guard. Angry people live in angry bodies.'[10]

The second rupture is a rupture in time. In this sense, the normal timelines of cause and effect, of past, present, and future, cease to have meaning. In the aftermath of trauma, the experience of that trauma in the past continues to invade the present. For some trauma survivors, this past invasion of the present occurs in the forms of nightmare and flashbacks; for some, it may even occur in trance-like hallucinations and repetitions of actions. For many, this rupture in time is the persistence of valid adaptations of trauma that persist in non-traumatic environments. What once kept the trauma survivor alive continues to run through their body, maintaining high-alert, fight-or-flight instincts and surfacing at the most inopportune of moments.

The third rupture is a rupture in cognition. The trauma survivor is unable to articulate what has happened to them. It may be that, due to the ruptures in bodily integrity and time, they do not even know what has happened to them. The connections between the brain and body are disrupted. Again, to draw on the wealth of van der Kolk's experience, he notes,

> Because traumatised people often have trouble sensing what is going on in their bodies, they lack a nuanced response to frustration. They either react to stress by becoming "spaced out" or with excessive anger. Whatever their response, they often can't tell what is upsetting them. This failure to be in touch with their bodies contributes to their well-documented lack of self-protection and high rates of revictimization and also to their remarkable difficulties in feeling pleasure, sensuality, and having any sense of meaning.[11]

Whilst highlighting these three ruptures is helpful for understanding some of the ways in which trauma impacts people, in reality, trauma is a messy, complex situation to live in. Simply knowing that these ruptures are likely to have occurred is not necessarily sufficient for successful post-traumatic remaking.

10 Van der Kolk, *Body Keeps the Score*, 100.
11 Van der Kolk, *Body Keeps the Score*, 99.

The Eucharist can be problematic

I argue in what follows that participation in the sacrament of the Eucharist, a central ritual of Christian life, can contribute to successful post-traumatic remaking. However, we must begin by acknowledging that the Eucharist is not a neutral ritual. Nor is it something that can only ever be characterised as a positive thing. Whilst Christians who are liturgical in worship style tend to be committed to the celebration of the Eucharist as something significant and even essential to their faith, not all Christians share in this ritual of eating and drinking together regularly or at all.

The Eucharist has a somewhat checkered history. Dramatically distorted in the medieval Church by the intense scrutiny of scholastic theologians and so contaminated by the anxieties of the clergy that most Christians received it in bread form only perhaps once a year (and then only after an intense period of shriving), receiving the Eucharist – then a very passive experience – was not the joyful celebration of a meal of Real Presence with co-believers. The Eucharist has been a tool of torment by the Church over the years. In her monograph, Marika Rose highlights the historical symbiosis of torture and the Eucharist in the Spanish Inquisition,[12] European anti-Semitism,[13] and even in the relatively recent experience of Latin America.[14]

Even in more contemporary times, inclusion in and exclusion from the Eucharist has been used as a form of church discipline and rebuke. Consider, for example, the LGBTQIA+ congregant denied a Eucharistic host in their outstretched hands as they come forward to participate. Or, in the Catholic tradition, the denial of the Eucharist to the divorced woman whose husband walked away from her and her children. Marcella Althaus-Reid notes, in the Latin American context, that there 'is no solidarity in holy communion . . . At its best, the sacramental ceremonies in the churches work as acts of exemplary colonial orderings.'[15] The Eucharist is still complicit, at times, in unjust practices around the world.

For the trauma survivor, participating in the celebration of the Eucharist has the potential to be problematic. In the first instance, participating in the Eucharist usually asks congregants to focus on the death of Jesus on the Cross, recalling perhaps (depending on the particular day and the

12 See, for example, discussions of the ways in which Eucharistic belief and practice was used to discover heretics, including Muslims (77–78) and Lutherans (102) in Helen Rawlings, *The Spanish Inquisition* (Oxford: Blackwell, 2006).

13 See, for example, the complex entangling of anti-Semitism and Eucharistic devotion in Jennifer Kolpacoff Deane, *A History of Medieval Heresy and Inquisition* (Plymouth: Rowman and Littlefield, 2011), 119.

14 Marika Rose, *A Theology of Failure: Žižek Against Christian Innocence* (New York: Fordham University Press, 2019). I am grateful to Marika Rose for sharing proofs of her forthcoming monograph with me.

15 Marcella Althaus-Reid, *Indecent Theology: Theological Perversions in Sex, Gender and Politics* (Abingdon/New York: Routledge, 2000), 92.

chosen Eucharistic prayers) not just the Last Supper but also Jesus's torture, abuse, and graphic, grotesque death on the Cross. They may be asked to dwell on Jesus's submission and obedience to the will of God. Participation in the remembering of this traumatic event has the potential to retraumatise a trauma survivor, making their own memories of abuse, violence, or terror very present and attempting to recast such event as positive, even necessary.

As a ritual, the Eucharist has the potential to replicate the three ruptures of trauma I outlined earlier. It is, or may be, a repeated ritual that ruptures. In the first instance, in the reception of the Eucharist the believer's body is ruptured by the presence of another: the body and blood of Christ. Participation in the Eucharist constitutes the Body of Christ, and thus, the believer is drawn into a new identity – Christ's. Whilst Eucharistic liturgies are primarily 're-membering events,'[16] they also have an eschatological character and so disrupt time. The sharing of the sacramental meal is a foretaste of the eschatological banquet to be shared by all at the end times. Thus, time is ruptured as the future and past are brought crashing into each other in the present. Finally, as with all sacraments, language and cognition fail in the face of the mystery of God. Centuries of theological endeavour can only hint at what takes place in the Eucharist. Understanding is ruptured, and the believer has to rely on faith to be assured on the effects of their participation in the ritual of the Eucharist.[17]

For most participants in the celebration, the Eucharist is not experienced as rupturing in the mode I have outlined here. For many, if they think about what they are doing at all, the celebration of the Eucharist is powerful and important, whether it is believed to be the Real Presence of Christ or a memorial of his Last Supper, Passion, and death. However, it would be a mistake to think that this is true for every person who approaches the altar, or for all those who stay in their pew because their approach to the altar will be denied. For some, participation in the Eucharist is (re)traumatising, rupturing, and potentially damaging.

The Eucharist and post-traumatic remaking

I have, in this chapter, foregrounded the intensely damaging experience of trauma alongside the potentially problematic nature of the Eucharist deliberately. Many theologians, clergy, and even lay Christians are very quick to turn to the Eucharist as a panacea – a cure-all – that will, of course (!), be helpful in post-traumatic remaking. Consider, for example, two relatively

16 I use this hyphenated term *re-membering* to indicate the twofold meaning of this word, both the remembering of the last days of Jesus's life and the rebuilding (or membering) of the Body of Christ.

17 I outline the relationship between sacrament and trauma more fully in my book: Karen O'Donnell, *Broken Bodies: The Eucharist, Mary and the Body in Trauma Theology* (London: SCM, 2018).

recent texts on the Eucharist and the ways in which the Eucharist is presented as not merely neutral but as almost uniformly positive. In *Torture and Eucharist*, William Cavanaugh claims that he is aware of the realities of the actually existing Church and the real, problematic practices that take place within it, but in claiming that 'torture is essentially an anti-liturgy,'[18] to which the Eucharist is a compelling contrast, he elides the ways in which the Eucharist has been historically associated with torture (as I noted earlier). Furthermore, although his monograph, *Material Eucharist*, is rich and nuanced in many ways, David Grumett similarly evades the association of the Eucharist with the abuses of the person. Nor does he acknowledge the trauma caused by the persistent exclusion of women from the Eucharist in a variety of modes.[19] Whilst I have, perhaps unfairly, picked out two texts that consistently frame the Eucharist as almost universally positive, these are by no means the only theological engagements with the Eucharist that approach it in this way.

It is important, I think, to foreground the ways in which the Eucharist can be problematic for trauma survivors before we approach the ways in which participation in the Eucharist might actually be able to contribute to post-traumatic remaking in a positive way, if only to acknowledge that not all Eucharistic celebrations will accomplish this, and certainly not by default.

The ancient liturgists, those who composed early prayers, who formulated the rites and rituals that we have handed down to the Church today, had an instinct for post-traumatic remaking. In those church traditions that follow ancient liturgies, there are remarkable similarities between different denominations and with the modes of post-traumatic remaking. The Eucharist is the kind of bodily practice that complements the talking therapies recommended for post-traumatic remaking.

Whilst post-traumatic remaking is a complex process, and one that does not follow a linear pattern that sees the completion of each stage of post-traumatic remaking before moving on to the next one, it is a process with some definable characteristics. Post-traumatic remaking will usually begin with the establishment of bodily integrity; that is to say, such remaking cannot begin whilst the trauma survivor is still in a place of danger. She must be in a place of safety where she has control over her body.

A key element of post-traumatic remaking is the construction of a narrative that enables the trauma survivor to move forward. This might mean coming to a point where the trauma survivor is able to recount a narrative of their trauma that does not retraumatise her in the telling but gives voice to her experience and begins to repair the ruptures in time and cognition that have dissociated her from her body and her bodily experience. It is a narrative of the traumatic experience that brings hope for the future.

18 William T. Cavanaugh, *Torture and Eucharist: Theology, Politics and the Body of Christ* (Oxford: Blackwell, 1998), 279.

19 David Grumett, *Material Eucharist* (Oxford: Oxford University Press, 2016).

The third element of post-traumatic remaking is some form of a reconnection with society. This enables the trauma survivor to overcome the isolation of the traumatic experience. Many trauma survivors reconnect by involving themselves in advocacy work or becoming a voice for those who have experienced similar trauma. It is not uncommon, for example, for rape survivors to become involved in rape advocacy or campaign for changes in the law.

These three elements of post-traumatic remaking are mirrored in the liturgy of the Eucharist.[20] Whilst the ancient liturgists had no language of trauma, nor were they specifically creating rituals to promote post-traumatic remaking, it seems they had an instinct for such a remaking. If one considers the traditional shape of a Eucharistic celebration, it begins with the welcoming of the congregation into the sanctuary of the church before leading worshippers through the confession of sins and the receiving of forgiveness. Both of these elements are focused on the integrity of the body. The worshipper is 'safe' in the body of the church community, and they are made clean before God through the confession of sins and the receiving of forgiveness.

This establishment of bodily integrity is then followed by the construction of a narrative that communicates to the gathered community the truth of who they are as Christians. In two parts, this narrative begins with the reading of Scriptures, the preaching of a sermon, and (usually) the saying of a creed. In this, the congregation hears and acknowledges the ways in which God is engaged in the world, as well as their own place within the divine landscape as Christians. The second part of this narrative construction is in the participation in the Eucharistic liturgy itself. Here, the presider recounts the narratives of Jesus's Last Supper, before bringing the gathered body of Christ together to share in the Body of Christ. The congregation become one new body because they all share in one bread. After chewing the word in the hearing of Scriptures, congregants now eat the *Logos* in the sharing in the Eucharist. Louis-Marie Chauvet, in the context of his analysis of the Eucharist and Eucharistic prayers, notes,

> In the sacraments, as in all other ecclesial mediations, it is always as *Word*, bitter and sweet at the same time, that Christ gives himself to be assimilated. Such a proposition opens up from within any sacramentality that would be tempted to close in upon itself: the efficacy of the sacraments cannot be understood in any other way *than that of the communication of the Word . . .*[21]

20 Whilst I am referring specifically to the Eucharist in this chapter, in my monograph I outline the ways in which sacraments in general are post-traumatic remaking rituals. See O'Donnell, *Broken Bodies*.

21 Louis-Marie Chauvet, *Symbol and Sacrament: A Sacramental Reinterpretation of Christian Existence*, trans. Patrick Madigan and Madeleine Beaumont (Collegeville, MN: Liturgical, 1995), 226 (italics in original).

Eating the bread and drinking the wine, assimilating Christ into one's own body, need not be experienced as a traumatic rupturing but as part of a narrative construction that contributes to the post-traumatic remaking of a trauma survivor.

The third element of post-traumatic remaking – that of reconnection with society – is the simplest element of the celebration of the Eucharist. It is evident in the fact that the congregation members do not stay in the Church but are dismissed into the world. They are released to be Christians in their communities, not to remain in the church building away from the other. Often, the words of the dismissal make this engagement with the world explicit. In the Catholic Mass, the dismissal follows one of three forms: 'Go in the peace of Christ'; 'The Mass is ended, go in peace'; or 'Go in peace to love and serve the Lord.'[22] These words are almost identical to those used in the Church of England.[23] After participating in the Eucharist, the congregation is dismissed to re-engage with the community outside the Church with the peace of God.

Whilst it is clear that one can read the ancient shape and words of the liturgy of the Eucharist as redolent with the imagery and flavour of post-traumatic remaking that would not become explicit until the 20th century,[24] it is important to note that the simple form of the words does not exact some magical recovery for a trauma survivor who happens to be at a Eucharistic service. For a Eucharistic liturgy to contribute positively to post-traumatic remaking requires, on the part of the presider and the gathered congregation, careful curation.

Healing in the B/body

A number of key ideas are made apparent through this consideration of the relationship between the experience of trauma and participation in the celebration of the Eucharist by a trauma survivor. It is clear from this approach to understanding trauma that I take an ontologically materialist perspective on the person. Rather than claiming that persons *have* bodies, I claim that persons *are* bodies. Even a brief reflection on the impact that the experience of trauma has on the trauma survivor is enough to indicate that one cannot hold to sharp distinctions between body and mind or body and soul in the face of such traumatic experience. The body is; the person is body. This is the overwhelming sense of the biblical texts which are best understood in terms of a monist anthropology.[25] Similarly, Wolfhart Pannenberg notes,

22 The Liturgy Office: England and Wales, 'The Concluding Rite' (The Liturgy Office: England and Wales, 2005), 4, www.liturgyoffice.org.uk/Resources/AYWL/AYWLConcluding.pdf.

23 The Church of England, *Holy Communion Service* (London: Church House Publishing, 2000), 178, www.churchofengland.org/prayer-and-worship/worship-texts-and-resources/common-worship/holy-communion#.

24 Herman, *Trauma and Recovery*, 7.

25 Joel B. Green, 'Three Exegetical Forays into the Body-Soul Discussion', *Criswell Theological Review* 7, no. 2 (2010): 4.

> [T]here is no independent reality of a 'soul' in contrast to the body, just as there is not a body that is merely mechanically or unconsciously moved. Both are abstractions. The only reality is the unity of the living creature called man.[26]

This is a significant distinction because the predominant imagery used to describe the Church is the Body of Christ. We do not *have* the Body of Christ; we *are* the Body of Christ. This is Paul's understanding of the body as a holistic entity both in terms of the church and the individual. Paula Gooder writes,

> Paul's use of the metaphor [the body] is revealing of his view of physical bodies. The one sure fact for him is that bodies are unified. Bodies are an integrated whole and cannot be separated into their component parts. This why this metaphor is so important for him. Just as we cannot split down our physical bodies, so we also cannot split down the body of Christ. Bodies are bodies – single, whole entities.[27]

This ontologically materialist perspective draws us into unity with one another and with the divine. Participation in the Eucharist, at its best and most carefully curated, draws the participants into both horizontal unity with one another and vertical unity with God. Whilst I have used the term *Eucharist* throughout this chapter, at this point I could well turn to its other name and call this ritual 'Holy Communion,' which would better describe the unity I refer to here.

This unity is essential in understanding the role of the gathered congregation in post-traumatic remaking. Whilst it is the prerogative of the trauma survivor to construct the trauma narrative that will allow them to move forward, this narrative is powerless unless it is heard and witnessed by others. To 'witness' simply means to observe or to look on. But this is too thin a meaning for what it is to witness trauma. Shelly Rambo notes,

> To witness to trauma is a complex and disorienting process. It is a process of witnessing death and life in a radical reconfiguration. Because trauma shatters so much of what we understand to constitute life, the very definition of life is in question.[28]

To witness, then, is to attend to not only the traumatic experience but also the ongoing experience of living in trauma, witnessing to what remains. In

26 Wolfhart Pannenberg, *What Is Man? Contemporary Anthropology in Theological Perspective* (Philadelphia, PA: Fortress, 1970), 48.

27 Paula Gooder, *Body: Biblical Spirituality for the Whole Person* (London: SPCK, 2016), 123–124.

28 Shelly Rambo, *Spirit and Trauma: A Theology of Remaining* (Louisville, KY: Westminster John Knox, 2010), 25.

this, Rambo draws our attention to Holy Saturday as a site of witnessing and remaining in the aftermath of death. She cautions against rushing to the Resurrection too quickly. There is a theological value in remaining in Holy Saturday, in witnessing the devastation of trauma.[29]

Drawing our bodies into the unity of the Body of Christ through participation in the Eucharist, in Holy Communion, draws us in as witnesses to the devastation of trauma. Whilst we *celebrate* the Eucharist, we should not forget to attend to the devastation of trauma visible for us on the Cross and in the broken bread and poured out wine that speaks of a body torn apart. To witness is to remain at the foot of the Cross for a while before turning our gaze to the Resurrection. This might be termed a vertical witness.

To witness horizontally, to witness to the trauma of the abused woman sat next to us in church, to witness to the PTSD of a veteran, decades since combat, to witness to the trauma that afflicts the bodies around us, is to accept that this is a complex and disorienting process in which the life–death boundary is complicated and ever shifting. But these bodies are our body. We declare after the Eucharist that 'we are one body because we all share in one bread.' To witness is to listen, to believe, to stand in grief and horror at the traumatic experience and to do so repeatedly, perhaps for a lifetime. There is no recovery from trauma but rather a post-traumatic remaking in which the trauma survivor reconstructs a self out of their own narrative and the witness of those around them.

The liturgy of the Eucharist offers both a model for post-traumatic remaking and the tools to witness to trauma. In the celebration of the Eucharist, we witness, again, the trauma of the death of Christ; we stand again at the foot of the Cross; we see again the broken bread and wine poured out. And then we repeat it. Daily. Weekly. For a lifetime. This is what living in the aftermath of trauma looks like.

Conclusion

When considering the relationship between the Eucharist and trauma, one can easily fall into one of two traps. Either one can have so high a view of the Eucharist that one believes that simply participating in the Eucharistic liturgy is so independently powerful that any trauma survivor is bound to find it helpful in their post-traumatic remaking. This perspective ignores the power of the Eucharist to (re)traumatise people and devalues the need for a careful curation of the sacrament of the part of the presider and the gathered congregation. On the other hand, one can have so low a view of the Eucharist that one cannot imagine how participating in such a ritual might have any tangible benefit for the trauma survivor. This perspective disregards the powerful contribution that participation in the Eucharist can make to post-traumatic remaking.

29 Rambo, *Spirit and Trauma*, 79.

Of course, the most helpful position is somewhere between these two perspectives. Recognising that participation in the Eucharist might offer the trauma survivor some of the tools they need for their own post-traumatic remaking can situate the Eucharist as a powerful ritual for such remaking. Similarly, recognising that for such an experience to be positive requires careful curation of the liturgy is essential. This careful curation might mean attention to the readings chosen and the ways in which they are framed by the celebrant as well as the language used to talk about the broken body of Jesus. Particular attention might be paid to services such as Good Friday or Remembrance Sunday, recognising that these are liturgies with the power to harm as well as to heal.[30]

Participation in the Eucharist has the potential to offer a context in which the tools for post-traumatic remaking are modelled for the trauma survivor. Drawing the individual into both a unity with God and with the gathered body of Christ might offer an opportunity for trauma survivors to feel safe, to construct a narrative of their trauma that brings hope and a future, and to reconnect to the wider society. The Eucharist might just be the place in which trauma can be witnessed and a future constructed.

Select references

Grumett, David. *Material Eucharist*. Oxford: Oxford University Press, 2016.

Herman, Judith. *Trauma and Recovery: The Aftermath of Violence – From Domestic Abuse to Political Terror*, 2nd ed. New York: Basic, 1997.

Jones, Serene. *Trauma and Grace: Theology in a Ruptured World*. Louisville, KY: Westminster John Knox, 2009.

O'Donnell, Karen. *Broken Bodies: The Eucharist, Mary and the Body in Trauma Theology*. London: SCM, 2018.

Rambo, Shelly. *Spirit and Trauma: A Theology of Remaining*. Louisville, KY: Westminster John Knox, 2010.

Van der Kolk, Bessel. 'The Body Keeps the Score: Memory and the Evolving Psychobiology of Post Traumatic Stress'. *Harvard Review of Psychiatry* 1, no. 5 (1994): 253–265.

30 See Jones's reflection on *The Mirrored Cross* at a Good Friday service in Jones, *Trauma and Grace*, 75–83.

Part V

Pastoral resources

Introduction to Part V

Part V draws the reader back to a focus on consideration of pastoral responses to traumatic events in a range of contexts.

Ruth Layzell's essay performs a significant role in relation to the collection as a whole. Layzell offers the opportunity to reflect on the range of themes and challenges already presented in the previous essays but in a collective sense, and from the particular point of view of the provision of pastoral care in congregational settings. Layzell reflects, for example, on the crucial questions that must be addressed by any minister seeking to make an assessment of the care required in a given situation: Who needs pastoral care? What kind of care should be offered, and by whom? and How should the carers themselves be cared for?

Mia Kyte Hilborn, whose hospital chaplaincy work has incorporated a strong focus on trauma response, offers two chapters. In the first, she considers the challenges of formulating disaster response that meets ethical tests. Disaster response must, by definition, be made in the context of chaos and the unknown. Bearing this in mind, Hilborn offers the concept of the 'good enough' response and focuses on six key ethical issues that need to be addressed by any minister responding to a trauma situation that has had an impact on a congregation or other community to which he or she ministers: truth-telling, competence, boundaries, money, confidentiality and evaluation/reflection.

In her second essay, Hilborn introduces the reader to the particular challenges presented for trauma response in chaplaincy settings, such as hospitals, universities, schools and prisons. She begins by tracing the beginnings of chaplaincy and follows the development of chaplaincy ministry over its history to chaplaincy practices in relation to trauma response today. One of the particular challenges faced by chaplains that do not concern most ministers is the fact that the chaplain is responsible for the pastoral care of individuals with a wide range of relationships to faith; while some will have strong faith, whether Christian or otherwise, others will have none at all and may even resent attempts to be cared for pastorally. Hilborn explores the ways in which this particular challenge is further complicated by the realities and variety of trauma response. This second essay also contains the volume's only specific focus on the special demands of ministering to children in the context of trauma.

In the final essay of Part V, Carla A. Grosch-Miller draws on her research and experience of working with church hierarchies on the handling of ministerial sexual abuse. She makes the case that this particular form of disaster presents challenges and injuries that are distinctive and unusually persistent. The cycle of trauma response phases tends to be, she argues, especially protracted and confusing in this context. Given the particular challenges here, Grosch-Miller considers what might be classed as 'best practice' in the context of sexual abuse with congregations.

13 Pastoral response to congregational tragedy

Ruth Layzell

They started so well, Job's friends. In the face of tragedy after tragedy, which had taken Job's wealth, his livelihood, his children (his future), his health, his reputation and social standing and even the support and understanding of his wife, they, as well as he, were rendered speechless. What could they say? What words could be sufficient for this? So they expressed their grief at his plight symbolically and ritually, in physical action and expression, and then sat with him for seven days and nights without uttering a word. They offered him the most appropriate and healing of things – their presence in silence – sitting with him in the dust of his misery (Job 2:11–13).

But like most of us when faced with terrible tragedy and unutterable grief, they could not hold that kind of space or manage that level of empathy and identification for very long, and after a week the words began – moralising words, credal statements, words which tumbled out from the way they had to believe the world worked and that God worked. And none of these words brought comfort to Job. Rather, they provoked anger, outrage, rebuttal, self-justification and questioning. After what he had been through, for Job nothing was now beyond question; nothing was immune from scrutiny, not even God.

This is what tragedy and trauma, disaster and death do. They plough up the settled fields of our experience in the most unsettling and outrageous way. In faith terms, they move us from praise for the order of things ('God's in his heaven, all's right with the world'),[1] which is possible, in settled times, to protest and lament in the turmoil of order disturbed.[2] But the problem is: Who will accompany those engaging in such radical questioning? Being alongside those whose lives have been unsettled and unseated in this way, even when we have not experienced the trauma or tragedy at first hand, is demanding work which threatens to unsettle and unseat us, as the questions they ask begin to become ours.

This chapter addresses the question of what kind of pastoral response may be appropriate in the face of a tragic situation which affects a community,

1 Robert Browning, 'Pippa's Song', in *The Oxford Book of English Verse*, ed. Arthur Quiller-Couch (2nd Ed.; Oxford: Clarendon, 1939), 869.

2 See Brueggemann's schema of orientation, disorientation and reorientation in Walter Brueggemann, *The Spirituality of the Psalms* (Minneapolis, MN: Fortress, 2002).

what pastoral care is needed and what counselling and psychotherapy may have to offer in such circumstances. I shall assume here that first responses have taken place, that the most immediate issues of making safe and stabilising have happened and that we are in the next phases of bringing down the threat response and processing the trauma.

Pastoral responsibility

The first issue to address is who has responsibility for the pastoral care of a congregation affected by tragedy. Those in positions of leadership within a congregation – the minister, churchwardens, the eldership, the diaconate – are those with the primary duty of care and, even if they are not involved directly with all the care of all those who need it, theirs is the responsibility for ensuring that pastoral need is identified and responded to – in other words, that there is a pastoral strategy. And this pastoral responsibility – the cure of souls – persists until such time as they relinquish the roles which confer the responsibility. In the case of congregational tragedy, the pastoral repercussions may continue for a long time.

The exception to this is where the minister or key lay leader is implicated in the traumatic situation affecting the congregation or is incapacitated by it. Then, as Carla A. Grosch-Miller outlines in Chapter 16, the wider church structures need to take responsibility for the care of the congregation and appoint those who will, first, give accurate and timely information, together with reassurance and support, and then enable the community to process the effects of the trauma over time. In the absence of the minister, the wider denominational structures need to work with those within the congregation who normally share responsibility for pastoral care (e.g., small-group leaders, pastoral coordinators, youth and children's workers) to devise a pastoral strategy, always being mindful of what the needs of members of such a team may be and whether there are those within the team who cannot take on these roles because they themselves are too closely involved in or affected by the situation.

Just as important as recognising the extent of pastoral responsibility is recognising where it does not lie. Our safeguarding protocols make explicit that it is the responsibility of the police to pursue criminal investigations and that of the local authority through social care teams to respond to allegations of the abuse of children or vulnerable adults and that of concerned members of society to report allegations and concerns to those agencies.

Assessment

The starting point in developing a pastoral strategy must be assessment.[3] This book considers a range of situations which might throw a community

3 For discussion of a particular method for making pastoral assessments, see Pamela Cooper-White, *Shared Wisdom* (Minneapolis, MN: Fortress, 2004).

into crisis, and it does not take long to recognise that an 'appropriate pastoral response' to the communities around the Grenfell Tower fire or the attack on the Manchester stadium might be very different from that to a congregation whose minister has been accused and found guilty of sexual abuse of children or one rocked by the suicide of a young woman who felt she had no place in her church community. Similarly, immediate responses will differ from ongoing or long-term responses (the limited nature of the information available in the immediate aftermath of a disaster plays a role in this). There is no 'one size fits all' in this, and careful assessment of the situation and its ramifications must be the starting point.

Such assessment needs to be well grounded in an understanding of how human beings work – in other words, it must take account of psychological, as well as spiritual and theological, factors and, in particular, the theories and processes of trauma and grief. However, a caution must be sounded here. Theories are helpful in giving us a general map of the territory but do not excuse us from the harder task of understanding the particular contours for particular people. Platitudes and assumptions will not do, and space must be allowed for the unique experience of each person to be recognised and understood so that it can be attended to.

A second awareness needs to be held by pastoral leadership: that one person's story may have resonated with and brought to a head another's and thus provoke unexpected responses (e.g. anger, depression, a crisis of faith) which may seem out of proportion without an understanding of the second individual's back story. Again, this is an area in which it is important not to generalise or categorise, pathologise or condemn, but to be willing to allow experience and response to be particular, influenced by an individual's history and context. This requires humility on the part of pastors, lay or ordained, to set aside an expectation to know how it is for the other and be open to learn from them – to 'stand under' their story in order to understand it.[4]

Assessment also needs to be ongoing, with periodic review as the situation unfolds, in order to address changing needs. Those with pastoral responsibility need to consider the following questions:

- What kind of situation are we dealing with, and what effects might it therefore have?
- Who needs pastoral care?
- What might they need?
- How might it be provided?

What kind of situation are we dealing with?

First, was this a natural disaster, or was it the result of human action? While natural disasters can be widespread in their effect and remove for survivors

4 William Hubert Vanstone, *Farewell in Christ* (London: DLT, 2007), 27.

that fantasy of the safety and reliability of the natural world which makes living in it possible, research has shown that where the tragedy is the result of human agency (either in acting or neglecting to act), the trauma and resulting anxiety are more profound and worse still where trust has been betrayed by those who have a duty of care towards those who suffer.[5] I wonder if for Job the most painful aspect of his trials was the response of his nearest and dearest and the loss of their companionship in his suffering (Job 19:13–19). In some senses, pastoral response to natural disasters may be more straightforward, as a community can be united in their horror or sense of loss and bereavement and more readily come together to support one another. Nevertheless, as Christopher Southgate observes in Chapter 7, faith communities may have to address for themselves what *God's* agency and responsibility might be in these situations and be prepared to be on the receiving end, as God's visible representatives, of the questioning, bewilderment or anger of others towards God.

Where human agency is involved, in situations where culpability is clear (for example the shooting of children at the primary school in Dunblane) and where the perpetrator can be pursued and brought to justice, this brings one element of psychological release for those affected – the issue of culpability and justice has at least been resolved and grieving and recovering from the trauma can begin. This is part of the process of making safe or restoring order which is the first task of recovery. To know that the perpetrator of crime, violence or abuse is locked up, or that the possibility of further such actions is either prevented or much reduced, takes a significant burden from the shoulders of survivors. Where, however (as in the Grenfell Tower case), culpability is unclear or (as in the Hillsborough situation) suspected but not validated through a judicial process, recovery and grieving may be suspended or postponed – certainly it will be more complex. It may be true that human beings can only bear so much reality, but more unbearable still is a disjunction between experienced reality and an 'official' narrative.

More problematic still are situations in which it is a respected, valued and influential member of the community who is accused of misconduct. Reports on the trial of Bishop Peter Ball make it clear that it was hard for those who knew him personally to believe that a man who gave every appearance of spiritual maturity and wisdom and had undoubtedly been a significant influence on the spiritual formation of a generation, could have committed the acts of abuse of which he was accused in relation to those who were most closely associated with him and for whom he had a particular duty of care. It is psychologically easier to either sanctify or demonise our leaders and much harder to acknowledge that great good and great harm can be done by the same person.

5 Judith Herman, *Trauma and Recovery* (London: Pandora, 1992), 55.

Finally, some situations, such as the recent wildfires in California, the flooding of areas of Sri Lanka or the Grenfell Tower fire, are a complex mix of accident, natural processes and human neglect or direct agency.

Where there is culpability, then, the discovery of truth and the pursuit of justice, discipline and such redress as is possible are important pastoral concerns and must not be avoided or curtailed through the protection of perpetrators or premature calls for forgiveness which bypass the reality of the harm caused by human action or inaction and which can be a form of denial. Therapy or pastoral care cannot be a substitute for these things, and the pastoral task here is to support with compassion those affected as the often slow process unfolds.

Who needs pastoral care?

A significant part of the assessment will be the questions, who was affected by the tragedy, and how? Usually there are circles of effect. Some will be intimately and directly affected while others will have been involved as rescuers, medical staff or witnesses to the event. So, in the case of the Grenfell Tower fire, the lives of the bereaved and injured will have been irrevocably changed through the loss of one or more loved ones or by the injuries sustained or illnesses caused by the tragic event. Others will have been traumatised by having witnessed the fire as helpless bystanders or by having put their own lives at risk in the attempt to rescue those in danger. Still others will have been involved in treating the injured or comforting the distressed, while some will have become (fairly or unfairly) the targets of the anger which is part of the expression of grief and shock. All will need to process the emotional impact of their role.

In the case of the suicide of the young woman who could not reconcile her sexuality with her faith,[6] the waves of shock and distress at the tragedy will have rippled outwards from parents and close family to school friends and teachers, minister and church community, the wider local community, the gay community and the wider church community and will have had a different kind of impact in each layer. The loss of a daughter, granddaughter, sister, or close friend will be experienced differently from the loss of a member of the church community or a little-known fellow pupil, yet the whole community will have felt the impact of the event in some way and to some extent. In grief after suicide, the aspect of grief which has been named as guilt often looms larger, articulated in questions such as 'Why didn't I see this coming?' and 'Wasn't there anything I could have done to prevent it?'[7] As the reasons for her taking her own life became known, this sense of responsibility for the young girl's well-being will have been different for

6 See Chapter 2 of this volume for further details.

7 See Edward Dunne, John L. Mackintosh and Karen Dunne-Maxim, *Suicide and Its Aftermath: Understanding and Counseling the Survivors* (New York: Norton, 1987); Carol Staudacher,

parents, youth group leaders, minister, schoolteachers and the local congregation. In addition, some people, even though not closely connected to the young person through family or friendship relationships, may have felt a connection with her story – perhaps because they too were gay and unsure how to reconcile their sexuality with their context, or because for other reasons they had considered ending their life, or because they had in some way felt alienated by their community. Because they are so personal, these effects may remain undisclosed for a long time, but sensitive pastors, parents and teachers need to be alert to the possibility of hidden narratives such as these and to be ready gently to ask the question about the impact the tragedy has had on an individual. A problem will be, Is it even all right to talk about it when I'm not the one who has died or lost a family member or friend?

In the case of the misuse of power by church leaders, whether this is expressed in sexual misconduct or bullying, the dynamics will be especially complex as the natural responses of shock and disbelief play out differently for different members of a community. There are several strands to bear in mind here. First, as Carla A. Grosch-Miller and Hilary Ison have noted elsewhere in this volume, a psychological understanding of the human predisposition to protect ourselves from information which threatens our trust in the order and predictability of the world, or which threatens our own or a loved one's safety and security, helps us to recognise that a difficulty in digesting unpalatable information is not recalcitrance but a survival reflex, which cuts in without the involvement of rational thought. This reflex response may take a good deal of time and effort to move beyond.

Another factor which links with this is what Poling describes as the creation of 'blind zones' by the 'ideologies and institutions of society' so that 'certain relationship systems are regarded as normative and therefore not open to scrutiny'.[8] So, in faith contexts, a high view of the sanctity of family life, of the status of the priesthood or a lack of distinction between the church and the kingdom of God all make it more difficult to 'see' the possibility that abuse may take place within these settings or by people of particular status. Ironically, or perhaps tragically, it may be those who have experienced abuse in other contexts who may be able to discern when the emperor has no clothes, and such voices are ignored at our peril.

Additionally, those who identify with the perpetrator in some way (e.g., because they, too, are clergy or of the same gender) or those who are personally close to him or her, may find it harder to believe the account than those who have more distance. In all these examples, to accept the accounts of abuse involves the shattering and reconstructing of the world, of relationships and possibly oneself as they had previously been understood, and as

---

Beyond Grief: A Guide for Recovering from the Death of a Loved One (London: Souvenir, 1988), 178–188.

8 James Poling, *The Abuse of Power: A Theological Problem* (Nashville, TN: Abingdon, 1991), 31.

Carla A. Grosch-Miller notes, spouses and families have the most at stake, particularly where home and livelihood are at risk.

What may those affected need, and who should offer it?

Within the congregation

Immediate follow-up

Depending on the nature of the issues, then, some individuals in the congregation will need immediate and obvious pastoral support following the tragedy because they are personally affected (through bereavement, injury or the loss of home or livelihood), because they have been involved as helpers, either voluntarily or professionally or because they have witnessed the events as concerned bystanders. Some of this follow-up, such as funeral or hospital visiting, will be familiar pastoral tasks for ministers and congregations which they are well equipped to offer. However, even here, an assessment needs to be made as to who is best placed to make a response, and it will not always be the minister. For witnesses and helpers, and for some of those personally affected, pastoral support may best come from the networks of relationship in which they are already involved, such as home or friendship groups within the congregation. Where direct involvement from those with pastoral responsibility is not indicated, their task will be to enquire whether those networks are able to respond appropriately, offer support where they are and follow up where they are not.

Corporate gatherings

As noted earlier, the impact of tragedy on others may have been more diffuse or distant yet still keenly felt for a variety of reasons. Here, corporate gatherings may be especially helpful to enable people to situate themselves in relation to the tragic events which have affected their community and to find a way to express the feelings evoked. The churches, with their long history in the practice of rites of passage around birth, marriage and death and, for the Church of England, its place as the established church of the nation, have often taken a lead in this way. It is striking how often people who would not usually be seen in church will be part of a gathering in church to express a community's solidarity in the face of suffering – whether that be in Lockerbie in 1988 or Manchester in 2017. This is one of the gifts communities of faith have to offer to the wider community in times of tragedy and crisis.

Good rituals, well conducted, hold and contain what is beyond reason and understanding and, through their containing structure, the calm presence of the minister and the solidarity of the community, attend to the first tasks of recovery after trauma (making safe and bringing down the threat response). If trauma and tragedy shatter our sense of the predictability of life or the goodness of humanity, one role of ritual is – like the plates and pins that hold a shattered bone together – to hold the pieces until what has been broken can find its way to healing.

But there is no room for complacency here. Ministers do have expertise to bring to the table, but good rituals, and the liturgy which expresses them, must attend to the reality of the experience of those who need them, and so worship leaders must be willing to be impacted by the situation and informed by those most closely involved. Finding authentic ways to hold together the polarities of anger and compassion, grief and solace, despair and hope which may be needed is hard emotional, as well as liturgical, work. Church people can learn much from the spontaneous symbols and rituals which people devise for themselves such as the laying of flowers and the lighting of candles at significant places or the singing of 'Don't Look Back in Anger' after the Manchester Arena bombing. There must be space for lament following loss and protest over injustice and inhumanity, as well as expressions of solidarity, compassion and hope, and at a time when people cannot easily find words, well-chosen liturgy, hymnody, music and Scripture may express the inexpressible for us.

Several things issue from good corporate events. First, they work in the opposite direction to trauma. If trauma is shattering, with a tendency to push people apart, community events allow for coming together in solidarity. Second, where the events can be spoken of frankly and accurately in public (within the bounds of necessary confidentiality) and a wide range of responses (e.g., numbness, anger, outrage, guilt, despair, helplessness) acknowledged as normal, understanding may be increased and permission given for that range of felt responses, opening the way for conversations to continue which express rather than deny the impact so that the necessary processing of what has happened can take place. This works against the tendency for trauma to silence voices or for certain reactions to go underground and, again, enhances the possibility for mutual support and compassion.

But not everything can find expression in this way. Some things are too personal, private and particular, too much out of step with everyone else or felt to be too shameful – or simply not ready yet to emerge from the inchoate sensory knowing of the limbic system to the more cognitive awareness of the cerebral cortex. So space and silence within corporate worship, to gather those who might otherwise be alienated and to contain what cannot yet come to voice, are vital for a very long time (arguably always, since leaders of worship can never know all of what those joining the congregation may be experiencing).

Small groups

The impact of all the tragic or traumatic situations described in this volume will be deep and long-lasting, disrupting understandings of God, the world, others and ourselves. The third task of processing the trauma – discovering and then responding to the shape of this disruption – takes time and cannot be rushed. There may be new information to assimilate as disciplinary, criminal or judicial processes unfold, hard theological questions to address, new learning about people to do and, in all likelihood, some reappraisal and reorientation of relationships within the community. These issues need smaller spaces where dialogue and discussion can take place and time can be given to allow old frameworks to dissolve and new ones to be found. People will talk anyway – there is a great need for it following a tragedy – but if such talk is to be productive rather than destructive, compassionate rather than scapegoating, conversation needs to be informed by accurate facts, well-founded knowledge and honest awareness of self and others. Church leaders have three responsibilities here: first, to set the tone of such conversations by the way in which they speak in public worship; second, to ensure that clear and accurate information is communicated in a timely way (and where there are disciplinary, criminal or judiciary processes, advice will be needed as to what can be communicated when); and, third, to consider whether existing groups are sufficient for this processing or whether others need to be convened.

External or specialist resources

So far we have considered the resources available 'in-house', but by the very nature of tragedy and trauma, there will be needs which a local community is not able to meet. Wise pastoral leadership will also be assessing what can and cannot be addressed within existing structures, given the limits of their own or the community's capacity or competence. Response from within may be compromised by the congregation's or denomination's involvement in causing the trauma, there may be a conflict of interest or incompatibility of role (e.g., when a leader needs to remain open to the needs of the whole congregation and is therefore not free to give focused support to one or another party in a dispute), there may be a lack of the necessary expertise or it may be that processing the impact needs more safety, focus, time or containment than broader pastoral care can offer. Wise leaders also recognise that there is no shame in seeking consultancy and advice from wider denominational structures or from specialists in legal processes, mediation, bereavement support, mental health services, psychotherapy or counselling and referring on when appropriate.

While some will be well cared for within the congregation or community, through the containing patterns of public worship or the more intimate context of group exploration, others will need the private, boundaried space that counselling or therapy can provide to help them come to terms with the particular impact to them of the tragedy or trauma.

For some, this will be because they are the most closely affected by it and need particular attention because of the depth and acuteness of a pain which cannot truly be shared by those around them. Some will find that the present situation evokes feelings and behaviours which neither they nor others can understand and which belong to a previous trauma that is well-buried or unprocessed (perhaps because amnesia was the only way to survive the earlier trauma and/or because there was insufficient support to make processing possible). Others are silenced within the church context because the reality of their experience puts them at odds with their congregation's dominant narrative or because they have such a sense of shame in relation to the situation (because they are victims of, or closely related to abusers, for example) that they cannot speak of it. Yet others may feel betrayed by church authorities and have lost faith in the trustworthiness of help offered in this context. Any of these may need the skilled attention of trained counsellors and therapists within the highly confidential space which counselling and psychotherapy offer.

It is important to note here that referral to other services does not absolve those in church leadership from their pastoral responsibility. Rather, they share that responsibility with others who are able to offer different skills and a different setting in order to help. Where a member of the congregation is undertaking counselling or therapy, they will still – and perhaps all the more – need to know that they are cared for by minister and fellow congregants in both practical and emotionally supportive ways.

Caring for the carers

It will be obvious from all that I have discussed so far that those who hold pastoral responsibility within congregations carry a particularly heavy and long-lasting load following tragedies which affect their congregation and community. Such a burden should not be carried alone, and where possible and appropriate, ministers need to involve lay leaders and ministerial colleagues in developing and implementing a pastoral strategy.

Beyond this, however, careful thought needs to be given to what their own needs may be as they seek to care for others. The following are some of the questions that need to be considered:

- How far have *they* (the potential carers) been traumatised by the situation itself, and has any previous trauma of their own been evoked?
- Have they considered the possibility of vicarious traumatisation or secondary trauma – in other words, being traumatised by bearing witness – either at first-hand or through people's stories – to the trauma of others?[9]
- Even where they have managed the initial crisis well, how have they coped when the psychological protection of the adrenaline rush has subsided, and they are in for the long haul?
- How are they working through the challenges to their theology, worldview and relationship with God which may be raised by the situation?

9 See Charles R. Figley, *Compassion Fatigue: Coping with Secondary Traumatic Stress Disorder in Those Who Treat the Traumatized* (London: Routledge, 1995).

- How far do they understand what is going on in their community?
- And who in the wider church structures is offering *them* pastoral care?

A range of responses to these needs might be appropriate:

- Carers may need to access therapeutic help for themselves to enable them to process their own reactions to the situation so that they do not spill out inappropriately in their interactions with those who need their care. This is an indication not of weakness but of strength and is part of their responsible provision for their congregation as well as for themselves.
- They will need to protect – and even increase – time off. Time away from the situation, and time for rest and recreation is vital both in the early days and in the longer term in order to be able to remain present for those in their care. A wise palliative care consultant of my acquaintance has the habit of taking one week in four off precisely to renew energy and perspective in order to continue to provide a high standard of care and prevent the burnout which could easily be the result of constant contact with death and bereavement. Ministers and pastoral carers dealing with tragedy would do well to emulate this idea and find ways to include healthy Sabbath practices appropriate to their context into their schedules and ensure that members of the congregation understand why this is necessary.
- Leaders may already be in a spiritual accompaniment relationship, but, if not, may need a space like this in order to address the theological and spiritual questions which arise.
- They may also, like many others in the helping professions, benefit from the regular space for reflection on their ministry which is provided by pastoral supervision.

Challenges

I have throughout this chapter advocated a psychologically as well as theologically and spiritually informed pastoral strategy. However, there are certain challenges in the UK Christian context in achieving this.

First, in much ministerial formation, little emphasis is given to studying the psychological theory which might inform good pastoral care or developing the pastoral skills to practise it proficiently. While some ordinands come with knowledge and skills from previous careers, not all do, and a question arises as to whether ministers are sufficiently informed and skilled to be able to make the kind of pastoral assessment which I have proposed. Alongside this, do those in church leadership recognise that this is a body of knowledge and expertise from which they can learn? Churches have been more inclined to seek financial, legal or business advice than to access the advice of pastoral consultants or the psychologically trained and skilled, yet this is precisely the kind of advice needed in the aftermath of a tragedy.

Second, this lack of emphasis on pastoral awareness and skills in training raises the question of whether those in pastoral leadership have the resources to recognise the limits both of their competence and their role in order to know when and how to refer on appropriately. Because those in leadership need to be mindful of and available to the whole congregation both pastorally and liturgically, and because most are not sufficiently trained to do so, they are unlikely to be the most appropriate people to offer counselling. However, they need enough knowledge of mental health and psychological services to be good general pastoral practitioners – able to recognise when the situation needs more than they can offer and competent to refer to an appropriate source of help.

Third, although Carla A. Grosch-Miller outlines in Ch. 16 the optimal situation of action from the wider structures when local church ministers are implicated in the trauma (which I have extended to include those who are incapacitated by it), in practice, all too often this extension of pastoral responsibility is not recognised by those who share the cure of souls with local ministers. There is a need for training of those in positions of diocesan or area oversight to understand the need for this kind of support and how to exercise it.[10]

Fourth, where will those who do recognise the need for advice or referral find competent therapists and practitioners who are at ease with providing therapy which not only respects but also understands and can engage with questions of faith? Such practitioners do exist, but it is hard to identify them in a secular society which mistrusts religion and whose emphasis is on broad spirituality or within specifically Christian organisations which accommodate a wide range of training, not all of which assures the depth of therapeutic skill which trauma work requires.[11]

Fifth, unlike a number of other helping professions for which clinical supervision is a requirement,[12] at present there is no culture across the churches of regular facilitated reflection on practice to enable pastoral practitioners to develop their awareness, knowledge and skills and be sustained in their work.[13] In the aftermath of tragedy, it is my contention that pastoral supervision is particularly indicated in order to help church leaders to reflect

10 Other churches could learn from the Salvation Army which has set up a Well-being Department for its officers and developed a critical incident debriefing protocol.

11 For a more expanded consideration of the points made earlier, see Ruth Layzell, 'A Case of the Baby and the Bathwater', *Practical Theology* 4, no. 1 (2011): 97–116.

12 This has been standard practice in professions such as social work and probation for decades and is mandatory in counselling and psychotherapy. See www.bacp.co.uk and www.psychotherapy.org.uk for codes of practice for counsellors and psychotherapists which stipulate supervision requirements.

13 There are, however, hopeful signs of change. The Methodist Church is currently implementing a policy (www.methodist.org.uk/media/1848/supervision-policy-290617.pdf) requiring all its ordained ministers to receive pastoral supervision on a regular basis. There are, additionally, indications that other churches are beginning to recognise the potential for this

on what has happened, consider what their responses need to be, check their own fitness to practise and be supported and encouraged in the demands of a difficult situation.

Conclusion

This chapter began by noticing how unhelpful Job's friends were in their attempts to 'comfort' him and by posing a question about who will accompany those whose lives have been unsettled and unseated by the tragic circumstances affecting them. Having considered all that we have in the preceding pages, what might characterise more helpful pastoral accompaniment than that offered by Job's friends?

First and foremost, accompaniers need to be able to acknowledge that, much as we would prefer it to be otherwise, tragedy, with its capacity to upend us, is part of the fabric of human experience. Helpful companions for those distressed by it will not rush to proclaim that all is well after all but will remain open to the reality of the lived experience of those they accompany. Next, and just as important, they will recognise the importance of continuing to 'be there' for those who suffer, hard though it may be to sustain such presence. They will need to have the courage to acknowledge the difficulty of doing this in practice, when the instinct is to run away because the other person's experience puts them in touch with their own vulnerability in the shape of memories of past hurts or fears for the future,[14] and the humility to seek support to enable them to continue to be present. Alongside this, in contrast to the certainties of Job's friends, they will need to be willing to relinquish cherished assumptions and preconceptions that do not stand up to the reality of these experiences in order to learn from those they accompany, recognising that this reshaping may be part of the work of the Holy Spirit, the Comforter,[15] whose strengthening of the faithful may come at times packaged as disturbance rather than consolation.[16] And, where they recognise gaps in their own understanding, they will be open to the wisdom of other disciplines and to learning and training which will help them fill in some of them. In other words, such accompanying will be characterised by humility rather than heroics.

But they will also be people resourced by our faith's defining narratives of enslavement and Exodus, exile and return, Cross and Resurrection, who hold fast during times of turmoil in trust that this is not the end of the story

---

discipline to enhance ministerial practice. See the Association of Pastoral Supervision and Education website www.pastoralsupervision.org.uk for further information.

14 Justine Allain-Chapman, *Resilient Pastors: The Role of Adversity in Healing and Growth* (London: SPCK, 2012), 100.

15 Comforters are those who make others strong by their presence.

16 Cf. the picture of the Holy Spirit given in Wm Paul Young, *The Shack* (London: Hodder & Stoughton, 2008), 130–131.

and that although long years of waiting or wandering, protesting, lamenting and grieving may be their experience, God has not forgotten them or ceased to work. There will not be a return to what was, because nothing will be the same for having walked such paths and nothing that emerges from it either justifies it or makes it all right – the dead child is still dead; the fire, the plane crash, the abuse has still happened; the awful experience is no less awful. However, part of the accompanier's task is to hold hope that what emerges from the turmoil will have the shape of resurrection.

As noted earlier, this is not easy, and there is a cost. Perhaps, as Allain-Chapman argues,[17] those who have walked similar paths themselves, and who have discovered that the light has carried on shining in the darkness, will have the courage and resilience to walk compassionately and faithfully alongside others.

Select references

Allain-Chapman, Justine. *Resilient Pastors: The Role of Adversity in Healing and Growth*. London: SPCK, 2012.

Brueggemann, Walter. *The Spirituality of the Psalms*. Minneapolis: Fortress, 2002.

Dunne, Edward, John L. Mackintosh and Karen Dunne-Maxim, eds. *Suicide and its Aftermath: Understanding and Counseling the Survivors*. New York: Norton, 1987.

Figley, Charles R. *Compassion Fatigue: Coping With Secondary Traumatic Stress Disorder in Those Who Treat the Traumatized*. London: Routledge, 1995.

Herman, Judith. *Trauma and Recovery*. London: Pandora, 1992.

Layzell, Ruth. 'A Case of the Baby and the Bathwater'. *Practical Theology* 4, no. 1 (2011): 97–116.

17 Allain-Chapman, *Resilient Pastors*, 53–55, 105.

14 The ethics of disaster response

Mia Kyte Hilborn

Disaster – something that traumatically affects a nation, a localised area, or a smaller group such as a church or family – can cast long and difficult shadows. These shadows may be physical, emotional, cultural, spiritual, political, or ethical, as people, after the disaster, attempt to come to terms with the impact on their lives and on their society. People are rarely unscathed; they may be naturally resilient or learn resilience, but due to the disaster, things will have changed. Christopher Brittain, in *Religion at Ground Zero*, compares life to a quilt, suggesting that it is made up of an intricate interweaving of different squares, with one overarching concept or meaning, the 'master-signifier', which he defines as an ideology or overriding principle through which all things are seen and nuanced.[1] A disaster is a manifestation of the 'real' in a potentially brutal or violent way. It is a manifestation that sends spasms or shockwaves into the ideology of the individual – that is, the holding principle or master signifier – and thence into all the aspects of the 'quilt', all the 'squares' of life.

Impact of the real

This impact of the 'real' can be highly disturbing, such as a flood or earthquake killing people and making others homeless. It can impact a core belief in which an individual has invested, and that has served as an overarching concept of life for that person. This might perhaps be belief in a higher power, which then has to be rethought in the light of the disaster. People may not lose their faith in a disaster; their faith may, in fact, be strengthened by it, and it may thus become be a robust, life-changing part of them which is sustained and developed throughout the crisis and beyond. For example, turning to prayer is a very common response post-disaster, and prayer may become more important for them in the process. At some point after the disaster people are likely to reassess their world- and faith-views and their impact upon the 'squares' of their life's 'quilt'; everything is likely to have

1 Christopher Craig Brittain, *Religion at Ground Zero* (London: Continuum International, 2011), 122–124.

taken on a slightly different shade of meaning, and this can have an impact on them spiritually.

Spiritual disruption

'Spiritual disruption' is a term used when an individual undergoes a life-changing event that leaves consequences for their personal spirituality. The person undergoing a disaster or trauma may find their physical environment has changed, and that this has had an impact on their emotional wellbeing. They may experience negative emotions such as fear, anxiety and over-vigilance, which are entirely understandable given the situation the individual has encountered. However, spiritual disruption occurs more specifically when the normal spiritual life of the individual has also been affected. Signs of spiritual disruption could include a misappropriation of prayer in such a way that it starts negatively to affect others or adversely to impact the individual's normal life, for example praying in the aisles of supermarkets and in the middle of conversations, and/or questioning family, work colleagues or friends about their prayer life to an intrusive extent. A person may find themselves unable to pray, perhaps accompanied by a fear that God is punishing the individual or society at large. Sometimes, response to a disaster may take the form of extravagant confession and visible atonement for sin – dressing like John the Baptist, for example – or avoidance of faith gatherings such as Bible studies, prayer meetings or church services. Such responses may highlight the conflicting spiritual impulses being felt by the individual in the wake of a disaster.

Sometimes the behaviour exhibited by a person with spiritual disruption could lead to an over-attachment to a saint, religious leader or religious artefact. The minister should view with some caution any tendency in someone who has been through a crisis to become obsessive about seeking pastoral care, for instance by asking very regularly to speak to the minister, or to any other pastoral professional. There could well be transference in such a situation, or the individual may be viewing the pastoral carer as some sort of transitional object. Commonly a person who undergoes a traumatic incident will seek a safe space or may be drawn back to a space that represents safety for them: indeed, a minister, priest or church may become that space. Ethically, the pastor or church leader would need to recognise when something like this is taking place and to ensure that appropriate psychological care for the individual is provided.

Ethical response post-disaster

Ethically, when one responds in a disaster or post-disaster, emotions tend to be heightened and discerning the right thing to do may be difficult. Weeks, even years, later, when caregivers or religious leaders look back on their response at times of disaster, they can feel uncomfortable with their reactions and may think that they did not give of their best. Psychology has a concept of the 'good enough mother',[2] and it may similarly be useful to consider what is ethically a 'good enough' for a church leader to be and to do at times of crisis and disaster. Winnicott talks about an inner reality of the individual that is disturbed through violent and traumatic acts – an inner reality that has an intermediate area in which the individual 'experiences'. This inner reality, in Winnicott's terms, can be viewed as the place where Brittain's ideology or master-signifier resides: thus, the intermediate area, if disrupted, has the potential to influence the squares of life.

Spiritual disruption that in one way or another reveals to an individual that their faith is the core spiritual, numinous principle of their life, can have a wide-ranging impact upon other areas of life, too. If the person in question feels that they have acted in an unethical way – that is, on reflection, if they feel they were not good enough and they did not meet their own high ideals – they may become ashamed of their behaviour. If left without reframing or ethical enquiry, this could be detrimental to their way of life. They may start to blame God rather than thanking God for getting them through, thinking that their new reality is painful – perhaps more painful emotionally or physically than the disaster incident itself. Their disrupted response could mean that they turn against fellow Christians due to survivor guilt, or they could exhibit anger, or might worry that they are not now good enough to do their job. Then again, some religious leaders may become overly proud of their own achievements at having helped at events where others experienced extreme tragedy, and this could cause separation between the helped and the helpers, which may, in turn, affect congregational harmony in years to come.

Disasters are real events which themselves have a disturbing effect on wider reality. Part of a church's emergency preparedness, in addition to standard operational requirements, would ideally be the planning of an ethical response. This should be drafted prior to any disaster event, and should, vitally, inform continued reflective self and group care processes built into the operational response to such an event. It should then be discussed and reviewed honestly in the wake of the event and in preparation for any future such events. Ethical sections are not normally found in the emergency services' protocols for disaster preparedness, or in immediate disaster response service manuals, but this might be something that the Church could bring to the emergency response agenda. This need not in any way divert from the disaster response as such; rather, it would address what needs to be done in anticipation of a disaster event – that is, what *should* be done rather than what *can* be done. It would also provide a pastoral and moral framework for reviewing responses to a disaster after that event has occurred – to help responders once they have finished their shift to reflect on what they did,

2 Donald Woods Winnicott, 'Transitional Objects and Transitional Phenomena – A Study of the First Not-Me Possession', *International Journal of Psycho-Analysis* 34 (1953): 89–97.

and what they wished they had done, and to thank them for their efforts. The ethical facilitator in this scenario could encourage an honest assessment of individual and corporate responses and motives to help reduce the risk of spiritual and emotional disruption, which could itself impact future responses to disasters and make it difficult for responders to function openly again in a spiritual environment.

Testing of faith in a disaster

When a disaster strikes, the individuals caught up in the situation, particularly religious believers and their leaders, will normally find their worldview tested. Such challenges to faith and conviction could be one of the most difficult things for them to deal with long term. Issues that hitherto had not been a problem can become vitally important as the reality of the disaster hits home. For example, a person who strongly believes that God is love and that God loves and protects families may find it very difficult to come face-to-face with the deaths of several family members; moreover, if other families have also been affected it is likely to become more difficult for the individual to process the disaster within their own belief system, particularly if that belief system is of a more rigid sort. Similarly, a person who believes strongly in the power of prayer and places a high value on miracles may be severely challenged if confronted by death and dismemberment after claiming prayer victories for the individuals concerned. Indeed, religious leaders who adopt this approach may be tempted to blame the victims by suggesting that by their own sin, they brought disaster on themselves rather than countenance that their own leadership, prayer method and understanding of faith has been in error.

Brittain reminds us that there is no such thing as the perfect human being – an echo of Winnicott's 'good enough' – and that it is a fallacy to assume that everything we know and believe is correct. This is not saying that the creeds and liturgy of the Church are to be viewed primarily with scepticism; far from it. Yet it is to recognise that they mediate a wealth of theological resources that can sustain and nourish victims of and responders to disaster in different ways, for different purposes. In fact, each individual might take from them something that might inform their relationship to God, their understanding of who God is, what Christ has done, or how God's purpose is worked out in the world, and then assimilate this into their inner core, 'sanctum' or spiritual centre – the devotional vantage-point from which they interpret and reinterpret the world.

For some, this interpretation will be highly emotional, for some highly intellectual – but it will be very personal for the individual concerned – what might be described as the spiritual 'patterning' on their soul. It will include what they believe about the world, how they see that world and how they consciously put their faith and life into practice. When a disaster strikes, anything that does not stand on rock will be blown away, and that which is hidden inside may come to the fore. A person who has been abused as a child may have sudden flashbacks when seeing real fear in a child's face, for example. Truth becomes very palpable, and unconscious biases can be exposed. For religious leaders, dealing with others who experience such truths being uncovered by the trauma they are undergoing can mean standing on sacred but difficult ground with them; the same leaders will also need to realise that those for whom they are caring may be disclosing hard and difficult truths about themselves.

There will be ethical issues that arise which are disaster-specific, and which will need to be discussed at an appropriate time afterwards, with behaviours adapted as necessary. For example, pre–Hurricane Katrina there were no ethical plans put into place for hospitals having to decide who should have any potentially rationed treatment.[3] Due to the hurricane, some generators in hospitals failed, and only certain patients could be evacuated and treated. Far-reaching ethical decisions were taken in the moment and without guidance, and some patients died directly as a result of those decisions. Yet despite the morally profound repercussions for the individuals making and carrying out those decisions, no-one was actually convicted of wrongdoing. The key decision-makers had no prior ethical guidelines to follow; rather, they had to decide in an emergency situation quite literally who would live and who would die.

Ethics and church communities in disaster situations

I suggest that there are certain key ethical issues that churches should discuss when engaging in disaster work at the preparedness stage, at and immediately following a disaster (of any size), and in the rebuilding and reflection stages. These issues are

1 truth-telling,
2 competence,
3 boundaries,
4 money,
5 confidentiality and
6 evaluation/reflection.

Christian leaders should be able to understand the fluid nature of an emerging disaster situation, as one in which decisions have to be made quickly, and in which the nature of the response has to be swift and immediate, but also in which decisions can be made incorrectly sometimes, and have to be changed as further information comes to light. The decision-maker may

3 Carrie Y. Barron Ausbrooks, Edith J. Barrett and Maria Martinez-Cosio, 'Ethical issues in Disaster Research: Lessons From Hurricane Katrina', *Population Research and Policy Review* (2009): 93–106.

not have the full information to hand at any given moment and so may not realise the complexity of the situation. The church, with its centuries of ethical practice to draw on, and with its Christ-like respect for human life to uphold, should have a voice even at times of greatest incident-stress – not 'getting in the way' but being a genuine helper and spiritual responder to the crisis at hand.

Truth-telling

The Church should, of course, always tell the truth, albeit not necessarily in bald, unfettered language. Theologically and ethically, it should not collude in telling untruths about a situation or in calming someone by keeping the truth at bay. Conversations at the preparedness stage of emergency work can be had about the levels of communication that can be shared, and about the importance of using accurate information when communicated to those who are caught up in a disaster. Questions can be asked about who will share news and with whom they will share it, and about how news will be conveyed, especially with people who may potentially be in shock, or frightened. How can news be given so that people who need or want to know are told enough to maintain calmness and to reduce the likelihood of panic or disorder? How can news be shared so that the news givers do not feel guilty for years to come about not sharing the truth? There may be circumstances that impinge on national security or personal safety, in which case the necessity to tell the truth may be curtailed for the greater good; even then, however, information that can be shared should be truthfully shared, even if it is not the complete truth. The concept of truth-telling and information exchange may emerge in conversations about emergency preparedness. Churches may wish to identify news giver(s) in the first place, as well as those whom they should share the news with, and with whom they, in turn, should share it.

The developers of Psychological First Aid (PFA), which is the World Health Organization– and Red Cross–recommended tool for use in disaster situations, advise telling news to affected individuals in a clear and truthful way in the aftermath of a disaster, at a level that they can cope with. Part of a disaster response, or indeed any response to a trauma, would include the relevant church or churches being able to respond in an appropriate way which does not reignite the trauma. PFA is an evidence-based tool that can be easily learned by church leaders to respond effectively in trauma situations. PFA is designed to 'reduce the initial distress caused by traumatic events and to foster short- and long-term adaptive functioning and coping'.[4] Part of churches' competence is to make themselves ready to be able to help in times of trauma and disaster, to be trained in psychological first aid and

4 Psychological First Aid, 'The National Child Traumatic Stress Network', www.nctsn.org, home/treatmentsandpractices/psychologicalfirstaidandSPR/aboutPFA, accessed September 17, 2018.

to ensure clergy and church workers have the necessary tools to maintain resilience in the face of trauma.

After the incident, telling the truth can be ethically challenging: What is the truth, and what is allowed to be told? Churches have been criticised after acute incidents, such as sexual abuse scandals, of covering up crucial details, and of not being as fully truthful as they should be about what has happened. There is a fine line between disclosure and confidentiality and the protection of victims. It is often best to use words victims have used themselves rather than putting words into their mouths. Church leaders can talk about the personal impact events have had on them, but they must be careful to avoid any public perception that the incident was more about them or their church than the wider community. Clergy, in particular, can be viewed in a negative light as their attempts to provide care may shine the spotlight on themselves too much, thus shifting focus away from trauma victims. In today's world of 24/7 news, social media and celebrity, surviving trauma could be viewed in a positive light, and churches need to use their communications officers to check that their support of victims does not become more emphasised than the plight of victims themselves. Clergy still, in some locations, are seen as local community leaders, and it is therefore appropriate that they not only lead with messages of comfort after a trauma and during times of remembrance but also ensure that their messages are truthful, compassionate and appropriate for hearers and victims alike.

Competence

At the preparedness stage, planning, competence training and tabletop scenarios are all useful ways to build both individual and group resilience and to encourage churches to look at their role within the wider religious response and with reference to civic and secular agency responses. Unless churches are properly involved in planning for disaster events, they might be missed off crucial lists and, if and when an incident happens, excluded from coordinated local responses. Churches have a tendency to extrapolate from previous individual pastoral cases to larger disaster events. Sometimes this works well and might be dubbed the 'Miss Marple' approach. However, a mass incident has consequences that are beyond ordinary local scenarios, and churches would be wise to take a different attitude for preparing for major responses or potential mass trauma.

A security chief at Morgan Stanley Dean named Rick Rescorla worked in the Twin Towers before 9/11, and was convinced that there would be a terrorist attack there. He insisted on practising escape drills every three months, with more than 40 floors of staff involved. As a result, he was able to lead more than 2,000 people out before the towers collapsed, although he himself died as he went back to find more people. Churches would do well to learn the competencies and skills of trauma response, as this would furnish them with transferable skills which can be used in a multiplicity of situations where 'mini' traumas are affecting their congregations. Some of these situations may mean boundaries are blurred, and for this reason, part of the requisite competence training entails understanding the nature, role and function of confidentiality.

When disaster strikes, the fault lines from a trauma echo throughout the lives of individuals. For some this will be dealt with quickly, for others not so swiftly. People who have suffered as children, people who have substance abuse issues, mental health issues, difficult financial or domestic issues are likely to have more difficulties than those who are living in stable, happy homes and relationships with steady and sufficient income. People are naturally resilient on the whole; in general, they are remarkably good at dealing with disasters.

Churches can act as a focal points for support – places where people can come to escape if their roads are closed or transport is down. Short-term, they can provide refreshments, toilets, pews or floors to sleep on, mobile phone chargers, boards to convey the latest news reports or where people can leave messages looking for loved ones, and generally serve as a place of information exchange. Ecclesiastical authorities would need to provide personnel to look after congregations in times of disaster, ensuring that all the work does not fall on one person, no matter how much he or she enjoys the responsibility. The ethical response would be to have a trained team who could respond to helping in times of trauma and who would have time off to unwind. The church would need to be aware of the news bulletins that come out in relation to the disaster and would need to display these bulletins, as not everyone would have mobile phones fully charged. Churches would need to keep offering public and private prayers and to ensure that they did not add to gossip but kept to the truth, as far as it could be known. Having prepared for these scenarios should ensure that churches would have a level of competence in traumas that would enable them to be useful colleagues to the emergency services.

Being competent in an emergency means that everything is ready, and that church leaders do not have panic attacks or act as if they would prefer the public did not come into their buildings when there is a local traumatic situation. If a church is prepared for disaster response as indicated above, the amount of stress it faces will be reduced as it seeks to fulfil its ethical and missional calling to be available in times of difficulty. Churches do not take over from the work of the emergency services and local authorities' emergency preparedness work, but they can complement existing structures. In particular, the most tangible thing they can offer in an emergency is their building, with people who can listen giving tea and coffee and offering a safe, pastoral, friendly space. This should be what churches are ordinarily excellent at providing, but it will need to be significantly scaled up and intensified in a disaster situation, and in the short term, church members are likely to be very busy. Indeed, it is asking a lot of local church members and clergy to offer befriending post-trauma, not least because they themselves are likely to be affected by the tragedy even as they help others. Hence, it is important that a supportive framework for caregivers should be established. This is where an archdeacon or similarly a senior lay- or ordained person with a wider perspective can step in and put support structures in place on the church's behalf, as it comes to terms with its own experience of the trauma that has had an impact on the wider community. Such a senior figure could contact the church minister or ministry team two or three times a day to check they are coping, to find out whether any supplies are needed, to ascertain whether the church is managing its personnel adequately, and to determine whether others should step in to help. Other local churches could be asked to provide additional supplies or teams of people, to give the local community church workers and volunteers some time off in what will often be an on-going incident. The archdeacon (or equivalent) would be a person to whom the local church's minister(s) could speak confidentially about what was going on and what was needed, and could advise on any issues regarding boundaries and confidentiality.

Boundaries

Boundaries can become blurred in traumatic times. It can be difficult to know how the proper professional response might relate to the authentic response of the Christian, and what responsibilities the church should bear more specifically pre-, during and post-trauma. A major trauma can become career-defining or life-defining: it can be so extraordinary that everything else is subsequently framed in response to it. After conversion to Christianity, particularly as an adult, the convert may consistently refer to their coming to faith, and redefine their life through that new-found faith, hopefully reconstituting that life for good, and for God. Looking back with God-tinted eyes supposedly brings into focus the truth of the situation as it always has been, but in a way that a person with no faith could not see. Trauma, on the other hand, can have a negative reframing effect, where the memories can be overwhelming and potentially lead to PTSD. Similarly, the reframing effect can add to bitterness or depression, in which the reality of the danger faced can strip away the standard comfort-blankets of life, and can harden internalised negative emotions. Preparation regarding boundaries, responsibilities, faith edges, life edges, places of support and overloading, if duly readied in advance, can go some way to nullifying potentially negative effects.

Caregivers can seek to offer too much when faced with overwhelming need, and part of the preparedness stage is to ensure everyone knows what is expected of them and of the church and are aware of how much they can and cannot realistically offer. The church cannot and should not deal with someone suffering severe mental health problems as a result of the trauma; rather, they should provide a safe, secure, unthreatening location and should call in a suitable health care professional as soon as possible. People may need somewhere to sleep – in which case they might be accommodated in a church's halls, or congregation members might offer sofas or spare beds. Either way, such people movements would need to be properly documented, and safety would need to be paramount for all concerned.

Money

Money is often a negative factor in disaster response since disasters are typically very expensive. Churches will need to decide in advance of a disaster where monies will come from to buy resources that can be used, whether monies will be given out to help people get home after a trauma, whether monies will be given to disaster victims to buy food, and so on. The disaster itself is not the time to have these conversations, but in advance, the church would be well advised to have discussions about what the church should provide financially.

Generally, pastoral support in an emergency is not specifically remunerated in the case of church workers; rather, it is typically considered part of their normal work. Indeed, it may actually be considered unethical to pay church workers to help traumatised people when they have no specialised professional skills in this field. In refugee camps, surgeons will often offer their services free of charge, while aid workers are trained and are paid, and volunteers who help and befriend victims are normally self-funding. The level of skill therefore does not equate to pay. Usually the co-ordinators of disaster chaplaincy response are paid, whereas the disaster chaplains themselves often self-fund. However, thought may be given to paying expenses and to providing food for caregivers in churches, with paid supervision and perhaps a paid retreat or quiet day sometime after the trauma has died down. When serving in disasters, the church could pay its helpers to hire a taxi home, if taxis are available.

Confidentiality

Confidentiality can be a casualty in times of disaster. Clergy and church leaders will need to explore ahead of time what can and cannot be shared and with whom, so that they have in place a framework of care ready for when disaster strikes. Careworkers in disaster situations can be encouraged to make a care wall or something written up which reminds them of what supports them – such as favourite Bible verses, a loved photo or film, a historic prayer which chimes at a deep level, a recipe for a cake or a list of phone numbers of suitably empathetic friends or associates who can be called for an off-load. However one chooses to prepare for tragedy, after tragedy strikes, the caregiver can be exhausted and empty, and a 'care wall' or some such pastoral tool, prepared when times are good, can remind the person that good times will come again.

The confidentiality of those being helped should be understood as essential, and care should be taken not to use names without permission in prayers, while caution should be advised about stories from the disaster being used in sermons and church magazines. Ethically, conversations about particular individuals should be kept to private reflective practice or supervision, and if the requisite facilitation skills do not exist within the local church, the wider church should step in to provide such sources of pastoral support to the caregivers.

In disasters, it is important that records are kept, and the type of record needs to be decided beforehand. Records may need to be handed over to the police or emergency services. They would include the person's name and contact details (e.g., email), why they needed help, and why they were in the vicinity when the disaster occurred. It could be that the person in question is looking for relatives, has got caught up in traffic chaos, or has witnessed a crime. Keeping contact details (should the person give permission) is important for later memorials and commemorations of disaster events, and it is useful to know who has come to these, at the very least for the private prayers of the clergy. Ethically, thought needs to be given about storage of such records and the length of time they are kept.

Evaluation/reflection

Congregations can engage in dry-runs of emergency preparedness and then evaluate their responses by asking themselves questions: 'Where did log-jams occur and why?' 'Where were problems arising?' 'Was everyone able to perform at the optimum for their jobs?' and 'Did the plans work?'. Although one cannot properly evaluate a full-blown disaster response, there can be an operational debrief soon after the traumatic event has ended, which will enable those involved to explain what did and did not work, and which will enable times for further supervision and support to be offered to caregivers.

An honest appraisal of how the church has been able to support those who have undergone trauma, and the impact it has had on caregivers can helpfully inform any future responses that might be made, thus ensuring that resources, training and support can be properly targeted, both for the individual community that has been involved and as a template for how other local church congregations elsewhere might be involved in disaster and trauma relief in the future, at both the macro- and micro-levels.

Conclusion

It is clear, then, that with due preparation and training churches can help give support to the traumatised in disaster events, that they can help those undergoing suffering in and after such events to find meaning in the midst of pain, and that they may be able to help people regain resilience with an understanding of God and a renewed faith after traumatic incidents. In order to do this, churches will need to have a well-defined ethical understanding of their role within the different stages of trauma and be able to respond truthfully and competently through the different phases of the trauma cycle.

Select references

Barron Ausbrooks, Carrie Y., Edith J. Barrett and Maria Martinez-Cosio. 'Ethical Issues in Disaster Research: Lessons From Hurricane Katrina'. *Population Research and Policy Review* 28, no. 1 (2009): 93–106.

Brittain, Christopher Craig. *Religion at Ground Zero*. London: Continuum International, 2011.

The National Child Traumatic Stress Network. 'Psychological First Aid'. www.nctsn.org, home/treatmentsandpractices/psychologicalfirstaidandSPR/aboutPFA. Accessed 17 September 2018.

Winnicott, Donald Woods. 'Transitional Objects and Transitional Phenomena – A Study of the First Not-Me Possession'. *International Journal of Psycho-Analysis* 34 (1953): 89–97.

15 Chaplaincy and responses to tragedy

Mia Kyte Hilborn

There have been many tragedies in the world, from wars and earthquakes to train crashes and car accidents to bombs and stabbings. Since its beginning, the work of chaplaincy has been focused on helping and supporting the people involved in such tragedies. The first chaplains served in the army, caring for and supporting soldiers on campaigns and praying for the relevant military campaign to succeed (cf. Deut 20:1–4). In the Middle Ages, 'hospitallers' went to look after pilgrims and those who had been injured fighting in the crusades (*hospitaller* derives from the Latin *hospitalis* – 'hospitable'). The Knights Hospitallers, in particular, established hospitals to care for the sick and injured and were instrumental in opening and running places of care for the sick in many regions of Europe.

Tragedy and trauma can lead to heightened anxiety and stress for those affected. Some of this can be spiritual distress and can have long-term spiritual consequences, with the individuals concerned falling away from their faith communities if not given appropriate spiritual support post-trauma.[1] Anxiety, which is often associated with trauma, may lead a 'collapse of everyday significance', and the person exhibiting it may become so traumatised that he or she looks towards death rather than enjoyment of life – what Stolorow terms a 'Being-toward-death'.[2] This means that when a person has experienced tragedy, he or she may be functioning, but the impact of the traumatic event could have a significant effect on his or her existential or spiritual self, whereby the individual concerned may be 'existing until they die' rather than enjoying life and relishing existence. As Stolorow goes on to depict it,

> [t]he appearance of anxiety indicates that the fundamental defensive purpose of average everydayness has failed, and that authentic Being-toward-death

1 Emily McClung et al., 'Collaborating with Chaplains to Meet Spiritual Needs', *Medsurg Nursing* 15, no. 3 (2006): 147–155.

2 Robert Stolorow, 'Phenomenological-Contextualism in Trauma', in *Trauma and Transcendence*, ed. Eric Boynton and Peter Capretto (New York: Fordham University Press, 2018), 53–69, 60.

> has broken through the evasions that conceal it. Torn from the sheltering illusions . . . we feel uncanny – no longer safely at home.[3]

When a person has undergone some form of tragic event, and when the experience has left him or her feeling deeply worried and unsettled, separated from their former sources of comfort and support, when there has been a profound distancing of the person from his or her faith, and when the love of God seems a memory rather than a constant – then, historically, the Christian chaplain has helped. Chaplains may be able to support such victims of trauma, offering an active listening, compassionate and prayerful presence, and using techniques which can reground the individual in regular faith-based sources of support.

History of chaplaincy

The first hospitals in England were created in the Middle Ages. From this period, the oldest surviving institutions are St Bartholomew's and St Thomas's, which were both established in London during the 12th century. St Bartholomew's was created by Rahere, a monk who fought in the crusades. He promised God that, if he survived, he would establish a hospital for the poor in London. On returning, he founded St Bartholomew's in Smithfield. To this day, a nurse from St Bartholomew's annually lays a rose on Rahere's tomb, which is in the church of St Bartholomew-the-Great, in commemoration of and thanksgiving for his vision.

Even before the formation of Barts, care was given to people who would walk for days or weeks to come to London, looking to make their fortune. Many collapsed and died at the gates of London Bridge, and partly in response to this, the Augustinians set up a priory called St Mary's Overie on the south bank of the Thames in 1105. The post of Hospitaller was created there to look after the sick, and those who visited the sick in a section of the priory called the 'hospital', and the hospital and the priory became two institutions, priory and hospital, during the following decades. Near the end of the 12th century the Archbishop of Canterbury, Thomas Becket, was murdered in Canterbury Cathedral by knights wishing to curry favour with the king. St Mary's Hospital changed its name to St Thomas's in homage to the murdered archbishop. St Mary's Priory eventually became Southwark Cathedral.

Modern-day chaplaincy responses to trauma

Modern-day chaplaincy provisions for trauma response vary from disaster response roles to chaplaincy in emergency departments of acute hospitals to military or emergency services chaplains to hospice or palliative care chaplains

3 Stolorow, 'Phenomenological-Contextualism', 60.

working alongside patients and their loved ones as they experience the challenge of a painful death or bereavement to street pastors to education chaplains dealing with the loss of a pupil in a school or a student in a university or college. As for the military chaplain, this role has adapted from praying for a successful outcome in conflict to supporting military families, providing moral and intellectual education, facilitating diplomacy and interacting with the local community on a religious and cultural level.[4]

As the role of the military chaplain is changing, so too are the roles of hospital and hospice chaplain, including those related to more specialised trauma or disaster chaplaincy work. Not least, chaplaincy is adapting to the decline in regular churchgoers in Western contexts whilst trying to meet the needs of people with underlying spiritual needs and spiritual distress who have no regular place or person available to them for spiritual support. The role of the chaplain has adapted to offer care for those who are more generally 'spiritual', as well as those who are more distinctively 'religious'. More specifically still, it seeks to be supportive of those who, in situations of trauma, may exhibit signs of what might be called 'vicarious religion' – that is, who might wish they had the assurances and comforts of faith whilst not desiring to be part of a regular faith community.

Vicarious religion

The concept of vicarious religion posits that a religious group with a 'hard' understanding of faith, can practise that faith on behalf of the wider group with the consent of the wider group.[5] The wider group is defined in this context as one in which faith and religious practice are essentially private – distinguished not so much by services of worship, organised outreach or regular engagement in the civic or political sphere, but through individual rites of passage or Occasional Offices associated with births, deaths and marriages, and also through support provided at times of national tragedy. Davie argues that this form of religion is particularly seen in Europe, although it is challenged from time to time in places such as Germany and in the United Kingdom, where there are significant numbers of religious migrants who practise their faith openly and may expect the public life of politicians in their host nations also to be more openly religious.[6] The regular continuing presence and growth of chaplaincy, particularly in response to trauma and tragedy, could be seen as a corollary of this concept of vicarious religion –

4 Dennis R. Hoover, 'For God and for Country', *Faith and International Affairs*, April 26, 2010, https://ore.exeter.ac.uk/repository/bitstream/handle/10036/3186/Vicarious%20Religion_A%20Response.pdf?sequence=3, accessed October 22, 2018.

5 Grace Davie, 'Vicarious Religion, a Response', *University of Exeter Bit Stream*, https://ore.exeter.ac.uk/repository/bitstream/handle/10036/3186/Vicarious%20Religion_A%20Response.pdf?sequence=3, accessed October 22, 2018.

6 Davie, 'Vicarious Religion'.

that is, an indication that the public still wants a designated religious person or persons to provide active support in traumatic and tragic contexts. Davie has compared the relationship of the British to religion in terms of an iceberg; that is, only a very small portion of their faith is made visible in public. Chaplaincy could be regarded as part of this 'visible' component.

Against this sociocultural backdrop, the chaplaincy response to tragedy can be viewed more precisely as a response to normally 'unseen' faith and spirituality which may be surfaced or exposed during traumatic or tragic events. An individual's public faith may be described as a veneer, similar to the dentine on a tooth, which 'hard' experiences of trauma or tragedy break down, thus exposing the 'softer' core. As a hospital, disaster and fire chaplain, I have seen this happen again and again. Families of children in an acute hospital ward, who have had no contact with churches for two or three generations, ask for baptism for their desperately sick child and wonder if their other children could also be baptised or blessed at the same time. There have likewise been many occasions when, after a difficult death at a fire or rescue, a firefighter has started a conversation with the words, "I am not religious but . . .". Indeed, the first posters that were used for London Fire Brigade chaplains, designed by a former police officer who was then working for the fire brigade, bore the caption 'You don't have to be religious to talk to someone who is'.

Vicarious religion could be interpreted as an outworking of the biblical doctrine of the priesthood of all believers and, more specifically, of the Lutheran interpretation of this doctrine in which all Christian people are called to be priests – praying for and serving the world – but not all are called to be pastors and teachers or leaders of congregations[7] As it is, a traumatic situation will typically require the chaplain to combine both priestly *and* pastoral functions, with the pastoral function often more prominent in both the immediate impact of the trauma and in the post-traumatic period, which may often last a very long time depending on the symptoms that the victim displays in response.

The traumatic reaction

The symptoms that a person manifests after a trauma or tragedy can be multifaceted. They will depend on the life history of that person, his or her previous experience of individual trauma, how the person has coped with past national tragedies, his or her all-around mental and physical health, his or her domestic situation, his or her faith and/or worldview, the person's friendship networks and community support structures and his or her financial situation, amongst other factors. Most people will experience some form of trauma reaction during their life, and most people will recover, eventually.

7 Timothy George, 'The priesthood of all believers', *First Things*, 31.10.2016.

The chaplain's role is to support people emotionally and spiritually through the natural responses to trauma. This might include guiding them towards faith community social support resources, such as befriending schemes at local churches, coffee mornings, Bible study groups and so on. In fact, social support offered by faith communities can particularly help the traumatised overcome the isolation that often forms part of the post-traumatic experience and which can aggravate post-traumatic distress.

Traumatic reactions can include arousal, not dissimilar to that associated with dangerous experiences such as combat, being chased or bungee-jumping; constriction; dissociation; freezing; and helplessness.[8] Post-trauma, arousal is often linked to fear, meaning that it might be consciously distrusted or denied.[9] Physical signs of hyperarousal can include increases in heart rate, tingling, or sweats; mental signs of it might include one's 'mind racing' and anxiety.[10]

For people who manifest such symptoms, Christian practices of meditative, contemplative and 'centring' prayer, which are closely attuned to the calming of breath, heart rate and mental processing, can be beneficial. Then again, a chaplain would need to be experienced and competent in these techniques to use them in a beneficial way. If someone is in a post-traumatic place and continuing in that place, some prayer techniques might be harmful. For example, seeking to deliver or exorcise demons from the trauma victim in a loud or aggressive way or deploying forms of confessional prayer that could arouse feelings of excessive guilt within the 'victim' might not be the most appropriate modes of prayer in a post-traumatic context.

Helplessness and 'freezing' are closely aligned and typically mean that the person experiencing post-trauma cannot move or indeed 'do' anything, so the helplessness defines both their inability to help themselves and others. Constriction in the body may affect breathing, whereby extremities of the body can go cold, and the muscles can become tense, ready for fight or flight.[11] Dissociation can protect people from reality, muffling their reaction to the full horror of a desperate situation. It may especially be present in adults who face trauma having previously experienced it in childhood.[12]

When a person is retraumatised, echoes of previous helplessness can remain.[13] The chaplain may facilitate the process of the individual's remembering who they are and what they have done, or who they can be and what they may do in Christ, with a bringing to mind of the promises of baptism and a reminder of the ever-living presence of God, and God's promises for the future.

8 Peter Levine, *Waking the Tiger, Healing Trauma* (Berkeley, CA: North Atlantic, 1997), 132–142.

9 Levine, *Waking the Tiger*, 128.

10 Levine, *Waking the Tiger*, 128.

11 Levine, *Waking the Tiger*, 135–136.

12 Levine, *Waking the Tiger*, 138.

13 Levine, *Waking the Tiger*, 143.

Powerful reminders gently made about the numinous or divine dimensions of life may bring a sense of relief and hope to a person who feels unable to respond in times of tragedy and may allow them slowly to regain control over their lives. In the process, they may come to an experience of being 'caught by God', even in the shadowy depths of their own despair and powerlessness.

Other symptoms which may be present in the initial stages of trauma include hypervigilance, intrusive memories, hyperactivity, mood swings and difficulties in sleeping.[14] After the initial traumatic phase, a person who is not recovering may start to experience panic attacks, blankness, avoidance behaviours, amnesia, difficulties in dealing with stress, problems with relationships and possible over-interest in dangerous activities.[15] Spiritual symptoms may include avoiding church, an inability to maintain Christian relationships and interest in the occult or in possibly harmful cults. Longer-term symptoms that could imply a serious post-traumatic condition may include extreme timidity, lack of commitments, very low energy and immune dysfunction, psychosomatic phenomena, serious relationship issues, inability to formulate plans, diminished interest in life and alienation.[16] Spiritual issues may include lack of hope, inability to experience joy, feelings of impending desolation, preoccupation with the end times and unusual spiritualised sexual activity. These psychological behaviours need appropriate skilled psychological or therapeutic referrals and are beyond the role of the chaplain or clergy, unless the chaplain or clergyperson is also trained to provide levels 3 or 4 in psychological support;[17] however, an experienced and skilled chaplain or clergyperson should be able to work with someone experiencing extreme spiritual distress.

Chaplaincy around children in times of trauma

Of particular importance to the Christian chaplain and to the church should be the impact of trauma upon children and young people. Indeed, the church and its chaplains can have a distinctive role in helping children grow and thrive in post-traumatic contexts.

Often an infant or child baptism or blessing can be a means by which a parent asks for the chaplain to pray to a God dimly remembered. Parents may feel that they have no skills to pray themselves, they may feel it hypocritical for them to pray when they have had no relationship with a congregation or place of worship, or they may be so traumatised that they simply cannot contemplate praying themselves. Often in such circumstances, the chaplain will offer prayers or a religious rite, which it is hoped will bring some sense of calm and reassurance to the family. Also, the chaplain will

14 Levine, *Waking the Tiger*, 147.

15 Levine, *Waking the Tiger*, 147.

16 Levine, *Waking the Tiger*, 147–148.

17 National Cancer Services, *Manual for Cancer Services: Psychological Support Measures Version 1.0* (NHS Crown Communications, 2011), Appendix A.

characteristically engage in skilled active listening, which should begin to reduce some of the pressures that can be built up while sitting in an intensive care unit. In these scenarios, the parent or parents will likely have had to make many phone calls, explaining to other family members and friends over and again the condition of their child. In the process, they will have had to deal with successive waves of shock and pain with each new person they contact. In the case of a single parent, there may be unresolved problems from a previous relationship or marriage breakdown. Other children in the relevant household may also be deeply traumatised as a result of the child's illness. If there are mental health or financial issues, these situations may be aggravated by the experience of illness. The chaplain may be able to depressurise the situation by their very presence as a representative of God, by their use of de-escalation techniques, by the deployment of prayers and rituals and by advising on simple spiritual techniques to use when the parent is alone at the bedside. Such techniques could include the placing of a small, blessed cross above a cot so that parents feel the children is protected by God even when they or the chaplain cannot physically be there. Parents may welcome being given a Gideon Bible, which they can prop up next to the cot or on the bed. They may also welcome being given a prayer card that they can stick onto any machinery by the cot or leave by the child's bedside. They may like to have double or more of everything to include the child and other family and friends in these actions – for example, giving a simple cross to the child as well as receiving one as a parent or parents. Blessing crosses at the bedside and then giving one each to every child in the family can be a very moving ritual, not only for family members but also for hospital or hospice staff. Afterwards, the children and the family can touch their cross, remembering that both they and the child who is sick is beloved by God. In highly distressing circumstances, touching a cross can itself be a prayer, and for people who do not come from religious backgrounds, such simple gestures can be spiritually uplifting and emotionally calming.

The level of distress experienced by the parent(s) and the rest of the family can be influenced by several different factors, such as previous experiences of trauma, mental health issues, relationship issues, sources of community and family support, monetary concerns, clear or mixed communications, level of severity of incident and so on. Soon after a disaster, the chaplaincy and responder staff can use psychological first aid, with the parents and with the children themselves, to assess where people are and what type of response might be most helpful. Psychological first aid is a useful screening tool to help in the first hours and days following a crisis, and there are specific interventions for children at their development stages which can also prove helpful.[18] Younger children (up to adolescent age) might be deemed

18 National Child Traumatic Stress Network and National Center for PTSD, Psychological First Aid: Field Operations Guide, 2nd Edition. July, 2006, www.nctsn.org and www.ncptsd.va.gov.

receptive to what some secular psychology has dubbed 'magical' thinking, which implies that they might be particularly helped by spiritual care and spirituality that make use of supernatural stories from the Bible as means of support and by prayers which talk about heaven and angels. Very young children may experience increased trauma if separated from their parents or people whom they trust; in such cases, spiritual care which encourages them to feel safe and loved should be fostered. Teenagers may prefer a supportive, open environment with the opportunity to absorb factual details, conversations or time alone to work out their feelings with art, poetry or music. Appropriate and sensitive interaction with peers or family is also very important in this context. Opportunities for teenagers to provide practical help may be welcomed by them, such as making a video on their phone of family or friends giving supportive messages or creating a playlist of favourite music which can be used at the bedside of a seriously ill child or a sick parent.

When working with children after a traumatic incident, distraction can be another useful tool. Indeed, the presence of the chaplain or church worker can, in itself, be a positive distraction, given that they will not be there to take blood or persuade the child to swallow distasteful medication. A simple distraction tool can be using a 'grounding' image, wherein the young person is encouraged to recall or think of a pleasant picture, scene or happy place which brings a sense of relief and safety. Often prayer can be useful for this, or a physical image of a sacred space, a cross or the sense of an angel's presence. A 'grounding' place may or may not be specifically 'religious', but in a chaplaincy, interaction will typically be one in which the child is guided to remember that they are loved by God and that love cannot be taken from them – a place of safety in the midst of shifting certainties.[19] In this sense, grounding places can be both material and spiritual in nature.

In the days, weeks and months following the traumatic period, work can begin to reframe some of the intrusive thoughts and potential misconceptions that may arise as the child tries to make sense of what has happened. Indeed, the child may be harbouring fears and anxieties that could mean maladaptation to life in the present; he or she may have difficulties with making friends or with trusting older adults or people of different cultures or ethnicities from their own. Children may become withdrawn, especially if they have not, at or close to the trauma, had a grounding place of sacred safety. For example, it can take a lot of painstaking, gentle work to rebuild trust within a child or young person after a church worker has sexually abused him or her or when a child has lost a parent or parents in a fatal car crash. Such careful and lengthy work by a chaplain or church worker will need take place in the context of offering supportive 'church friendship' alongside a specially trained and experienced psychotherapist or specialist

19 Helen Kennerley, *Overcoming Childhood Trauma* (London: Robinson, 2009).

paediatric therapist, who will monitor and work with the child over the medium to long term to regain trust or intimacy at the emotional and psychosocial level.[20]

Phases of disasters and tragedy

Whether working with children, young people or adults, the different phases of a disaster or tragic event mean that spiritual care work needs to adapt to the relevant phase:[21] otherwise, much helpful work could be wasted or even be harmful on some occasions. Chaplains, if properly trained and deployed appropriately, can occupy slightly different roles at each stage.

Impact phase

The impact phase may occur when a person has had an accident and is brought into the emergency room in a hospital. As the full scale of what has happened is being made known, there may be further surgery required, and the person concerned may not know, for instance, whether a limb or limbs will be saved. That person might have been involved in a fire or a major disaster, and family and friends could still be missing. The person might be moved into theatre, and the chaplain is likely to be sitting with a relative or relatives who do not yet know the full implications of what will happen. In the impact phase, some of these early responses can be described as spiritual, such as guilt and shame, with those affected potentially feeling that they are somehow to blame for what has happened, and/or that they are being punished by God. The person being treated in these circumstances could feel angry with God for what has happened, or might deeply question their faith and the effectiveness of prayer, on the basis that the tragedy has occurred or is ongoing despite prayers to prevent or mitigate it. The impact phase may also involve the person's questioning concepts of redemption or eternal life, in which case the chaplain might feel it appropriate to reassure them that God still loves them despite their sense of isolation or abandonment by God. Beyond these questions, the person might have others that range in content and depth, and the chaplain will need to listen at this stage without judgement and often without profound theological answers, recognising that queries such as 'Why has God allowed this to happen?' 'Why has God abandoned me to this?' or 'Why did this occur when I was happy?' are typically as much expressions of shock and pain as metaphysical enquiries. They should be allowed to be expressed in a safe and 'held' way but are unlikely to need a detailed doctrinal response there and then as to, say, the purpose or meaning of suffering. Rather, they will more characteristically be viewed at

20 Kennerly, *Overcoming*.

21 For descriptions of the phases or disaster and tragedy, see the essays of Kate Wiebe and Carla Grosch-Miller, Chapters 2 and 4, respectively, in this volume.

the time as anticipating a future lived response to the question which might take much longer to process.[22]

It is hoped that the Church will be part of the answer to the existential cries that emanate from the impact phase, as its supportive and loving presence in the form of chaplains and others can serve as embodied proof that God has not abandoned the person or people affected. In the impact phase, a victim or loved one may begin to recite prayers from memory, may sing hymns and may call out to God. The chaplain's role is sit alongside them, to listen and discern if a more formal liturgical response is required and, if so, to use traditional or well-known and well-loved devotional formulae that will bring comfort to the person, whether a hymn such as 'Great is thy faithfulness', the Lord's Prayer, the 23rd Psalm or other familiar, suitable biblical and liturgical responses. Prayers might often also be appropriately offered for any family members or friends who are missing. At the impact stage, a person may experience great fear and anxiety until reunited with family, and every effort should be made to bring reassurance and comfort to the individual here, both spiritually and practically. In time, the Impact phase will lead to the heroic and honeymoon phases.

Heroic phase

This is the phase when adrenaline flows in the process of seeking to mitigate the initial impact of a tragedy. In the case of natural or human-made disasters, it can involve search and rescue missions that generate great delight when a survivor is found and made safe – for example, when earthquake victims are dug out or plane crash victims are retrieved alive. After the London terrorist stabbings in 2017, finding relatives alive and being able to reunite families was a wonderful part of otherwise difficult and deeply troubling days. Such experiences of survival, hope and healing amidst wider tragedy may be perceived by those involved in miraculous terms, because they have pulled through or witnessed loved ones pulling through when they might not have done so. Often, after a disaster, a lot of injuries take place in this phase as people rush to help or to look for loved ones, paying less heed than normal to their own safety. The chaplain's role in such cases is to help with processes of thanksgiving and, if necessary, to speak words of thanksgiving on behalf of a community or an individual in formal circumstances. The heroic period can be quite short-lived, so the words of thanks that are used, and the circumstances of their use, may be time-limited. Sometimes, relief for having personally survived can lead to words being used which can be deemed inappropriate with hindsight; for example, giving fulsome thanks

22 Stephen B. Roberts, 'Defining Disaster and Its Impact on the Community', in *Disaster Spiritual Care: Practical Clergy Responses to Community, Regional and National Tragedy*, ed. Willard W.C. Ashley and Stephen B. Roberts (2nd Ed.; Nashville, TN: SkyLights Paths, 2017), 28.

to God for having survived a major fire and then finding out children and babies were killed in that same fire can lead to complicated emotions and challenging theological dilemmas. The chaplain should be able to express and confirm words of thanksgiving while ensuring that extravagant claims to God's special favour or miraculous work on behalf of particular survivors are weighed in relation to the devastation of perhaps equally faithful peoples' death or bereavement. The chaplain should also be careful not to ignore a survivor who, due to his or her belief that God has miraculously saved him or her, could put him- or herself in danger.[23]

In the heroic phase, the chaplain's main role is actively to listen and to provide comfort, allowing people to repeat what they have experienced as they, in their repetition or recital of events, come to terms with what has happened. Not everyone will want or need to tell their stories; not everyone works out their emotional and psycho-spiritual responses by verbalisation. For those who do, however, the chaplaincy presence can be invaluable and unique in making sense internally and externally, existentially and in the present moment of their faith and their lived experience. Techniques that may be engaged by the chaplain at this stage include repetition, ensuring communication is being effectively processed, clarifying and checking, summarising and allowing the person concerned to process both current information and the reality of what they have been through at their own pace. However, in the heroic phase, the chaplain may do little more than affirm that the person is alive, help him or her find loved ones and feel safe: it may not be the right time for longer conversations or explanations; the person may welcome the silence of a chaplaincy presence or prefer not to have contact; it is up to the person to make his or her own decisions about the support required. The chaplain must not try to do too much for the person or justify his or her own presence. Rather, the role is spiritually, emotionally and pragmatically to assess the situation and then gently but firmly to be a supportive Christian pastor in the ways that will best help the one who has undergone a traumatic experience.

The heroic phase may morph into a 'honeymoon phase', where some people may be feeling joyful and thankful for some time until the reality of what has occurred sinks in, and low moods may result. This latter stage is called the disillusionment phase – a phase in which God most particularly may be blamed for tragic events which have occurred.

Disillusionment phase

After the immediate services of thanksgiving for survival, there usually follow times of mourning, when painful memories of loss become real and the euphoria of survival or rescue slides away. The Christian chaplain and

23 Roberts, 'Defining Disaster', 27; Kevin Massey, 'Impact and Heroic Phases – Small Disaster', in *Disaster Spiritual Care*, 79–90.

related Christian communities should still regularly offer opportunities for individual and collective gatherings, but in this phase, these tend to become more reflective and may include times of mourning for losses to be publicly acknowledged. Here, sermons, talks, newsletters and one-to-one and family conversations will often focus on individual Christian resilience and on building up the body of Christ. Through such discourses, people can be reminded of the losses and pain they have experienced and may be helped to recognise and reuse positive coping mechanisms from the past while learning new ways to ensure a healthy future. Individuals will experience these times of constructive mourning and resilience building in accordance with their own personalities, their previous experiences, their individual ways of coping and their particular domestic circumstances, but on the communal level, there should be opportunities for coming together for both appropriate liturgy and testimony. This period may take several months, if not years, depending on the severity of the tragedy and the numbers involved. Suitable, duly boundaried times need to be found for people to express any pain, anger or frustration at God and at the church in this context, carefully demarcated with respect to location and time and topped and tailed by prayer, a safe place to let go and to the use of techniques of self-control to enable a return to normal life.

Chaplains, clergy and church workers will usually be of most help if they are around for the long haul to aid communities in their recovery from potentially devastating tragic events. The designated chaplain is likely to hand over to the local clergy for the majority of this work in due course, although the chaplain should be acting as the faith and liturgical lead for the organisations for whom they work, such as hospitals, prisons, schools, and emergency services. In the United Kingdom, most people do not have a local faith leader whom they would automatically approach for support following tragedies, so the chaplain will usually step into the vacuum and offer pastoral and liturgical support for the institution as colleagues recover together from career-defining traumatic events.

Chaplains should generate opportunities for people to talk, whether to themselves or to trained professional counsellors who can offer skilled therapeutic frameworks for those suffering from post-traumatic symptoms. However, the impact on chaplains and clergy can be very high:

> As the clean-up process dragged out . . . and as the demands to pastorally serve members' emotional needs, to participate in community recovery efforts, and to rebuild resulted in role confusion and the introduction of new priorities, signs of excessive stress among the clergy have become evident.[24]

24 William V. Livingston, Myrna Matsa and Beverly Wallace, 'From Honeymoon to Disillusionment to Reconstruction', in *Disaster Spiritual Care*, 142–151.

Clergy and chaplains can show signs of severe stress in the disillusionment phase, and depression can sometimes follow for the caregiver as well as for the victim and for loved ones. The chaplain or clergy can hopefully stay the course while encouraging others to do likewise. They will also need to support colleagues and community members who have come to be part of the community or family post-trauma, despite not having shared in the initial traumatic event. This can be an exacting situation but is part of the rebuilding and normalisation process. The tragic event, no matter how serious, has happened and is in the past – although some, of course, may bear mental, spiritual and physical scars for years to come. The family and/or the wider community that bore the tragedy has to look forward, with God still on their side and alongside them: as they do so, the presence of those who did not experience tragedy can be an important part of normalising the present and the future for those who did.

The disillusionment phase can include the additional stress of chaplains or clergy supporting others, or themselves, while trying to decide whether to stay or find homes and work elsewhere for the sake of family and themselves. As people reassess their priorities in the wake of a traumatic event, some will leave their current job. Chaplains and chaplaincy support staff should not feel guilt or shame if they decide to leave and move on. Clergy who do this can experience negative emotions from congregations who are not yet recovered from a tragedy: the feeling may be expressed that they should not be leaving their flocks in such difficult times. When this occurs, the senior leadership of church denomination, diocese or regional network will have an important role to play in supporting both clergy and congregations. If a key church leader does depart during the disillusionment phase, it may lead to a more complicated recovery if they, with a congregation, have shared together in a traumatic event. Even so, it is common in these situations for people to leave, clergy included, and recognition of this can also, in fact, enrich the overall recovery process.

After the death of a firefighter in active service, some members of the watch or fire station can decide to leave in the months or years of the aftermath. Families of current firefighters will talk and discuss the consequences for them, not least for any children involved. Life plans are often reassessed in this period and, in moving from the disillusionment phase to the reconstruction phase, decisions can be taken to relocate and start afresh. After the 7/7 bombings in London, many health care workers left Central London hospitals, putting considerable strain on staffing for those hospitals. After the 2017 London terrorist attacks, some National Health Service trusts (Guy's and St Thomas's, in particular, under the leadership of the chief nurse, Dame Eileen Sills) put great emphasis on supporting staff in the days, weeks and months following. Such support included chaplaincy and counselling and noticeably fewer staff left than might have been anticipated, with staff turnover remaining around the same as normal.

Signs of suboptimal coping during the disillusionment phase could include difficulties in communication with others and with God in prayer, frustrations and limited concentration, anger with God and with the church, mood changes and despair, sleeping problems, substance abuse or abnormal sexual practices, declining working performance, overwhelming negative emotions such as guilt, preoccupation with sin or the demonic, psychosomatic problems such as headaches or stomach upset and fears such as of being alone or in crowds[25] Chaplains and clergy need to be aware of the difficulties that people they support may be undergoing in such cases and should make referrals appropriately. They should also demonstrate self-awareness with regard to the potential that they themselves might experience such symptoms. Recognition, acknowledgement and commitment to working through these difficulties can mark the beginning of the reconstruction phase, as the individual or the community approach a stronger place – perhaps even stronger than the place they occupied before the tragedy struck.

Reconstruction phase

There may be immense confusion and difficulties as individuals and communities try to recover following a trauma – that is, as they enter the reconstruction phase. Circumstances are experienced as irrevocably different, and people and communities will behave differently compared to how they did before the trauma. Chaplains, clergy and churches will need to be careful not to overpromise or to overprovide in this context and will need to give people the opportunity to grow for themselves rather than simply relying on others to stimulate growth. Just as a mother who has seen one of her children killed in a car accident may become overly protective of any surviving children, particularly around roads, the church must ensure it does not overcompensate in cases of trauma and do so much that the individuals affected rely on the church or the church workers rather than themselves, such that their post-traumatic growth is stunted.

In the reconstruction phase, chaplains and churches need to have clear expectations of their own roles, and should not do so much that they suffer burnout. They should provide prompt and respectful care and communication and be flexible, just as they should expect other colleagues and bodies to offer and exemplify the same.[26] People who have undergone a trauma and are beginning to rebuild their lives are unlikely to be able to keep to rigid schedules or standard routines or to have robust expectations in the same way as before the tragedy. A family may want a service at the event site of a fire; an individual may want prayers said at home on the anniversary of a person's death; a planned service in a church may be cancelled at the last

25 William V. Livingston, Myrna Matsa and Beverly Wallace, 'From Honeymoon to Disillusionment to Reconstruction', in *Disaster Spiritual Care*, 142–151, at 150.

26 John Robinson Jr., 'From Honeymoon to Disillusionment to Reconstruction', in *Disaster Spiritual Care*, ed. Willard and Roberts, 185–208, 186.

minute as the family cannot cope – this is all OK and should be understood with intelligent and compassionate kindness by clergy.

There is no absolute blueprint for recovery from trauma. The phased model summarised earlier offers a generalised pattern of lived experience, response and rehabilitation, but trauma changes people in diverse ways, and part of chaplains' and clergy's response will be to ensure that God is recognised variously within this diversity and that the wishes of victims are respected as they seek in different ways to relate to God as part of their recovery. It also needs to be recognised that such intelligent, compassionate and empathetic spiritual care can come at a considerable cost for the chaplains, clergy and Christian leaders involved.

Self-care and resilience

While emphasising that work with people who have experienced traumatic incidents can take a significant immediate toll on chaplains, clergy and caregivers, we also need to recognise that there can be secondary traumatic distress which may have an impact on their working and domestic lives in the longer term. Crucial though it is to behave compassionately towards people who have experienced trauma, it needs to be stressed that this can lead to vicarious suffering on the part of the caregiver or chaplain. Listening to the details of the traumatic experience, especially when the listener is potentially a person with highly developed empathetic skills, can be draining. It is therefore crucial that those who enable victims in recovery are themselves enabled to work through the strains they face as they offer care and support – something that may be realised through peer review, appraisal, mentoring and group and individual therapy.[27]

Compassionate care

One caregiver and clinical psychologist defines the imperative of compassion thus:

> Compassion is really total immersion, becoming part of the suffering of another person . . . It's about saying that is not something you would wish anyone to experience . . . I have sensations about it; you may either acknowledge this, not be aware about it or even minimise it by reassuring yourself that things are fine: it's not a problem . . . I believe [compassion] is an inherent adaptive human emotion that develops very early and in intra- and inter-personal relationships. While one can feel compassionate with the inanimate world, it is with the animated life of humans that this is truly expressed . . . You're trying to give

27 For further discussion of the care of caregivers see Chapter 17.

> back what you have received through others being compassionate to you. I definitely believe that for any average human being, compassion should come naturally, beginning with the early mother-child reciprocal attuned manner of relating.[28]

This sense of compassion towards others, and particularly towards the child or young person, should be practised habitually by the chaplain and should be understood as such by the child and the adult or adults caring for the child. Compassion is a core-communicable attribute of God himself and as such may be stirred into recognition by the calm presence of the chaplain.

Conclusion

The chaplain has an important role to play in individual and group responses to tragic events, particularly for those people who do not normally have access to faith communities. Chaplains and clergy need to be prepared for and trained in the stages of disaster response described earlier, from impact to reconstruction, so that they are able to recognise the phases that people are moving through in recovery and thereby respond appropriately. Chaplains have different roles to play at each stage of a disaster and its aftermath, and chaplains, clergy and churches should be important figures and places in that context, providing compassionate care at every turn.

Select references

Ashley, Willard W.C. and Stephen B. Roberts, eds. *Disaster Spiritual Care*, 2nd ed. Nashville, TN: SkyLight Paths, 2017.

Boynton, Eric and Peter Capretto, eds. *Trauma and Transcendence*. New York: Fordham University Press, 2018.

Bruce, Steve and David Boas. 'Vicarious Religion: An Examination and Critique'. *Journal of Contemporary Religion* 2, no. 25 (2010): 243–259.

Davie, Grace. *Religion in Britain, a Persistent Paradox*, 2nd ed. Chichester: Wiley Blackwell, 2015.

Levine, Peter. *Waking the Tiger, Healing Trauma*. Berkeley, CN: North Atlantic, 1997.

Parry, Sarah. *Effective Self-care and Resilience in Clinical Practice*. London: Jessica Kingsley, 2017.

28 Sarah Parry, ed., *Effective Self-care and Resilience in Clinical Practice: Dealing with Stress, Compassion Fatigue and Burnout* (London: Jessica Kingsley, 2017), 62–63.

16 Sexual scandals in religious settings

Carla A. Grosch-Miller

In recent decades, the uncovering of sexual abuse committed by religious leaders has rocked faith communities. The revelation that a beloved priest, minister, rabbi, imam or spiritual teacher has molested a child or had sex with congregants sends shock waves through a congregation, triggering predictable responses from disbelief to anger and distress. As the shock wears off, not only are people's assumptions about religious leaders in tatters, but their very understanding of the divine can be shaken. Such is the depth of the betrayal of trust that it may be a very long time before a congregation can be said to have recovered from the trauma of clergy sexual abuse.

Focus on church congregations

Religious leaders of all kinds have stepped outside the bounds of appropriate sexual conduct, engaging in a range of behaviours from sexualising pastoral relationships and harassment to assault and rape. In the 1980s and 1990s, work aimed at responding to this kind of sexual violence came out of two church-related organisations in the United States: the Center for the Prevention of Sexual and Domestic Violence (now FaithTrust Institute)[1] in Seattle, Washington, and The Interfaith Sexual Trauma Institute at St John's Abbey and University in Collegeville, Minnesota. (The latter organisation is no longer active, although its website remains a valuable resource.) Since the early 2000s, FaithTrust Institute has become a multifaith organisation equipping religious communities to address sexual and domestic violence inside and outside their communities. Whilst clergy sexual abuse happens in diverse religious settings and the principles discussed later may have broad application, this chapter focuses on Christian churches and denominations.

Moreover, the chapter highlights the congregational impact of clergy sexual abuse. Many are the victims when a minister commits sexual misconduct:[2]

1 'FaithTrust Institute Hopes Religious Institutions Will Be Sanctuaries of Safety', *The Fig Tree*, November 2008, www.thefigtree.org/nov08/110108faithtrust.html, accessed July 10, 2018; Carolyn Waterstradt, *Fighting the Good Fight: Healing and Advocacy After Clergy Sexual Assault* (splatteredinkpress.com, 2012), loc. 586.

2 The words *minister* or *clergy* are used in this chapter to cover the category of ordained people that includes deacons or elders in some denominations.

the person(s) who were the focus of the sexual behaviour, family members of the primary victim(s) and of the minister, the congregation and the credibility of the institution and of the faith in the wider community and world. As the phenomenon of clergy sexual abuse began to be recognised and the institutional failure of the churches' response to be documented, attention was first drawn to the needs of primary victims and survivors of sexual abuse. In 2002, the organisation Churches Together in Britain and Ireland published *Time for Action: Sexual Abuse, the Churches and a New Dawn for Survivors*,[3] an ecumenical report commissioned and written to address the failure of the churches to respond pastorally and adequately to the needs of individuals who have been sexually abused. Congregations are regarded in *Time for Action* primarily as communities that can learn to provide support and safety for direct victims, not victims themselves of clergy sexual abuse. The purpose of the immediate chapter is to shine a light on the impact on the congregation which may be neglected in the aftermath as denominational structures work to address the needs of those more obviously victimised.[4]

Prevalence

For all the shock engendered when it is revealed, clergy sexual misconduct appears to be surprisingly prevalent. It is difficult to assess the full scope of the problem. Surveys require self-awareness and honest self-reporting. Assessment is further complicated because of the range of behaviours covered under the subject matter of sexual misconduct and the closeness with which institutions hold information about reported incidences. Numbers of cases adjudicated in church disciplinary actions may be the tip of an iceberg given the barriers and costs to victims of reporting.[5] There is, however, evidence

3 Churches Together in Britain and Ireland, *Time for Action: Sexual Abuse, the Churches and a new dawn for survivors* (London: CTBI, 2002).

4 The congregation is often the forgotten entity: Nancy Myer Hopkins, 'The Uses and Limitations of Various Models for Understanding Clergy Sexual Misconduct: The Impact on the Congregation', *Journal of Sex Education and Therapy* 24, no. 4 (1999): 268; Peter Mosgofian and George Ohlschlager, *Sexual Misconduct in Counseling and Ministry* (Eugene, OR: Wipf & Stock, 1995), 181. The focus on the congregation in this chapter is not intended to diminish the trauma experienced by primary victims or by family members. Spouses of clergy offenders may be particularly badly traumatised and are underserved by the current literature. Broken Rites (www.brokenrites.org) supports and advocates for clergy spouses who have experienced marriage breakdown.

5 Candace R. Benyei, *Understanding Clergy Misconduct in Religious Systems: Scapegoating, Family Secrets, and the Abuse of Power* (New York/London: Haworth Pastoral, 1998), 81. Benyei observes that 'disbelief, disenfranchisement, scapegoating, isolation and abandonment by the family of faith are the real possibilities of bringing forward a complaint of sexual misconduct'. The failure of denominations to deal adequately and sensitively with such cases contributes to a reluctance to report. Even under optimal circumstances, making a complaint is very difficult for victims. Margo Maris, '"that which is hidden will be revealed"

that clergy may be more likely to exploit those in their care than secular therapists.[6] In a survey of Church of England clergy reported in *Time for Action*, almost a quarter of priests surveyed had inappropriate sexual contact with someone not their spouse in the course of their ministry.[7] Earlier American surveys report from 6 to 39 per cent of surveyed clergy being involved sexually with people in their care.[8]

An abuse of power and a betrayal of trust

To understand how best to assist congregations to recover from the trauma that clergy sexual abuse causes, it is important to understand the nature of such abuse. Clergy sexual abuse is first and foremost an abuse of power.[9] With training, skills and resources and by ordination, ministers are powerful people in the church. Leading worship, administering sacraments, preaching and providing pastoral care, ministers can be identified with God in the mind of a church member.[10] This identity with the divine intensifies normal, unconscious processes of projection and transference and amplifies the impact of the abuse.[11] For some victims, it can feel as though God is

---

(Luke 12:2)', in *Restoring the Soul of a Church: Healing Congregations Wounded by Clergy Sexual Misconduct*, ed. Nancy Myer Hopkins and Mark Laaser (Collegeville, MN: Liturgical, 1995), 9. See Waterstradt, *Fighting the Good Fight*, loc. 1244 ff., for stories of church collusion with offending ministers and the impact on victims.

6 CTBI, *Time for Action*, 83. The report concludes that high levels of clergy sexual abuse can be attributed to personal susceptibility, the stresses and a lack of boundaries in the work, inadequate training, non-existent supervision, and an ecclesiastical culture 'dominated by sexual shame and endemic secrecy' (99).

7 CTBI, *Time for Action*, 84, citing T. Birchard, 'Clergy Sexual Misconduct: Frequency and Causation', *Sexual and Relationship Therapy* 15, no. 2 (2000): 127–139.

8 Stanley J. Grenz and Roy D. Bell, *Betrayal of Trust: Confronting and Preventing Clergy Sexual Misconduct* (2nd Ed.; Grand Rapids, MI: Baker, 2001), 22–25. See also Waterstradt, *Fighting the Good Fight*, loc. 362. For the scope of child sexual abuse in the Catholic Church in the U.S., see Karen J. Terry, 'Stained Glass: The Nature and Scope of Child Sexual Abuse in the Catholic Church', *Criminal Justice and Behaviour* 35, no. 5 (2008): 549–569.

9 Jason M. Fogler, Jillian C. Shipherd, Stephanie Clarke, Jennifer Jensen and Erin Rowe, 'The Impact of Clergy-Perpetrated Sexual Abuse: The Role of Gender, Development, and Post-traumatic Stress', *Journal of Child Sexual Abuse* 17, nos. 3–4 (2008): 349; James Poling, *The Abuse of Power: A Theological Problem* (Nashville, TN: Abingdon, 1991), 23.

10 Nils Friberg, 'Wounded Congregations', in *Restoring the Soul of a Church*, 57. Note also that in Roman Catholic theology a priest is *the alter Christus*, another Christ, contributing to incomprehensibility and isolation for victims. Robert Orsi, 'Praying Angry', *Reverberations* (The Social Science Research Council Forums, August 27, 2013), http://forums.ssrc.org/ndsp/2013/08/27/praying-angry/, accessed July 9, 2018.

11 E. Larraine Frampton, 'Conflict Management: Selecting the Right Tools', in *When a Congregation is Betrayed: Responding to Clergy Misconduct*, ed. Beth Ann Gaede (Herndon, VA: The Alban Institute, 2006), 29; Nancy Myer Hopkins, 'Congregational Intervention When the Pastor has Committed Sexual Misconduct', *Pastoral Psychology* 39, no. 4 (1991): 249.

implicated in the abuse;[12] at the very least, God stood by while it happened. The power of the role of clergy person cannot be overstated.[13]

Ministerial power conferred by ordination and role can be amplified by the gender, race or age of the minister. The great majority of clergy perpetrators of sexual abuse are male;[14] most victims are women or children.[15] These demographics reflect the strongly patriarchal nature of Christianity,[16] and of the wider culture. James Poling focused his study of the abuse of power in the Church on 'the two groups silenced by present patriarchal structures of society: children and women'.[17]

With power comes a fiduciary relationship: the minister holds his or her congregation in a sacred trust, with a duty not to exploit them.[18] In recent years, this duty has been more explicitly set forth in professional guidelines for the conduct of ministry, including more explicit references to sexual activity.[19] Because of the power dynamics inherent in the pastoral relationship and the minister's duty not to exploit, sexual contact with a congregant is a betrayal of trust.[20] A minister's sexual behaviour with an adult who is not his or her spouse is not an 'affair', as may be claimed by offending clergy;[21] meaningful consent on the part of a congregant is not possible.[22]

12 Kenneth I. Pargament, Nichole A. Murray-Swank and Annette Mahoney, 'Problem and Solution: The Spiritual Dimension of Clergy Sexual Abuse and its Impact on Survivors', *Journal of Child Sexual Abuse* 17, nos. 3–4 (2008): 403: 'when a clerical figure violates his or her ordination, responsibility, and privilege as a representative of God in a human relationship, it is as if God himself has committed the violation'.

13 Jason M. Fogler, Jillian C. Shipherd, Erin Rowe, Jennifer Jensen and Stephanie Clarke, 'A Theoretical Foundation for Understanding Clergy-Perpetrated Sexual Abuse', *Journal of Child Sexual Abuse* 17, nos. 3–4 (2008): 307.

14 Fogler et al., 'Theoretical Foundation', 304; Pamela Cooper White, 'Foreword', to *When a Congregation is Betrayed*, x.

15 Fogler et al., 'Impact', 331–332, who also assert that male children are particularly at risk.

16 Fogler et al., 'Theoretical Foundation', 306, 314; Poling, *Abuse of Power*, 30. Poling notes that gender and race relations are structures of domination in which women and non-white people have fewer resources and choices to protect themselves from abuse.

17 Poling, *Abuse of Power*, 14.

18 Darryl W. Stephens, 'Fiduciary Duty and Sacred Trust', in *Professional Sexual Ethics: A Holistic Ministry Approach*, ed. Patricia Beattie Jung and Darryl W. Stephens (Minneapolis: Fortress, 2013), 24–25.

19 See, for example, 'Guidelines for the Professional Conduct of Ministry (revised 2015)', The Church of England, www.churchofengland.org/sites/default/files/2017-10/Clergy%20 Guidelines%202015.pdf, accessed June 1, 2018. The guidelines articulate the relationship of trust (1.2) and power dynamics attaching to the role (2.4). Sexual activity is covered in 2.8, 10.2, 11.9 and 12.4.

20 Robin Hammeal-Urban, *Wholeness After Betrayal: Restoring Trust in the Wake of Misconduct* (New York: Morehouse, 2015), loc. 310; Fogler et al., 'Impact', 331.

21 Patricia Liberty, 'Why It's Not an Affair', www.advocateweb.org/publications/articles-2/ clergy/affair/, accessed June 1, 2018. Fogler et al. note that 'affairs' with women in a congregation are a particularly insidious type of clergy sexual abuse, with women who believe it is an affair for which they are partly culpable more reluctant to report it. Failing to recognise the inherent power differential impedes a woman's ability to name what happened and to heal. Fogler et al., 'Impact', 348–349.

22 Stephens, 'Fiduciary Duty', 29. For a discussion about the implications for single ministers who may wish to date someone in the congregation, see pp. 31–32.

Any sexualised behaviour destroys the pastoral relationship and its potential for good. It is always the minister's responsibility to maintain the boundaries of the pastoral relationship and to protect the integrity of individuals in their care.[23]

What is damaged, then, when a minister abuses power and betrays the trust rightfully expected of them by sexually exploiting a child or adult in their care? Ken Wells characterises clergy sexual abuse as 'a trauma which denudes the soul of the basic sense of trust'.[24] Kenneth Pargament *et al.* describe clergy sexual abuse as destroying the most sensitive parts of an individual's identity, a sacred role and relationship, the sacred institution that legitimated the minister, a set of rituals and symbols, and the individual's understanding of God as loving.[25] They describe clergy sexual abuse as 'an earthquake . . . that creates spiritual havoc'.[26]

Amongst direct victims, spiritual grounding is disrupted, vulnerability and innocence are stolen, and the ability to trust is gravely undermined.[27] The betrayal of trust can also be devastating to congregations, impacting not only personal and collective identity and spirituality but also the structure of the community of faith and its shared fundamental assumptions about God and life.[28] Nils Friberg observes that there will be a diversity of responses among congregants to an occurrence of clergy sexual abuse depending on the context, the quality of the pastoral relationship and personal attributes of the congregant. When a minister has attended the personal and family crises of the congregant, the sense of betrayal can be immense: 'The basic fabric of life gets torn. God seems to have let us down . . .'.[29] People question the legitimacy of sacred moments involving offender ministers; places of worship are soiled; new encounters with clergy are seen through the lenses of the prior abuse.[30]

The trauma can be multileveled: there is the original trauma to the direct victims; trauma to others, including the congregation at the point of disclosure; and inadequate institutional response which increases the trauma, as does the absence of adverse consequences or clear accountability for the

23 Patricia L. Liberty, 'Power and Abuse: Establishing the Context', in *When a Congregation is Betrayed*, 26.

24 Ken Wells, 'A Needs Assessment Regarding the Nature and Impact of Clergy Sexual Abuse Conducted by the Interfaith Sexual Trauma Institute', *Sexual Addiction and Compulsivity* 10 (2003): 206.

25 Pargament et al., 'Problem and Solution', 403–404.

26 Pargament et al., 'Problem and Solution', 404.

27 Maris, 'that which is hidden', 4.

28 Alexander L. Veerman and R. Ruard Ganzevoort, 'Communities Coping with Collective Trauma', Paper for the International Association for the Psychology of Religion (Soesterberg, The Netherlands, 2001), 5.

29 Friberg, 'Wounded Congregations', 58.

30 Paul M. Kline, Robert McMackin and Edna Lezotte, 'The Impact of the Clergy Abuse Scandal on Parish Communities', *Journal of Child Sexual Abuse* 17, nos. 3–4 (2008): 298. See also Barry O'Sullivan, *The Burden of Betrayal: Non-offending priests and the clergy child sexual abuse scandals* (Leominster: Gracewing, 2018).

offender.[31] The latter, unfortunately, has been common. The 'automatic' institutional response is to 'shoot the messenger', misname the problem and blame the victim.[32]

Past institutional failure

In previous decades, the institutional response to clergy sexual abuse protected the offender and the reputation of the institution rather than protecting the victims. The remedy was 'the geographical cure': male clergy who abused women or children were offered treatment and financial assistance and moved to another ministry setting, without consequence for the clergy or warning for the new setting.[33] This phenomenon reflects the patriarchal nature of the Church, ignoring the suffering of women and children whilst maintaining the power of the minister.[34] The experience for the victim who reported abuse was that they were abused twice: the first time by the offender and the second time by the Church.[35]

From the 1980s, however, there have been concerted attempts to redress the Church's inadequate and injurious handling of cases of clergy sexual abuse. It began because victim-survivors successfully asserted claims in criminal and civil courts in North America.[36] The stories of individuals who had survived clergy sexual abuse fuelled the search for answers to the problem.[37] Articles and books were published, and policies and procedures promulgated as advocates and churches sought to right the wrong and equip a

31 Deborah Pope-Lance, 'Trauma Intervention: Planning Strategies for Recovery', in *When a Congregation Is Betrayed*, 48.

32 Marie M. Fortune, *Is Nothing Sacred? When Sex Invades the Pastoral Relationship* (San Francisco: Harper San Francisco, 1992), 120. See also Ken Wells, Ralph H. Earle and Marcus R. Earle, 'Outpatient and Inpatient Intensive Treatment Models', in *Clergy Sexual Misconduct: A Systems Approach to Prevention, Intervention and Oversight*, ed. John Thoburn, Rob Baker and Maria Dal Maso (Carefree, AZ: Gentle Path, 2011), loc. 1393, who observe that denial and minimisation are well-established patterns for the Church in such cases.

33 Nancy Myer Hopkins, 'Best Practices After Betrayal is Discovered', in *When a Congregation Is Betrayed*, 3; Poling, *Abuse of Power*, 150–151; Hopkins, 'The Uses and Limitations', 268.

34 Poling, *Abuse of Power*, 14, 123: 'Power and privilege become organised in institutional forms that resist change, and these forms are protected by powerful ideologies that promote the power of some groups at the expense of others. Unjust ideologies create a state of affairs in which adults are privileged over children, men are privileged over women, whites are privileged over people of color, and rich are privileged over poor.'

35 Melinda, 'A Bent-Over Woman Stands Up', in *Victim to Survivor: Women Recovering From Clergy Sexual Abuse*, ed. Nancy Werking Poling (Cleveland, OH: United Church, 1999), provides a compelling testimony about church leaders protecting abusive male clergy and seeking to silence women who have been abused.

36 Hopkins, 'The Uses and Limitations', 268.

37 Marie M. Fortune's *Is Nothing Sacred?* is the groundbreaking publication that alerted the wider Church to the problem. It tells the story of Revd Dr. Peter Donovan of First Church of Newburg, who groomed and exploited a number of women in the congregation.

better response to victims of clergy sexual abuse.[38] Nancy Myer Hopkins, drawing on her experience of working with wounded congregations, began publishing articles and editing and contributing to books on the topic.[39] Hopkins's work, alongside that of others, is drawn on later in this chapter.

First responses

When a congregation learns that its minister has been accused of sexual abuse, everyone in the congregation is victimised to some extent. The impact on a particular individual will be shaped by external factors – the intensity and severity of the abuse, the identity of the victim(s), the congregation's history and the means of disclosure – and by internal factors such as their relationship with the minister and the church, personal history and personal skills and characteristics.[40] The trauma is collective not only because of the number of traumatised individuals involved in the congregation but also because of the injury to the congregation's structure and shared fundamental assumptions.[41]

Within this variability, however, there are some predictable responses.[42] The first is *shocked disbelief* and *denial*. In the face of the shocking news, the system goes into overdrive to throw up defences and protect itself from harm.[43] The strength of this response should not be underestimated – it is

38 Early publications, with Marie Fortune's *Is Nothing Sacred?*, include Mary D. Pellauer, Barbara Chester and Jane Boyajian, eds., *Sexual Assault and Abuse: A Handbook for Clergy and Religious Professionals* (San Francisco, CA: Harper San Francisco, 1987) with one chapter on responding to clients sexually exploited by clergy; Karen Lebacqz and Ronald G. Barton, *Sex in the Parish* (Louisville, KY: Westminster John Knox, 1991); Richard M. Gula, S.S., *Ethics in Pastoral Ministry* (New York and Mahwah, NJ: Paulist, 1996); and Nils C. Friberg and Mark R. Laaser, *Before the Fall: Preventing Pastoral Sexual Abuse* (Collegeville, MN: Liturgical, 1998).

39 Nancy Myer Hopkins, *The Congregational Response to Clergy Betrayals of Trust* (Collegeville, MN: Liturgical, 1998) is a helpful handbook for congregations in distress. Published in association with the Interfaith Sexual Trauma Institute, it is no longer in print. Other Hopkins publications include Nancy Myer Hopkins and Mark Laaser, eds., *Restoring the Soul of a Church: Healing Congregations Wounded by Clergy Sexual Misconduct* (Collegeville, MN: Liturgical, 1995) and chapters in Beth Ann Gaede, ed., *When a Congregation Is Betrayed: Responding to Clergy Misconduct* (Herndon, VA: The Alban Institute, 2006).

40 Veerman and Ganzevoort, 'Communities Coping', 4; Friberg, 'Wounded Congregations', 55–57.

41 Veerman and Ganzevoort, 'Communities Coping', 9.

42 Hammeal-Urban, *Wholeness After Betrayal*, loc. 422–438; Mosgofian and Ohlschlager, *Sexual Misconduct*, 182. Mosgofian and Ohlschlager list common responses noted by the Minnesota Interfaith Committee on Sexual Exploitation by Clergy. The authors observe that 'consistent with trauma theory and the denial/shock response, most church organisms are thrown into immediate disarray and act to protect the rest of the body, or parts of it, from further harm' (p. 183).

43 Friberg, 'Wounded Congregations', 58–59. Veerman and Ganzevoort, 'Communities Coping', 2–3, observe that the congregation's efforts to protect the minister are actually efforts

particularly intractable in cases of clergy sexual abuse because of the power of the ministerial role.[44] Here, trauma theory helps to explain the phenomenon: when a person is traumatised, the more primitive parts of the brain take over and the individual's capacity to receive information and process it is impaired.[45] What is happening is the body's coping mechanism in response to information that is overwhelming spiritually, emotionally or psychologically. As discussed in the 'Best Practices' section, what people need upon receiving the shocking news is to express their emotional responses and thoughts in a safe and accepting environment. Given the impaired cognition and enflamed emotional state of people in the congregation in early trauma, confrontation will get those seeking to assist the congregation nowhere and may be further damaging.[46] After the shock abates, the provision of accurate information that is repeated over time along with the sensitive acknowledgement that the information is hard to hear and hard to accept is the only thing that will counteract disbelief and denial.[47] It is important to note here the importance of an initial sustained listening exercise in which feelings are accepted and validated without censorship or judgment.

Connected to denial is anger. The focus of the anger is usually first directed at the bearer of the bad news: the denominational leader who delivers it[48] and the unnamed person(s) who made the complaint, particularly if that person is female.[49] Again, this emotional response is protective of the congregation. But anger is also a normal and necessary stage of grief, and the congregation is not only betrayed but also bereaved. One of the tasks for the leadership of the congregation is to facilitate the safe expression of anger. People who have been victims of abuse in the past may react particularly strongly as displaced anger bubbles up from prior experiences.[50]

It is common that denial and anger get focused on blaming the victim, especially if the victim is female.[51] Adult victims are frequently scapegoated by some or most of the congregation because believing that the beloved minister could do such things is unbearable.[52] Not only is the victim blamed,

---

to protect themselves. See also Chilton Knudsen, 'Understanding Congregational Dynamics', in *Restoring the Soul of the Church*, 97.

44 Patricia L. Liberty, 'Grief and Loss: Dealing with Feelings', in *When a Congregation is Betrayed*, 40; Hopkins, 'Congregational Intervention', 249, 251.

45 Bessel Van Der Kolk, *The Body Keeps the Score* (London: Penguin Random House, 2014), 51–73.

46 Liberty, 'Grief and Loss', 40.

47 Liberty, 'Grief and Loss', 40.

48 Harold Hopkins, 'The Effects of Clergy Sexual Misconduct on the Wider Church', in *Restoring the Soul of the Church*, 128, 132–133; E. Larraine Frampton, 'Conflict Management', 35. Harold Hopkins notes that for denominational executives, dealing with cases of clergy sexual abuse is second only to the death of a spouse in the degree of stress.

49 Kline et al., 'Impact', 293–294; Hopkins, 'Congregational Intervention', 248, 252.

50 Hopkins, 'Congregational Intervention', 252.

51 Hopkins, 'Congregational Intervention', 252; Wells, 'Needs Assessment', 206.

52 Benyei, *Understanding Clergy Misconduct*, 95.

but female spouses of offending clergy are also blamed.[53] Like denial, scapegoating and victim-blaming protect fundamental assumptions.[54] They are normal responses to the trauma of clergy sexual abuse and necessary first stages in the move towards recovery.[55] The congregation is an emotional system that, like all others, aims towards homeostasis. The collective process requires that some people defend the minister.[56] Nonetheless, as time goes on, victim-blaming prevents individuals from grappling with what has happened. Moreover, it can be persistent, leading to divided loyalties and conflict within the congregation, and is resistant to change.[57] Hopkins asserts that blaming the victim must be challenged: the congregation needs to be reminded that the source of their pain and chaos is a result of the offender's behaviours, not because victims came forward or a spouse was not paying attention.[58] Again, this is a message that will need to be given sensitively at the right time and possibly repeatedly, without demonising the offender or his supporters. Not only will such a message aid the recovery of the congregation in time, but it will also prevent further suffering to those blamed.

In the maelstrom of emotion surrounding the disclosure of clergy sexual abuse, it is important that everyone involved – the alleged perpetrator, the victim(s), congregational members – be treated as people deserving of dignity and care. The congregation's recovery will be aided if they are assured that both the alleged perpetrator and the victim are being provided with pastoral care and support. When an alleged perpetrator is accorded dignity, as well as being held to account for his or her actions, it helps the victim (who may have complex feelings which may include guilt that they felt special receiving the minister's attention).[59]

In the weeks and months thereafter . . .

After the initial shock begins to wear off, the congregation's recovery begins by grieving the losses sustained as a result of the betrayal of trust. As will be discussed in the 'Best Practices' section, a guided intentional recovery process

53 Friberg, 'Wounded Congregations', 67; Grenz and Bell, *Betrayal of Trust*, 151, 155.

54 R. Ruard Ganzevoort, 'Scars and Stigmata: Trauma, Identity and Theology', *Practical Theology* 1, no. 1 (2008): 29. Ganzevoort draws on psychologist Ronnie Janoff-Bulman's theory of basic assumptions, which posits that individuals have assumptive worlds or systems of meaning that hold together our life and identity. These assumptive worlds shatter in the face of trauma but retain some resilience as defences are thrown up in self-protection. See also, R. Ruard Ganzevoort, 'Religious Coping Reconsidered, Part Two: A Narrative Reformulation', *Journal of Psychology and Theology* 26, no. 3 (1998): 286.

55 Personal conversation, Angela McKean, mental health professional, July 2018.

56 Personal conversation, R. Ruard Ganzevoort, practical theologian, November 2018.

57 Friberg, 'Wounded Congregations', 60, 72–73.

58 Nancy Myer Hopkins, 'Congregations: Further Steps in Healing', in *When a Congregation is Betrayed*, 65, 143; Friberg, 'Wounded Congregations', 61.

59 Personal conversation, Lynn Stoney, co-founder and facilitator of 'Constellation Workshops', November 2018.

with emotional, educational and spiritual elements best serves a traumatised congregation which has begun a journey that could last years. It is impossible to predict how long a congregation will be in recovery; the damage done by clergy sexual abuse is subtle and deeper than people will expect. The crisis phase usually lasts six months or longer, depending on diverse variables.[60] If there are legal proceedings involved, the congregation will not be given sufficient information until the conclusion of the proceedings and will be further traumatised by a conviction or civil judgement.[61] Long-term recovery, which includes integration of the event and behavioural change in the congregation that will prevent further abuse, can take 10 years.[62] Recovery will not be linear. There will be setbacks and challenges, as well as movement towards recovery, and what people will need to further recover will change. The new or interim minister who leads the congregation in the aftermath of an offending minister will pay a particularly high price in the process. Called "afterpastors" in the American literature, these clergy face bewildering behaviours and distinctive stresses as a result of the original offences.[63] Their average tenure is short, and their need for support is high.[64] The good news is that congregations who face into the trauma and work intentionally on recovery can experience renewal and strengthening.

Basic care in the response to any trauma revolves around three elements: calming, communicating and caring.[65] In the first weeks after a traumatising disclosure, people are trying to cope with the pain of what they have heard. The leadership's primary tasks are to make safe spaces for the expression

60 Nancy Myer Hopkins, 'Living Through the Crisis', in *Restoring the Soul of a Church*, 201. Variables that impact recovery include the congregation's history, whether it is an open or closed system, the health of key leaders, the presence of the offender in community and whether he is recovering, the status of family members of victims and offenders, and the support of the denomination (see pp. 225–231). Glenndy Sculley, 'Judicatory Leaders: A Resource for Healing', in *When a Congregation is Betrayed*, 110, recommends one to three years of recovery work before the congregation calls a permanent minister.

61 Hopkins, 'Living Through the Crisis', 202.

62 E. Larraine Frampton, 'Response Teams: Laying a Foundation for Recovery', in *When a Congregation is Betrayed*, 114; E. Larraine Frampton, 'Reassessing the Recovery of the Faith Community', in *When a Congregation is Betrayed*, 137; Matthew Linden, 'Managing Situations That Might Never Be Good', in *When a Congregation is Betrayed*, 178.

63 See, for example, Knudsen, 'Congregational Dynamics', 82–91.

64 The average tenure of afterpastors is three years (Linden, 'Managing Situations', 178). The work is difficult. Linden remarks (at 177) that 'ministry in the aftermath of a fire is a walk in the park compared with being an afterpastor'. For more resources for afterpastors, see Deborah Pope-Lance, 'Afterpastors: Restoring Pastoral Trust', in *When a Congregation is Betrayed*, 53–63; Candace R. Benyei, 'Psychological and Spiritual Resources for Afterpastors', in *When a Congregation is Betrayed*, 162–170; Darlene K. Haskin, 'Afterpastors in Troubled Congregations', in *Restoring the Soul*, 155–172; Nancy Myer Hopkins, 'Further Issues for Afterpastors', in *Restoring the Soul*, 165–172; and Hammeal-Urban, *Wholeness After Betrayal*, loc. 470–484.

65 Laurie Kraus, David Holyan and Bruce Wismer, *Recovering From Un-Natural Disasters* (Louisville, KY: Westminster John Knox, 2017), xiv, 5, 7.

of feelings, to reassure people that what they are going through is a normal response to an extraordinary and difficult situation, to provide clear and accurate information about what has happened, and to plan a recovery process. If there are limits to what information can be disclosed, it is helpful if a law enforcement officer or lawyer explains to the gathered congregation why that is and what they can expect as time goes by.

In these first weeks in particular, leaders themselves may be traumatised, so it is essential to have the support of the denomination.[66] As time goes by that support continues to be important: the leadership will be called on to exercise responsibilities well outside of its prior experience for potentially a long time. There will be resistance and reactivity in the congregation. Conflict and divided loyalties often arise, and leaders (especially afterpastors) may become the target of displaced anger and mistrust. Feelings of shame, fear and self-doubt may emerge as the lay leadership copes with the prior minister's deceit and manipulation.

The congregation's journey in the aftermath of clergy sexual abuse has been described as a grief process.[67] It is a complex grief process, made all the more difficult by the nature of the harm caused by the betrayal of trust. Numerous individuals are making the journey in different ways and at different rates, and there is the possibility of further traumatisation as the situation continues to develop and as people cope with the strong reactions of others. Leaders are tasked with attending to individuals with different needs and with attending to the community as a whole. It is good to remember that the congregation's ordinary practices of worship and service will root and ground it, providing both a foundation and food for the journey for individuals and for the community. Recovery for individuals is highly dependent on the support of the congregation,[68] a fact that should never be far from the leadership's collective mind.

Distinctive elements of congregational grieving in the aftermath of clergy sexual abuse include pressures to 'forgive and forget' and to 'get over it' in order to do the work of the Gospel. The reality is that the work of recovery *is* the work of the Gospel. Learning to be calm, communicate and care in a traumatised congregation and to accept the diverse reactions of fellow church members builds the community for the sake of Gospel. Pressure to forgive is often an unconscious ploy to cover up denial or to put a plaster on the deep wound of betrayal. It can be strong, as anxiety and discomfort drive an effort to begin to feel better. But it untenably places the burden of responsibility to make the situation right onto the injured party. Moreover, premature forgiveness will not work and does further damage to victims

66 Kraus et al., *Recovering*, 57, emphasise the need for skilled assistance from outside the congregation in the aftermath of clergy sexual misconduct.

67 Liberty, 'Grief and Loss', 40–45; Laaser, 'Long-Term Healing', 232–250.

68 R. Ruard Ganzevoort, 'Religious Coping, Part Two', 285.

and the offender.[69] Rather, more in-depth exploration of forgiveness – in sermons or small groups – will give people the opportunity to work with their discomfort and deepen their understanding of true reconciliation that includes accountability alongside compassion.

As individuals' strong feelings fade, they will begin to be able cognitively to process information that will enable them to make sense of what happened and how best to respond. Because of the variability in individuals' reactions and recovery, to be effective, information will need to be clear and offered at different times. Education that will help with sense-making includes the normal processes involved in trauma and grief, the power dynamics inherent in the ministerial relationship and the minister's duty of care, and the impact of clergy sexual abuse on the direct and secondary victims, including the congregation.[70] Seminars on sexuality and spirituality may be useful to dispel paranoia about sexual matters and to equip people to talk more openly; shame and secrecy about sex foster the possibility of abuse. In due time, the congregation will be ready to do the hard work of examining the unwitting complicity of its structures or attitudes that may have permitted the abuse to evolve. New practices, policies and procedures can be developed that will strengthen the community and prevent the possibility of future abuse.

A word about worship and spiritual nurture

While the normal worship practices of the congregation will significantly resource recovery, there will be special needs in the aftermath of abuse that will shape those practices. Church rituals are containers for both pain and grace. Acknowledging the pain and confusion that people are experiencing in prayers and liturgy enables safe passage through difficult feelings. As discussed elsewhere in this volume, psalms of lament may be particularly helpful. Lamentation places the grievance at the foot of God and demands a response. The whole of the mess is thus entrusted to God – the injury to victims, the deep sense of betrayal, the violation of the sacred.

Through worship, Bible study and prayer groups, the congregation may be resourced to see its own journey of recovery as a faith journey. Drawing on the stories of the faith, a period of unknowing becomes a wandering in the wilderness,[71] feelings of isolation mirror the exile, sharing in the suffering of victims is a communion with Christ, and the experience of new insight that brings new life is a resurrection.

69 Liberty, 'Theological Reflection: Naming the Problem', in *When a Congregation is Betrayed*, 19; Nancy Myer Hopkins, 'Remembering the Victim', in *When a Congregation Is Betrayed*, 143; Laaser, 'Long-Term Healing', 249. Laaser testifies that consequences for the offender and justice for the victim enable healing and reconciliation.

70 Hopkins, 'Further Steps', 66–69.

71 See, for example, Hammeal-Urban, *Wholeness After Betrayal*, loc. 1733ff.

The sacred stories, places and symbols of the faith are precious resources, as is the congregation itself. If they have been defiled, they may be restored. Places or objects within the church may be ritually cleansed and rededicated; children may be blessed; litanies of healing and commitment may be created and recited to a resounding Amen.

Best practice in aid of recovery

The experience of those who work with congregations that have experienced clergy sexual abuse is that careful disclosure and an intentional, structured healing process best serve the long-term health and well-being of congregations.[72] In contrast, failing to disclose the abuse to the congregation has effects that are far-reaching and long-lasting.[73] Robin Hammeal-Urban observes that

> in the wake of misconduct, there is often a sense of separateness, broken relationships among members, unhealthy power differentials, secret keeping and displaced anger . . . without a timely and appropriate response to the misconduct, these unhealthy dynamics can become the way a congregation operates for decades.[74]

The essential elements of a disclosure and recovery process as identified by practitioners are the following:[75]

1 *Disclosure*. Recall the three strategies for coping with trauma: calming, communicating and caring. Timely disclosure of accurate information fulfils all three and sets the congregation on the road to recovery. Information must be available to everyone in the congregation at the same time;[76] a prepared disclosure statement that is read out at the beginning of a disclosure meeting can be emailed or posted to members of the congregation who do not attend. A disclosure meeting can last from two to five hours and should be led by facilitators not from the congregation, with denominational participation and support. After the disclosure

72 Chilton Knudsen, 'Congregational Dynamics', 78, 97–101; Hopkins, 'Best Practices', 2–13; Hammeal-Urban, *Wholeness After Betrayal, passim*.

73 Hammeal-Urban, *Wholeness After Betrayal*, loc. 662–720. See also Knudsen, 'Congregational Dynamics', 75–93, for a description of predictable behavioural symptoms that mar congregational ministry and mission when clergy misconduct has not been faced and worked through.

74 Hammeal-Urban, *Wholeness After Betrayal*, loc. 484.

75 These elements are drawn from the practices described in Hopkins, 'Best Practices', 2–3; and E. Larraine Frampton, 'Critical Incident Stress Management', in *When a Congregation is Betrayed*, 214–217. Hammeal-Urban, *Wholeness After Betrayal*, includes in appendices sample disclosure statements for the congregation and for the press, an outline of responsibilities for a disclosure meeting, and a checklist for care of victims and offenders.

76 Hopkins, 'Further Steps', 65.

statement is read, it is important to give people the opportunity to ask questions for clarification. Note that victims are never named. Disclosure and clarification are followed by an opportunity to react.

2 *Small-Group Listening*. People need to express their thoughts and emotional responses in a safe environment. Small-group facilitators from the congregation can be trained, and guidelines for the conduct of the group can be provided.[77] Strong emotions should be expected, along with the first responses discussed earlier: shock, denial and disbelief, anger and blame. The purpose of the small-group listening is not to set things right or debate the matter but to allow individuals to express themselves.

3 *Education*. Although people will have varying abilities to process information cognitively depending on their state of traumatisation, it is never too early to begin providing clear and accessible information that will help them to make sense of what has happened. What information is needed will depend on the context and offending behaviour. Fact sheets may be helpful, highlighting the information provided, so that people can take it home to review later. Topics that will be useful from the beginning are ministerial power, the communal journey through trauma and grief, and the impact of clergy sexual abuse on victims.

4 *Next steps*. Informing people what will happen next is another calming strategy. They have been given shocking news and an overload of information. A map of the way ahead reduces anxiety and sets expectations that timely updates will be given and that thought and prayer will guide the congregation through the valley of the shadow. It is recommended that a task force be set up for six months to a year with the express aim of assisting the recovery of the congregation.[78]

5 *Spiritual reflection*. Ask people, in the gathered group or in small groups, to share with each other where and how they know God to be in their midst. Hymns may be suggested; Bible stories or prayers offered. Ending the meeting in this way has been reported to be very positive, and it sets the tone for the work of recovery and integration.

In the weeks and months that follow, a recovery task force can take the temperature of the congregation, consider the needs of vulnerable groups in the church such as children, prayerfully discern what additional listening or educational tasks may help recovery, draw in experts from other fields as needed and implement events in consultation with the leadership. It can also intervene in any resistance or reactivity among members by listening to those who are struggling to accept what has happened, asking what they need and communicating the task force's role and commitment to recovery for the whole congregation. The work of a task force will vary enormously

77 Hopkins, 'Best Practices', 8–9.

78 Advice for the organization and equipping of a recovery task force can be found in Hopkins, 'Further Steps', 69–71.

depending on the offending event, the context and available resources. The work of recovery can enable people to face personal issues as well as invigorate congregational life.

Further down the line, the task force or another group can assist the congregation to do the hard work of looking at its structures, attitudes and behaviours to ask if there were ways that it unintentionally allowed the offending behaviour to evolve.[79] Are there clear lines of communication and accountability? Do the unwritten rules of the congregation (*don't rock the boat; the minister is always right*) make it impossible to confront unacceptable behaviour? Are safeguarding policies and practices up to date, and are staff and others trained? Is the minister adequately supported? Or is he or she expected to work all hours to the detriment of well-being and family relationships? Having experienced what can happen without care and attention, the congregation is in a place to reshape the way it does things to prevent the possibility of future abuse.

It is also important that the leadership communicates a willingness to receive and respond to any concerns individuals may have about a past or present, ordained or lay, leader's behaviour or activities. Finally, as trauma often reveals a multitude of other sins and because clergy sexual abuse is more likely to occur where congregational systems enable it, it is advised that a financial audit be undertaken.[80]

Integration and post-traumatic growth

As with any trauma, the end goal of recovery is not a return to things as they were. The congregation has experienced a profound event that may have shattered their world view and their understanding of the trustworthiness not only of clergy but also of God. Integration of the experience requires not only the recovery work described earlier but also the reweaving of one's story of the nature of God and how God interacts with humanity. Human beings are storytelling creatures; we write and rewrite the story of our selves throughout our lifetimes, making sense of our experiences.[81] When a crisis happens, the framework of the story of one's life is shattered. As one gathers the fragments, makes meaning of events and reframes the story, there arises the opportunity to gain new, more realistic and more durable understandings of God and of human beings.

79 Benyei, *Understanding Clergy Misconduct*, 153; Benyei, 'Systems: Identifying the Roots', in *When a Congregation is Betrayed*, 37–39. See also Nancy Biele, 'Creating Safer Congregations', in *When a Congregation is Betrayed*, 147–155, for areas of congregational life to review in order to enhance congregational health and ministry whilst preventing future abuse.

80 Biele, 'Safer Congregations', 151.

81 Antonio Damasio, *The Feeling of What Happens: Body, Emotion and the Making of Consciousness* (London: Random House, 2000), 224–226; Ganzevoort, 'Religious Coping, Part Two', 284.

The task of reassembling the story begins almost immediately and inchoately. Experiencing the trauma with the community of faith and making the journey of recovery together, individuals begin slowly to make meaning. Theological reflection and spiritual nurturing through the church's life together (worship, small-group work) facilitates this. But the most important factor is the experience of the support of the congregation. Meaning-making is a social process; spiritual support from the community is one of the strongest correlates of successful integration. As Ruard Ganzevoort reports, '[s]imply and boldly put, the experience of a supportive social context is a prerequisite for the experience of a supportive God'.[82]

Meaning-making is corporately supported but highly personal. Not everyone will have the same interpretation of what happened. Acceptance of the event – the final stage of grief – is evidenced not by an agreed interpretation of events but rather by agreement that the congregation has suffered and now has a renewed commitment to mission and ministry.[83] What is important is that the truth has been told, the facts disclosed, and people understand and accept that not everyone will respond to such events in the same way or come to the same conclusions.[84]

For some, the event will have required a reframing of their understanding of how God works in the world. Crises are significant moments for faith development. The meaning horizon is broken open, and new possibilities arise.[85] Beliefs accepted in the innocence of childhood come face-to-face with the realities of human existence and may be found wanting. In the aftermath of clergy sexual abuse, an appreciation of sometimes neglected biblical images for God can resource reframing. An all-powerful Father may be re-imagined as a nurturant Mother Eagle carrying people on her wing; a distant transcendent God uninvolved in the sorrows of the world may become an immanent God suffering with God's people and strengthening them.[86] Individuals may come to see God and humanity as working in partnership and to re-imagine their own role in the unfolding kingdom of God. Faith is a journey. The earliest Christians were called People of the Way, a name well suited to a learning, growing community seeking to walk the way of Christ in a world where violence and betrayal happen even in the community of faith.

Conclusion

How does a congregation know that it has integrated the experience of clergy sexual abuse and is on the other side? Laurie Kraus *et al*[87] posit that, as a

82 R. Ruard Ganzevoort, 'Religious Coping Reconsidered, Part One: An Integrated Approach', *Journal of Psychology and Theology* 26, no. 3 (1998): 270.
83 Liberty, 'Grief and Loss', 45.
84 Hammeal-Urban, *Wholeness After Betrayal*, loc. 2397–2424.
85 Ganzevoort, 'Religious Coping, Part One', 269.
86 Pargament et al., 'Problem and Solution', 410.
87 Kraus et al., *Recovering*, 101–103.

congregation moves forward on the journey of recovery, they move towards wisdom. A post-traumatic community of wisdom has a deeper acceptance of both the gifts and the limitations inherent in human life; there is a willingness to accept human fallibility, yielding up shame to a more generous and gentle life together. The trauma may have awakened a new sense of calling, based on what has been learned. After a period – maybe a long period – of survival and self-examination, a post-traumatic community of wisdom will be keen to reach out to serve others. Congregations that have looked hard at their internal workings will have crafted new ways to assure accountability and transparency and to safeguard the vulnerable. As they live into these new ways and slowly rebuild the capacity to trust God, they may reclaim the joy of faith and the hope for a new day when no child, no woman, no man need fear abuse by another.

Select references

Benyei, Candace R. *Understanding Clergy Misconduct in Religious Systems: Scapegoating, Family Secrets, and the Abuse of Power*. New York/London: Haworth Pastoral, 1998.

Churches Together in Britain and Ireland. *Time for Action: Sexual Abuse, the Churches and a New Dawn for Survivors*. London: CTBI, 2002.

Fogler, Jason M., Jillian C. Shipherd, Stephanie Clarke, Jennifer Jensen and Erin Rowe. 'The Impact of Clergy-Perpetrated Sexual Abuse: The Role of Gender, Development, and Posttraumatic Stress'. *Journal of Child Sexual Abuse* 17, nos. 3–4 (2008): 329–358.

Gaede, Beth Ann, ed. *When a Congregation Is Betrayed: Responding to Clergy Misconduct*. Herndon, VA: The Alban Institute, 2006.

Hopkins, Nancy Myer. *The Congregational Response to Clergy Betrayals of Trust*. Collegeville, MN: Liturgical, 1998.

Hopkins, Nancy Myer and Mark Laaser, eds. *Restoring the Soul of a Church: Healing Congregations Wounded by Clergy Sexual Misconduct*. Collegeville, MN: Liturgical, 1995.

Kraus, Laurie, David Holyan and Bruce Wismer. *Recovering From Un-Natural Disasters*. Louisville, KY: Westminster John Knox, 2017.

Poling, James. *The Abuse of Power: A Theological Problem*. Nashville, TN: Abingdon, 1991.

Part VI

Implications for care and self-care of ministers

Introduction to Part VI

In this last section of the book we consider the implications of traumatic experiences for clergy care, self-care and training. We do so through the medium of an extended interview with an experienced practitioner whose career has been devoted to the care of ministers and their families in varying degrees of distress, from tiredness and burnout to post-traumatic stress disorder.

The interview brings out many of the themes we have explored in this book, in particular the whole-body, physiological character of trauma, the triggering of past experiences and the contrast between the 'heroic' phase of response to a shock event and subsequent disillusionment. The importance of narrative, and of having someone witness to that narrative, also resurfaces. Valuable principles of care are offered, including the need to lower levels of arousal, the need for wisdom in the use of email and social media and the very physical needs of the body if it is to relax.

The Christian churches do not have as good a track record of ministerial care as might be hoped of such organisations, and the interview shows how easily even help that is offered may be misconstrued. Also, how pernicious the concept of resilience can be if wrongly deployed, even implicitly.

The interview then turns to the question of how individual ministers may grow through the emotional learning derived from trauma and recovery, and how they may best care for themselves. The inevitable question arises, as to where God is in these experiences, and the reader will want to ponder what more can be said in this area.

Finally, there is a consideration of what can be offered to ministers in their initial training, which takes the conversation back to the all-important question of the resources on which the new minister will draw.

Part VI

17 Annotated interview with Sarah Horsman

Christopher Southgate

Members of the Sheldon (Mary and Martha) Community run a retreat and education centre in Devon. Their primary work is to provide support resources to people in Christian ministry at times of stress, crisis, burnout or breakdown. For 30 years, they have been aiming to provide effective, affordable, confidential, short-term help.

Dr Sarah Horsman was one of the founder members of the Society, and was elected Warden in 2014. She came to Sheldon after completing basic medical training and has followed an eclectic learning path along a range of approaches to mental and physical health.

She is interviewed here by Christopher Southgate, and the text has been edited for ease of reading.

Sarah begins by reflecting on the particular issue of sudden congregational tragedy that has been the focus of the project. She begins,

R: We tend to see people who have been through some sort of personal trauma or tragedy and we don't have a particularly wide experience of people going through things like the bigger congregational tragedies that you're talking about – which is maybe interesting in itself.

I: **It's often the case though, isn't it, that there are things that have happened in ministry which may not be particularly huge in themselves, but they knock against personal stuff in ways that amplify it.**

R: Absolutely. One that came to mind, when you were asking about how people present, was somebody whose brother had died completely unexpectedly. She'd heard the news in a situation where she had no support, came home to cover for her colleague who was on holiday, and was straight into a sudden death in the parish and supporting somebody else. She put on her professional hat, she got on with it, but two or three months later she was really struggling. This is slightly more hidden than the flamboyant, 'Oh, this is the big thing that's happening now.' It's often those sorts of things that I think we most notice in our work here.

I: **Can you think of times though when people have come, maybe not in crisis, but needing the space because something unexpected had happened in their church?**

R: We've certainly had situations where people have been dealing with a murder in the parish or a body found in the parish or somebody from the parish who has been murdered. Situations where a colleague has been accused of child sex offences, situations like a multiple road crash or an air crash or something like that. We would not necessarily be seeing people in the immediate aftermath of those, we're much more likely to be seeing people a few months, six months, a year, a couple of years down the line when they're processing and reorienting, having coped in the moment, because people so often do pull out what's needed in the moment. Another thing I notice – and maybe it's why those particular people end up here or maybe it's a more general thing – the number of times people will say, 'I was already over-stretched and then this came along.' You never get to choose when the big things happen to you, do you, they just happen – they do by definition happen unexpectedly and it's a strong argument for not living in permanent over-stretch.

I: **So people find they've coped in the moment, because people do, but then they've somehow recognised the need to take stock or to process further this disruptive event?**

R: How would people get to know that they need to do something? It can be quite varied. For some people it can be a progressive loss of energy, focus, sense of aliveness, wellbeing, a sense that that's just gradually grinding down or winding down. Sometimes it can be feeling anxious, maybe flashbacks, maybe not sleeping, maybe self-medicating – alcohol, whatever. Sometimes it's other people noticing, particularly with depression and depressed mood and flatness and not quite being with it. I would say it's as often colleagues or family who will pick up that side of things. The anxiety distress is often more like, 'I can't tolerate this, I'll go and get help', whereas the sort of going flat is harder to see from the inside. It's more often people around you that notice, and that again is a good sort of self-care thing to know that there are people around you who you trust well enough and they know to be able to say to you, 'Are things really okay?'

I: **Yes. So I'm just wondering whether we could make a connection with the diagram of the dynamics of congregational response in the book *Recovering from Un-natural Disasters,*[1] which contains the heroic phase of response to a shock event, followed by the so-called disillusionment phase of a congregation, when the heroic phase is over and the squabbling and confusion and disorientation that sets in after that heroic phase can be very painful. So what the project team say, rightly or wrongly, is that that's the time clergy are most likely to need support and least likely to seek it. Does that ring any bells with you?**

1 Laurie Kraus, David Holyan and Bruce Wismer, *Recovering From Un-Natural Disasters* (Louisville, KY: Westminster John Knox, 2017).

R: I like the term *the heroic phase*, because it captures one of the things that's both useful and so potentially dangerous about adrenaline. It actually feels very good, that initial stepping up and responding, almost to the extent of a high, and I don't mean that at all critically because I've been through that myself. And I know that you actually need it at that stage, but that it's also dangerous – partly because it can make you over-confident and partly because you don't factor the cost of it. It's overdraft energy, it's not part of your running budget. You're going to have to pay for it in due course.

I: **And yet the desire to regain the high can be very strong, can't it?**

R: Yes, because it's nice, it feels nice. However ghastly the thing that you're dealing with, there is a paradoxical feeling – is pleasure too strong a word? There is something that is desirable within that experience.

I: **As in that disastrous quote after the fire at Grenfell Tower, where a cleric, when asked how the last 24 hours had been, called them 'exhilarating'.**

R: Ouch, yes. Because you're needed, you're the focus of attention – that exactly encapsulates it. And, of course, it looks so totally off-key. This can also happen in a more chronic sense if you're just in chronic overload and you're struggling more and more to stay on top of things. You might just sort of slide off into depression, but it's also quite common to get a bit of a high and overconfidence before you crash. I think we would save ourselves and other people an awful lot of misery if we actually understood a bit more of how that feels like from the inside and how the high is a warning sign, not a sign that it's all okay. Certainly, I learnt that the hard way, absolutely the hard way. I think most people do because we don't understand that it's a short-term gift for a specific need, but that it's a gift with dangers. It's overdraft energy.

I: **Can you say just a little bit more about that, getting a high before one crashes?**

R: The human function curve – basically the amount of effort you're putting in against the amount of performance you're getting out, can be drawn as effort along the X axis, performance along the Y axis. And we grow up knowing that in order to do better, we have to try harder. That is a fundamental rule of life and because it's so fundamental, we imagine that we are infinite pieces of elastic and so in order to do really, really well, you have to try really, really hard. But, of course, it's not an infinite straight line. We're humans and so we have a human function curve, not a human function straight line. There is a point at the top of that curve, before you start going down from the anabolic build-up phase into the catabolic phase of struggling and things starting to not work so well, physical behaviour or health or whatever starting to disintegrate. That bit just before you start to go down can just feel great and you might feel you're juggling plates, you're doing really well, you're keeping all the balls in the air, you're fantastic. 'The rules don't apply to me, gosh, most people wouldn't be coping with this, but look at me, I'm just doing so fantastically well.' We all have our different ways of saying that.

I absolutely say this from the inside, with huge empathy. It's that well-worn aphorism that pride comes before a fall. It's like 'Mere mortals can't do this, but I can'. It's just by the nature of our biology. I always come back to biology because biology is morally neutral. We can beat ourselves up so much for our perceived (and real) weaknesses. But actually, biology is morally neutral; it's about understanding it and then harnessing it and not being tripped up by it.

I: **Absolutely. So we were talking about the people coming to you in the second phase of processing stuff that has happened and finding themselves with a range of possible symptoms – loss of energy, anxiety, flashbacks and so on. So, what's good aftercare for such a person?**

R: Starting generically from the biology side; withdrawal to a place of safety and allowing arousal levels to settle. Really an awful lot comes down to that. The body and mind need space to stabilise. You've been in sympathetic arousal for a long time, you need the rest, healing, growth and repair of the parasympathetic nervous system. We can switch on the high arousal, sympathetic nervous system in a nanosecond. But with the parasympathetic nervous system, we don't know where the switch is. There are techniques, but we don't have that same instant access to it. So it's more a case of getting out of our own way in order to have that healing space. The components of the environment that we try to create here at Sheldon are about getting away from being got at. It may not look like being got at, but just away from the vigilance, the availability, the stuff coming into you. And that was much easier twenty years ago, before we had electronic communication always available. Back then you could create safe space for people much, much more easily. And so one of the things that we try to do now while people are with us and needing to stabilise is check in with them. Who has access to you? Are you going to have the Wi-Fi code? Is your phone going to be switched off? We don't tell people what to do, but we see people getting hijacked over and over again and it's more challenging than it used to be, even in the middle of Devon, to create that safe space.

I: **Yes, I was walking in Scotland with my son last month and we didn't have any Wi-Fi. And when I got back, I had a very strong sense that now I was receiving my life from other people who were bombarding me with stuff, rather than my living my life out of myself.**

R: Yes, I think that's a very common feeling generally. I was saying earlier about the thing of living at full stretch and then the big thing happens. I think an awful lot of us feel we are on that hamster mill of just trying vaguely not to be miles behind and it's a miracle when you see the end of your inbox or bottom of your in-tray. So, going back to the thing of the needful environment, it's about reducing the risk of hijack as far as possible. So that the autonomic system can rebuild trust that the world is going to turn safely on its axis for the next hour, the next half-day, the next day. Because when you have a highly disruptive thing happen, all your alarm systems are set to permanently 'on', permanently on a hair-trigger. And it takes a while to rebuild visceral trust that normal expectations are going to apply. Having a stable environment helps.

Of course, it's all an illusion anyway, because of any one of us can drop dead at any minute. But we actually can't live in the full knowledge of that. We have to live with a basic expectation that life is tolerably predictable. To live otherwise is an extreme spiritual discipline.

It has biological costs to not know that the sun is going to rise tomorrow. It has biological costs and so we have to find ways of reducing our arousal levels. We have to regain trust that the sun will rise tomorrow, or come to an accommodation within ourselves that if the sun doesn't rise tomorrow, I'm still fundamentally loved, fundamentally okay, and fundamentally the universe is a good place to be.

I: **So you create here, and in places such as this, a place of safety, a place of low arousal?**

R: Yes, that's what we're trying to do. So the timetable is gentle, the décor is gentle, the environment is gentle, including the social environment. That's why we have our 'no clergy shoptalk' house-rule, because it's so easy for somebody that you know to be here. An awful lot of this is about safety – that biological sense of safety that I'm not going to have to respond to somebody else's need or demand, that this is about my space and my need. Also vital is our rule about no ministering to other guests. Because many of the clergy we see have a very, very strong helper reflex. It's no good just saying, 'Well, you can if you want to, but you don't have to', because unless you ban it, the reflex has kicked on before you're even aware.

So we try to provide those basic physical and social aspects of safety, and then some people also want to access one-to-one time. That might be massage for reconnecting, restoring that physical sense of safety. For some people it might be the opportunity to tell their story. Often people haven't told the story as a whole in any context. They might have told bits of it, whether as evidence or in a line management or accountability setting, or they might have told bits to their doctor if there are health issues. But there may be a strong need to just tell and hear myself tell the story in its entirety. Which isn't necessarily every little detail of what happened, but more how this whole thing was for me.

I: **That can often be a helpful way, presumably, in which people come to evaluate what the cost of the story was for them.**

R: Yes, sometimes people find themselves with tears at an unexpected point, like 'Blimey, I didn't realise that bit was what was really troubling'. So that experience being seen, having another person witness your story, matters hugely when you've been a witness to other people's stories. You've been holding other people's stories, you've been holding that space for those others – and it's hard for clergy to find people who will hold that space for *them*. With family and close colleagues, the people that you're going through it with at the time, you sort of assume that they know – you're unlikely to stand back and tell the story as a whole to those people. So there is value in doing that with a stranger, I think, because you tell it from the beginning – tell the whole thing in a way that you don't tell the people who are going through it with you.

The telling of a story matters, the making of meaning matters. There is a very fundamental human yearning to make meaning. These big events change us, and very often there are choices around – will the events harden our hearts? Do we allow our hearts to be enlarged by them or do they shrivel our hearts? There's an element of regaining agency in understanding what the event has done to us, because whatever the crap that's being thrown, we do have some choices in how we use that, what can we do with that base metal, if you like. Sometimes those questions need to be made explicit, what are we actually doing with it? Because we're all doing something with our responses, but until you get that reflective space, sometimes you don't know what you're doing with it, or what you want to choose to do with it.

I: **That does seem to be a really powerful question – does this event shrivel our hearts or enlarge them?**

R: What do we want and what do we need to do as a result of that choice. Yes. Often people need help with understanding basic biology, because we are biologically very illiterate with some of this stuff. Sometimes I will tell people's story back to them from a biological perspective – not so much the detail of the story that I've heard, but '[t]his is what I heard your amygdala experience (the amygdala is the threat detector in the brain that processes emotional responses). This is what triggered some of the feelings you experienced and the things you did'. Sometimes people find that enormously reassuring. When I've seen the need for that biological retelling, the most common response is, 'Thank goodness, I thought I was going mad'.

That fear of disintegration can be very real and very secretly held, because there's disintegration all around you. That's the last thing you want to be doing yourself. So just putting experiences into context can be very helpful. You quoted that response to Grenfell, where the cleric maybe feels shamed for having said that ministering there was exhilarating. Maybe somebody like him needs to be given reassurance that although the response was off-key for the people who had experienced death and injury, there is also truth that that *was* what it was like it for you, and here's why. The person shouldn't be shamed for having had the experience, even if it was problematic to have said it out loud in an unprotected context.

Sometimes people need very specific help with relaxation, so I might do audio tapes for people. It depends what language they are comfortable with, but you might call it relaxation or self-hypnosis or for comfort, healing or sleep. Sometimes they hit the spot, sometimes they don't, but they're a useful tool to have.

Sometimes also people need to be able to forgive themselves. This is very common after a personal bereavement, where there are always things that we wish we'd done better. And actually to be able to name and forgive ourselves for the things that we did, which were the best we could with the knowledge and the resources and the whatever we had. With hindsight we may know they weren't the best possible response, and we would have liked to have done better, Processing that sort of thing can be really hard.

I: **But perhaps we didn't do the best we could?**

R: That's even harder, isn't it? Yes. Particularly if we misread a signal or ignored a signal, or took one priority where, with hindsight, we wish we'd taken a different priority. They're hard things to live with.

I: **Ministry seems to me to be full of failure, and maybe we don't teach people about that in training.**

R: No. We certainly don't teach doctors that either.

I: **And maybe there are connections with the question about shrivelling or enlarging one's heart. Whether living with the extent of failure, whatever it is, is a learning and growing thing or a lasting hurt.**

R: I'm sure you're right. I suppose bringing that into the context of this project, this topic, this conversation, is partly about the preparation. How can a minister best be prepared through formal training and personal development for the crisis when it comes, and how can that minister use what has happened as a trigger for further development?

I: **But maybe there are events that people actually can't learn and grow out of, something may happen where a combination of underlying personal stuff and the weight of whatever happened is going to be too much. And someone ought not to continue in ministry.**

R: Yes, some events can break people. It's important however that no decisions are taken too early potentially for the wrong reasons. People may sometimes try to make decisions to get out when they're not in a fit state. And that's where supervisors and senior clergy need to really be on the ball, recognising if people haven't had enough support yet to be able to make a wise decision, because sometimes the day to day stuff is too much.

But also, the learning that comes out of an event is not necessarily predictable, in fact it almost certainly isn't predictable. One form of good supervisory care that we sometimes see is a 'diary forward'. So the line manager makes a diary note for four months or six months later to offer that processing space provide the resources (like funding or cover) to make it possible.

When that offer is made a week after the thing happened, the minister may be neither ready for it nor able to take it. The big event, and the minister's response, will be yesterday's news in six months. After staying upright and breathing and keeping the show on the road, it may be very valuable to be encouraged to take that growing point space at that point.

But how we express the possibility to taking growing point space is crucial, because 'You must be exhausted' or 'You probably need some recovery space', may well be perceived as a criticism that 'I'm not coping'. So a routine expectation that growth is healthy and needs times of reflection is culturally important.

I: **I suppose it is possible that the growing point would be to leave the ministry.**

R: Yes. It may be that the person's work there is done.

I: **I'm not sure churches as institutions are very good at that, because there's a sense that we must all buckle down and continue.**

R: Oh yes, there are no proper exit routes for people, particularly with the tied housing and the way that your CV just diverges further and further from the rest of the world in terms of skill sets that other people know they might want. I think we really need a proper track to support people out of ministry. Because if you can't get out, then you can't stay with your whole heart, can you? I think the military may do it more, at least at the officer level, give people training and preparation for leaving.

I: **Is there anything else that occurs to you about the sort of aftercare that you would provide or recommend in this sort of situation?**

R: We haven't talked about specifically about trauma therapies and I think people need to know what sort of things are available. One of the things that I sometimes offer is the Human Givens Rewind Therapy. It a way of helping the brain to separate out the factual content of a traumatic experience from the emotional content of it. So it's not a way of forgetting, but it's a way of enabling the memories to be filed as normal memories rather than having a high emotional tag to them.

I think it's really important to know that sort of thing is available. There can be a voyeuristic element in some people's offers of help, wanting to know about the shock event. And if you've been in a traumatising setting – at a personal level it might have been a very distressing death of a loved one, or an assault or a rape. In a public setting, something like being present at a fire or a terrorist attack, we don't necessarily want to be talking about the details of those experiences, because it can be retraumatising. So to know that it's possible to have therapies that are non-voyeuristic, that don't require you to be verbalising and rehearsing the detail of what happened, but that can give relief from the symptoms of anxiety and distress – particularly the flashbacks and sleeplessness, etc. – is really important. I really think that that sort of thing needs to be funded, because it's so essential for people whose roles may put them in the front line.

If someone broke their leg at a scene of an incident, you wouldn't expect them to go away and pay for their leg to be put together. I don't know much about the other types of trauma therapy, but there are techniques like EMDR [Eye Movement Desensitising and Reprocessing]. And it is important to remember that a traumatic event can awaken or echo a previous trauma. I'm thinking of people who find themselves in a situation which reactivates a childhood trauma such as accident, loss, abuse. If the reaction seems excessive for the context, then it may be that there's a historical component. It may be valuable to look out for this in colleagues and family members, as well as ourselves. But we tend to be quite pejorative in our judgment of ourselves and others. 'Well, come on, the rest of us are getting on with it', or, 'The rest of us are coping', or, 'Why aren't I managing this?' And just being aware of the possibility that there's an invisible factor complicating the picture is important with trauma.

I: **Yes, so Hilary Ison gives the example of the recent suicide at St Paul's Cathedral and how the worst affected staff member was somebody who didn't even witness it, but for whom it had brought up buried experiences . . .**

R: Yes, that sounds like a classic. We all take away emotional learnings from the experiences of our lives and we're quick to assume what our own and others' emotional learnings would be, but they're precisely not rational. So going back to the phases of response – in the heroic phase, people just get by. They just do what's got to be done and they're very much acting on instinct at that stage. If their instincts are well trained, well prepared, then hopefully they come good at that point. But there's a useful question to be asking afterwards: are there hidden people, or hidden parts of me, that are affected in ways that aren't rationally obvious?

Pathologising traumatic responses as being in some way a weakness or 'something wrong with me that needs fixing' is problematic and may reduce the likelihood of accessing effective help.

Resilience

I: **The church uses the dreaded word *resilience* of course.**

R: Well it is becoming something of a bad word because it's used as a stick to beat people with; 'Why aren't you more resilient?' You don't need to hear it said out loud if those appear to the assumptions around you. That's why it's really important to work hard at building healthy cultures. You can say one thing with your policies and your documentation but if you're not giving people the lived experience of support then it won't amount to much.

I: **So in the training context actually it's the lived stories of the teaching staff that are hugely influential. But I was interested in your response to the word *resilience* which is so much part of the currency these days.**

R: I do think it's a very important concept but it is already being degraded because of the wider messaging within the Church which is that what matters is numbers and money. And, of course, we do have an organisation to run here so I know that if you can't balance the books your organisation may not survive. But if that numbers focus becomes out of kilter with real care for persons, then . . . There's that lovely quote from Ian McEwan; human beings are 'a material thing, easily torn and not easily mended',[2] and we need to remember that.

The risk with the resilience agenda done badly is that it becomes about making each individual person solely responsible for not getting torn or pretending not to be torn or doing their own mending when they get torn, and neglecting the communal and community element of care for and responsibility for each other. I don't just mean in a top-down way – although that matters very much in terms of the signals that are sent and the culture that is created – but also in a mutual and a peer-to-peer way.

Resilience training is essential, but I think it can be toxic if the concept is misused within an organisation. Certainly there are some conversations on the Sheldon Hub (www.sheldonhub.org) to the effect that ministers are experiencing it as a stick to be beaten with rather than as a resource to be thankful for.

Learning from experience

I: **We were talking about the emotional learning from trauma being highly unpredictable. Where does that leave us then?**

R: Yes, our rational cognitive function can't so easily access or understand the emotional learnings that we take out of experiences. Here's what I'm reading just at the moment: *Unlocking the Emotional Brain*.[3] Ecker, Ticic and Hulley are talking about the psychological and neurological research showing how the mind has this extraordinary five-hour window in which significant emotional learnings can be unlocked, re-orientated and re-locked. All the good trauma therapies seem to be utilising this whether they are aware of it or not. This ties in with my experience of the rewind therapy – you don't necessarily have to go on and on battling the trauma symptoms: sometimes it's possible that once it's resolved it's resolved. I don't want to go too far down that road because then there's the risk of people thinking, 'I haven't been fixed in two sessions so what's wrong with me?' But I find it encouraging that good therapies are being developed that are both short-term and able profoundly to resolve trauma. Otherwise it can be a counsel of despair can't it – a bad thing has happened to me so that's the rest of my life ruined, or I'm going to have to spend years in therapy to recover.

2 Ian McEwan, *Atonement* (London: Jonathan Cape, 2001), 287.

3 Bruce Ecker, Robyn Ticic and Laurel Hulley, *Unlocking the Emotional Brain: Eliminating Symptoms at Their Roots Using Memory Reconsolidation* (New York/Hove: Routledge, 2012).

I: **We've talked about what might happen when a minister gets to a place like Sheldon or when they get the help that they need, but what in the person's own attention to themselves do you think would be healthy after they've faced something that was big and overwhelming for themselves or people they were with?**

R: A gentle and forgiving expectation on timescales would be top of my list. The timeframes we live in are already inhuman, you know, the speed of news cycles and turnaround of emails and that sort of thing. It's a bit like convalescence from an operation – just because it's safe to drive after eight weeks doesn't mean you've actually recovered at eight weeks. It might be a year before you're really feeling, 'Yeah, I'm back at the top of my game again.' With a lot of these things our culture has lost track of human timescales, and when the culture is out of whack it's harder to honour your own needs for your body and your mind and your spirit to heal to catch up with yourself. We very quickly turn round and say, 'What's wrong with me? What's wrong with you?' because you're not fixed or fine after one holiday or eight weeks. I think it changes the feeling of pressure if you say to yourself something like, 'Okay, between now and Christmas it's basically, if you like, convalescent time, and between Christmas and Easter is basically thinking about what I want to do next time. And then between Easter and the Summer is starting to put out feelers and implement that and then I can look to be fully back on track next autumn.'

That sort of gentle mapping of the road ahead can make the journey feel more do-able than just being stuck in the middle of 'I'm struggling, I don't know where I'm going, I don't know what to do'.

I: **It's interesting about holidays because there's often an unspoken assumption that once someone has taken their holiday they will be fine then. When you unpack it it's a very odd expectation.**

R: Yes, very odd. But also there may be a whole group of people all struggling. Maybe there isn't just a single identified person who everybody else could look after, but a whole group of people, in their different ways and at their different paces, needing recovery time. And then maybe all you can do is together step back on the non-essentials and be careful about choosing what your priorities are, because the things that seemed terribly important to be progressing and driving ahead with, and achieving this, that or the other objective, might need just binning completely because actually this thing was so big that it made you realise they weren't important. Or it might be that they need to be scaled down, or it might be that the timescale needs to be extended so that together we can all walk this path that's been unexpectedly put our way, because otherwise it's just that on top of everything else (which was probably to capacity anyway).

And I think it's a very key responsibility for people with access to the levers of power – whatever they are in that environment. So if a leader keeps their foot on the accelerator too hard through a period like this, other people may have less choice. So the leader needs to try and be aware of his or her own needs, aware of what's going on for other people, and taking decisions on the priorities and workload. That is all hard work in itself. And don't think I've got this one cracked by the way – I'm feeling my way as much as anyone! Some things can be postponed or abandoned, but others will bite you on the bum and cause bigger problems if they don't get done. Discerning the difference can be hard from inside the situation, and getting an outside perspective may be helpful.

I: **The question was about self-care after a shock event, and then you pointed us particularly to timescales, generous wide timescales.**

R: And stepping stones. So, putting in the diary stepping stones or oases so that you know that you're travelling from one to the next to the next. You know that they are there and you know that you are prioritising putting them in place. Sometimes with people I do what I call a 'canary in a coal mine' exercise:[4] What are your personal and particular symptoms that are warning signs for you that you're not 100% okay? The more specific you can be the better. So, I did the exercise with somebody once and he said, 'If I've eaten fish in the last week that's a good sign for me and if I've not eaten fish in the last week that's a bad sign for me.' And it wasn't the fish *per se* but it represented a whole load of other things that, 'I'll have been shopping, I will have prioritised buying a healthy thing when I went shopping. I will have cooked', so that one thing which was very easily identifiable, 'I have eaten fresh fish in the last week', actually identified a whole load of other health-giving behaviours but also symptoms of being healthy because I was doing that level of self-care.

Another example that somebody gave was, 'If I can remember a time in the last week where my husband and I have laughed together'. Again, it's a very specific thing but it's symptomatic of a whole load of other things. And just having your oasis slots, getting out your 'canary in the coal mine' questions and answering them quietly – sometimes people find it helpful to be accountable to another person for answering them, because it's so easy just to make up. You might commit to another person to do this and just report back that you have done it, or you might ask them to ask you the questions and help you reflect on your responses.

These sort of specific yardsticks, warning signs or measures can be helpful, because most of the time we just get on with living life and things creep up on us. They are an accessible self-care thing, which you don't

4 A 'canary in a coal mine' is an advanced warning of some danger. The metaphor originates from the times when miners used to carry caged canaries while at work; if there was any methane or carbon monoxide in the mine, the canary would die before the levels of the gas reached those hazardous to humans.

have to depend on a professional delivering to you. You can be responsible for setting up and implementing it yourself or in a peer-to-peer relationship if you want.

And, of course, another thing that can often happen in the intensity and focus of the big thing, the shock event, is that you miss out (because you have to) on a holiday or retreat. Doing your best to reinstate the lost holiday or retreat or days off is very important, because you need it more not less. The resource needs to be carried over, rather than just, 'Well, I lost that'.

Implications for God-talk

I: **We've spoken very much and very helpfully in physiological and psychological terms . . .**

R: Yes I know, you're going to ask me 'where's God in all this?'

I: Yes.

R: I think both in my practice and in my personal path I would say God is more often implicit than explicit. And it's quite common for people to have to ask me to make it explicit! For me a lot of this stuff is precisely about our spiritual path, about our becoming fully human, which of course is the glory of God.

I had a breakdown myself twenty years ago and I spent six months away from home on a very challenging journey of recovery of physical, emotional mental health. At the end of the time I came to write in the guest book where I was staying. Completely unexpectedly I found myself writing that it had been a profound and extended retreat, with my body as my retreat-giver. And I realised that it had been a deeply spiritual and meaning-making experience all along, but I had been too busy with the detail of going through it to realise it at the time.

That's not something I preach to people but I do file it in the back of my awareness and if I observe happening with other people then just occasionally I will say, 'I wonder if this is what's going on'. And people generally resonate strongly with that. It's common for people to say, 'God's gone away, I can't pray'. We seldom give people spiritual exercises, but might just say, 'Go and walk the Labyrinth or show up in one of the chapels now and again and don't try to pray, but just physically get yourself there, wait around for a few minutes and then go away again'. Because God has this habit of showing up; and when we are doing our properly human thing of opening ourselves in truth and honesty to these big experiences of life, they can't help but be spiritual and I don't think we necessarily have to go looking for that dimension specifically.

I guess people with a more theological training than me might naturally use those portals of entry more spontaneously than I do. I tend to assume that there are more people who have got those skills than have got my skills, so I fill in the gaps. Sometimes people are spontaneously explicitly spiritual, especially when telling the whole story for the first time, integrating and joining the spiritual, the emotional and the physical. That integration is of itself healing.

For me God is just in it all and woven through it and inseparable from these processes. The physiological is simply the portal of entry that I'm most familiar with and people tend to be less familiar with it, so I harness it. But if everybody was doing this I would probably be going off and doing other things.

I: **It strikes me that a lot of God-talk is actually dualistic and neglects or demeans the body implicitly or explicitly.**

R: Yes. And we can be over-anxious to put up the banner proclaiming where God is. But I think God actually can be quite quiet, that sometimes the banners are too superficial. We have to go to the depths to find out what's really happening, and the depths are quite quiet – I'm going to cry in a minute – and maybe very seldom are there words there. Maybe by reaching too readily for words and reaching too readily for our cognitive function to explain or theologise we risk missing the whole point. We haven't even got to where it matters that God emerges in and through this, rather than giving us a nice big template saying, 'follow this/do that and you'll be fine'. It's reaching to the places which are profoundly not fine and really not at all okay, yet we discover God there in unexpected ways. That element of surprise is so often a marker of genuineness in healing – something unexpected coming into fresh focus and new perspective.

And in a one-to-one context you so often have that tender sense of treading on holy ground together – it's a shared endeavour and yes, as the professional or therapist you're bringing particular resources to the table but that it is profoundly a shared endeavour I think. That's enough about God!

I: **That was a profound reflection so thank you for it. Theologians were well and truly put in their places.**

R: Sorry, I wasn't intending to diss theologians! I'm glad there are theologians doing that work and it's important. But at the end of the day with these big things we're naked aren't we, totally naked. All our learning affords us nothing. We need it, but we need it freshly . . .

I: **Freshly exposed to the bar of real experience. I vividly recall those times long ago when in the mornings I would lecture on divine action up at the University and then in the afternoons I would go down to my work as a mental health chaplain on the psychiatric wards and realise that all those theories seemed so much straw.**

Implications for ministry training

I: **One more area of questioning, which would be about training: we've spoken about self-care within ministry and particularly after a significant**

incident. It strikes me that when people are in training they're not in touch yet with the kind of particular weight and dynamic of how ministry will be and they have I think typically very over-optimistic impressions of how it would be. I can imagine one could tell ordinands a whole bunch of this stuff and they might not hear it at all, so what will be the real core things that you would want people to take away from training in this sort of area? How should people be started out on their ministry in the light of all these things that we've said?

I: I think the biggest gift we could be giving to ordinands would be a fundamental expectation that life and ministry will serve up things which I cannot learn about in advance. But when they come, I can reach out for resourcing and I will be supported to do the necessary learning and reflecting and healing, rather than it being a sign of weakness or something wrong with me.

Also, I would like for people to be a bit more biologically literate. To know some of the stuff that I've spent the last thirty years pulling together from all over the place like a magpie. These biological understandings need to be part of our vocabulary, and to some extent some of it is creeping in.

But I fear the church is in the slow lane on this because we prioritise the spiritual over the physical. We seem to have a profound misunderstanding of the place of the body which for an incarnational faith seems entirely bizarre.

My original professional training was in medicine, 30 years ago, and that had all the same flaws really. A friend committed suicide in our final year and another student said, 'Well, perhaps it was best if she went now if she wasn't going able to cope with the job', I still find it deeply shocking that somebody going into a healing profession could even entertain a thought like that let alone say it out loud. But that was the mentality, the air we breathed, that training was about toughening us up and ultimately dehumanising us.

I hope theological training is very different from medical training but maybe there is a parallel divorcing from deep human encounter as well as promoting it. I'm not sure we really understand what it means to be in a healing profession, how we need to prepare ourselves, learn from our own and others' life experience and grow and in body and in spirit. I think we've missed something about the whole trajectory of what that growth is.

There's something about hearing or having access to other people's stories and using story as a vehicle for increasing empathy, both for other people but also for ourselves until our life pattern matches to the stories that we've heard. I was telling you earlier about the human function curve. I wrote a book including that at 22; at 35 I had an inkling of what it meant; at 55 I'm just beginning to understand it. The facts alone don't cut it do they? We can only learn what we have hooks in our experience to hang our learning onto. By definition at the early stages of training we don't have the hooks. And maybe nobody would ever get ordained if they did! I was talking to a theological educator the other day about trainee ministers having access to the Sheldon Hub where people in ministry are talking about experiences, struggles and the rest. And he said – 'Well, we don't want anything that will put them off.' 'Really?'

I think that actually having that access to people's lived experience in a truthful and unfiltered and real way is a precious gift. This isn't about learning facts, it's about learning a willingness to learn from the experience of life itself and a willingness to learn from the experience of ministry itself, and to know that that is good and where to seek it when you need it.

If you've learned that, then whatever your path in ministry, stuff will happen and things will be thrown at you and they might be internal, they might be external, but you have a basic template that says: I recognise that this is one of those times that they were talking about and that it would be a good idea to reach out and be resourced at this point.

Post-script

The interviewer ends this chapter by noting the famous prayer of St Ignatius of Loyola:

> Teach us, good Lord,
> to serve you as you deserve,
> to give and not to count the cost,
> to fight and not to heed the wounds,
> to toil and not to seek for rest,
> to labour and not to ask for any reward,
> save that of knowing that we do your will. Amen.

More than once he has heard discussion of clergy care and self-care followed by prayers that include that prayer. The whole burden of this conversation with Sarah Horsman is the vital importance of ministers heeding wounds, and knowing when to seek for rest.

In Southgate's chapter on God's involvement in tragic events he rewrites – very controversially – David Blumenthal's prayer deriving from his reflection on the suffering of the Jewish people. Here is a Christian prayer much in need of rewriting.

The reader is invited to consider what a 21st-century version would look like in the light of our contemporary understandings of trauma and resilience and the burden for clergy, in particular, of giving without counting the cost.

Conclusion

Megan Warner

As I sit down to pen some concluding thoughts, news is coming in of a horrific terrorist attack at two mosques near the centre of Christchurch, New Zealand. Forty-nine people are reported to have been shot dead, and scores more injured. One gunman, an Australian citizen, has been charged with murder and a number of others arrested.

During the course of the Tragedy and Congregations project, Christopher Southgate visited Christchurch to talk with clergy about their experiences of the earthquake that struck their city on 22 February 2011, destroying the city's iconic cathedral and some city churches, and of the aftershocks that have continued to traumatise the city in the years since. He writes about these conversations in Chapter 7.

These conversations, together with the countless interviews that the project team have conducted with ministers and lay members of congregations that have experienced traumatic events, suggest to us the shape of the painful terrain likely to be travelled by the people of Christchurch in the coming days, months and years. First reactions are likely to be a heady cocktail of shock and community solidarity, as the 'heroic phase' kicks in. Already we are hearing about New Zealanders' shock that an attack of this kind could have happened in their country. New Zealand has not previously experienced a mass shooting, and it has long prided itself on its peaceful stance. Just as the attack on New York's Twin Towers shocked Americans, who had long considered New York to be invulnerable (pretty much as the ancient Israelites had considered Jerusalem to be inviolable prior to its destruction at the hands of the Babylonians), New Zealanders will be experiencing the radical disillusionment that comes with a shattering of assumptions and identity. New Zealanders will no longer be able to construct their collective identity as they have done in the past. Reports suggesting that the Australian gunman charged with the murders chose New Zealand because he saw it as a 'soft target' will only serve to complicate this, and comparisons with Australia, which in 1996–1997 conducted a national arms buy-back and has not experienced a mass shooting of this magnitude in the intervening years, are inevitable.

By the time this book has been published, today's New Zealand attacks will almost inevitably have been eclipsed by some new horror, somewhere in the world, and may be only hazily remembered by non–New Zealanders. Nevertheless, today's attacks offer a convenient, if appalling, focus for drawing together the various themes presented in this volume, even as the reader's imagination will inevitably have been caught by some yet more recent, or horrific, public trauma.

One of the reasons that the Christchurch experience is compelling is that our research into the theory of trauma, and the stories we have heard, suggests to us that Christchurch's history of recent trauma is likely to mean that today's attack will hit locals and the community as a whole even harder than would otherwise have been the case. We know that unprocessed and unhealed trauma, whether stored in the bodies of individuals or communities, means that new shock experiences are likely to have a greater impact. It may well be that the people of Christchurch have learned a great deal about resilience over the last eight years (more about resilience later) – they undoubtedly know what it means to come together in a crisis – but it is equally undoubtedly the case that the city is still engaged in a process of recovery and the repair of damaged relationships, buildings and identity. Some of the services of mourning for those killed in today's attack will no doubt be held in the city's cardboard cathedral, erected after the destruction of the stone cathedral in 2011, and this will add an extra layer of pathos to the observances of a city thrust back into mourning.

Once the heroic stage has passed, the city will begin the long descent into the valley of the shadow of death and the disillusionment phase. Here is where identity questions will really come to the fore, and New Zealand may find itself undertaking an extended project of soul-searching. Relationships of all kinds will be sorely tested over this time, as connections of all kind are shattered. The relationship between New Zealand and Australia can be touchy at the best of times,[1] but the Australian nationality of the arrested gunman will no doubt lead to an intensification of ordinary tensions. Also inevitably, the religious focus of the attacks will lead to increased inter-religious discomfort and mistrust as people cast around to find scapegoats for the disaster and find themselves unable to resist apportioning at least some of the blame to the victims. An upside of Christchurch's trauma legacy is that inter-denominational and inter-religious relationships and allegiances are likely to be strong. These networks will be called into play in the coming months for the purposes of mutual support, displays of solidarity, multi-religious religious observances and the like. Our experiences in the team have impressed on us the importance of these relational links and the crucial importance of establishing them *before* disaster strikes. 'I didn't really know why I was doing it', said Dean of Southwark, Andrew Nunn, of his work getting to know the religious leaders and business owners around Southwark Cathedral prior to the London Bridge and Borough Market attacks.[2] He knows now.

1 I write as an Australian.

2 See Chapter 16 in this volume.

What is the likely impact for churches in Christchurch? Churches throughout the city, but especially those near the mosques where the attacks took place, will be dusting off their disaster-response plans. Across Christchurch churches of all traditions are likely to be turning on their lights and opening their doors, becoming gathering places for people in shock and mourning, and this one symbolic action may well register itself, as it did for the vicar of St Clements Church, near Grenfell Tower, as the most important action in a career of ministry. Most churches will have congregation members who were witnesses of the attacks or knew victims, and people will have gathered in churches today, as the news got out, to embrace, to cry, to light candles, pray and remember and to ask over and over again, 'Did that really happen?' 'Why?' and 'Where was God?' It will be the role of ministers to help their people wrestle with these questions and to help their congregations finally to be able to say, over time, 'What happened to us has happened'. In the more immediate future, however, some churches will become makeshift tea emporiums, counselling centres and warehouses for overwhelming donations of money, food and clothing. While some congregations may relish these roles – and perhaps it may remind some of the heroic phase following the earthquake – others will feel overwhelmed and long for a time when they can get back to normal again, even if 'normal' may include a good dose of wondering when and what the next disaster might be.

It is vital for ministers that, in the very early stages of a disaster that looks to have the capacity to generate long-term consequences, they book *and pay for* a holiday for between 6 and 12 weeks in the future. As Sarah Horsman stresses in her interview with Christopher Southgate,[3] self-care must be a top priority for ministers responding to trauma events. To carry on selflessly in the face of disaster is, at best, ultimately unhelpful and, at worst, dangerous for the ministers and for everyone around them.

Over time, members of congregations will find themselves divided about the attacks and about the changes they have wrought to relationships between Christians and Muslims and with secularists. In some congregations, other shock revelations may emerge: the treasurer has been engaging in creative accounting, the youth leader has been too close to a member of the youth group or respected couples within the congregation are having marital difficulties, for example. These sorts of external traumas have a tendency to expose internal traumas and to cause new rifts or to amplify their impact. Some congregation members will want to 'get past' these internal difficulties quickly and perhaps to deny that they have anything to do with the congregation at all. Others will want or need to address the tensions and divisions at length. All need to be encouraged to undertake the walk through the valley of death together, neither denying what has happened nor focusing on it to the exclusion of all else. Lamentation is likely to help for a time, and ritual and liturgy will be of great assistance. The attitude that will

3 See Chapter 17.

most help congregation members in all camps is one of 'warm resonance', combined with 'the three Cs' – calming, caring and the clear communication of accurate news. Over time, this attitude, together with prayer and ritual observance, is likely to have the result that most congregations, and most congregation members, will find themselves eventually emerging out of the valley and entering a period of gradual recovery and wiser living, in which a process of remaking (which may be largely unconscious) builds a new normal that holds together the injury of the trauma with the costly wisdom that has been born of it.

How can ministers and congregations prepare for traumatic events?

The short answer, of course, is that they cannot. The very definition of a traumatic event is one that overwhelms all available resources and preparedness. Nevertheless, the project team is convinced that some background knowledge of how trauma works, and how it typically impacts individuals and communities, can help ministers and laypeople alike to shepherd their energies and resources, to respond to one another with compassion, and to understand that the strange and unpleasant things they are experiencing in the wake of a disaster are perfectly normal. These are the three things that will best help communities to survive trauma and to grow through the experiences.

There are, of course, some very practical pieces of preparation that can be done before the disaster happen, things like keeping a checklist of people to be contacted (with contact details) and of actions to be taken when disaster hits and afterwards, having first aid facilities and trained responders, having some media understanding or a representative to delegate to, and becoming familiar with long-term sources of support such as emergency-response and trauma counsellors. These may not be easy to identify in the stress of the moment – and especially not if you hope to find professionals who are sympathetic to the Christian faith. Working through one's understandings of theodicy, becoming comfortable and familiar with the rich biblical resources available and practising the skills of lamentation are also very helpful things to do by way of preparation. The single most important piece of preparation that we would recommend, however, is the building of relationships – as many as possible. Individuals, we have learned (sometimes to our own chagrin), require at least six close, supportive relationships in order to flourish. As we have stressed throughout the book, trauma shatters connections, and so it is important to have built as many beforehand as possible. In particular, ministers can prepare by building close relationships with other clergy in their area and with interfaith leaders. As the Christchurch experience suggests, and as the Grenfell Tower and London Bridge/Borough Market experiences demonstrate, other faith leaders and communities are vital sources of support and partnership, and tensions around relationships between faith groups may be highlighted or even implicated in disasters.

It has been a privilege for the project team, over the last two years, to travel around the United Kingdom, visiting churches, dioceses, mission areas, theological colleges and the like and teaching ministers, those preparing for ministry and laypeople about trauma and how best to respond to it. Our overwhelming experience is that what we have been offering has been welcomed with open arms, even hunger, as people increasingly realise the truth that has struck Christchurch today – the impossible can, and will, happen – and it is better to be prepared than not. One minister was reported to have said after the Grenfell Tower fire, 'This is the stuff they don't teach you at theological college'. We hope that for those we have not been able to reach, and perhaps for some we have, this collection of essays will become a valuable resource, both in preparing congregations for disaster and in helping them survive it.

Where next?

There are strong indications in several of the essays in this volume that trauma experiences can, given appropriate responses, lead to increased wisdom and well-being, as well as to injury and diminishment. Some of the essays describe a fourth 'stage' of trauma response, sometimes called the 'wiser living stage'. The 'wiser' in this title reflects the idea that when a person or community emerges from a crisis having survived it, and having learned that life can be painful yet also holding hopefulness, they are better equipped to respond well to potentially overwhelming events in the future – to 'bounce back', if you like. The cultivation of the ability to bounce back is often referred to today as 'learning resilience'. *Resilience* is one of today's buzzwords. Even guidelines for selection for ordained ministry for some denominations now require that candidates demonstrate 'resilience'.

It can hardly be disputed that anything that can help a person to recover, and to recover quickly, from a setback can only be a positive thing, and it is therefore right that churches, as well as secular organisations, are devoting resources to teaching resilience. However, the current enthusiasm for promoting resilience is not without its shadow side. *Having* resilience to cope with unfortunate and unavoidable setbacks is a definite advantage. However, what is *not* helpful is for a person to be expected, or required, by others to display high levels of resilience. This is most particularly so when the 'other' is an employer or local authority and so on, which uses an expectation of resilience on the part of employees or citizens to relieve itself of the obligation to provide appropriate and safe working or living conditions.

The current focus on resilience in business settings, for example, has parallels with the corporate world's flirtation with mindfulness in recent years. On one hand, it is admirable for businesses to make mindfulness training available to employees if their true concern is for the well-being of those employees. However, if an underlying motivation is to build strength in employees so that they are able to manage what would otherwise be considered inappropriate working conditions or excessive production targets, the enterprise is potentially abusive.

What we know about trauma and hardship is that it impacts different people differently. Some people seem to brush off difficulties and setbacks that cripple others, as Hilary Ison demonstrated in her story about the suicide in St Paul's Cathedral.[4] We are learning that previous experiences of trauma can play a major role in this and that previous exposure to trauma is likely to cause a person to respond more dramatically to a new traumatic experience. We are also continuing to learn and understand that trauma response is the body working properly by taking action to protect itself. It is only when trauma response becomes 'stuck' and prolonged that it becomes pathological. Both of those things being the case, it is not only unrealistic to expect all people to be able to achieve a certain level of resilience; it is also inequitable to expect everybody's resilience levels to be uniformly strong.

Having noted that reservation, and, given the increasing complexity of life in the United Kingdom and the apparently rising incidence of major disasters, it strikes the Tragedy and Congregations project team that helping people to boost their levels of resilience (without demanding that they do so) is an important enterprise. We are hopeful that resilience, and helping people to increase their levels of resilience, will be a future focus for our work, and we look forward to being able to offer more training in that field, as well as the closely related field of trauma recovery, and more written resources, in coming years.

Further resources

Each of the essays in this volume is accompanied by a list of select references to scholarship that readers are likely to find most helpful, and readers are encouraged to pursue that scholarship as their individual needs and interests dictate. The Appendices, containing liturgical resources, may also be of assistance, as will the Select Bibliography at the end of the volume. Those readers who have a particular interest in the Tragedy and Congregations project will be able to learn more by accessing the project website at tragedyandcongregations.co.uk. They will also find an extensive bibliography, links to other helpful sites and contact details for project members.

On behalf of Christopher Southgate, Carla A. Grosch-Miller, Hilary Ison and myself, I wish you shalom in any current trauma you or your congregation are facing and God's grace to grow in and through it.

Megan Warner
London
15 March, 2019

4 See Chapter 4.

Appendices

Liturgical resources

These appendices contain a collection of liturgical resources that supplement the discussions in the collected essays and which are introduced in those essays. See Chapter 10 in particular.

Appendix 1

Text of the sermon preached by the Dean of Southwark, the Very Revd Andrew Nunn, in Southwark Cathedral on Trinity Sunday 2017, the day on which it was possible to reopen the cathedral, a week after the terrorist attack on London Bridge and in Borough Market[1]

'I am with you always'

Saturday night last week was like a living nightmare. It's the kind of experience that only happens to other people, not to you, not on your own doorstep. But it happened to us, it happened on our own doorstep, literally; it happened in our own community that we love and that we've served in Christ's name for over 1400 years. Those years have seen their share of war and pestilence and fire but I doubt that ever before has the church been inaccessible to worshippers for a week, inaccessible as the place of peace and contemplation that people expect and need, inaccessible as the place of welcome and embracing, radical hospitality and love that we seek to be. But it happened.

When I first heard that something was happening in the London Bridge area I put on my dog collar and headed down Bankside to try and open up the Cathedral so that we could be a place of refuge. But initially I didn't get far.

So I went through the back alleys and got as far as Park Street and Neal's Yard Dairy and the Market Porter. But heavily armed police barred my way and forced me back. 'Run, run' was all they shouted. I was directed on to Southwark Street and there saw people lying on the pavement being cared for by the emergency services. 'Run, run' was all I could hear through the sound of sirens and helicopters and I was forced on and on until I got back to the Deanery and shut the door behind me on the living nightmare.

Around midnight I received a text from Amir Eden, a young man who lives on Park Street, a lawyer who was a pupil at Cathedral School, a practising Muslim who's the chair of the Bankside Residents Forum. 'Could I come to yours? I can't really go anywhere.' was his text. I texted back 'Of course' and so he arrived and with 8 other people spent the night in our house.

The rest I suppose you know about. 8 brutally killed, 48 horribly injured. The Cathedral was forcibly entered by the police searching for more attackers,

1 The text of the sermon is reproduced with the kind permission of the Dean of Southwark, the Very Revd Andrew Nunn.

doors broken down, glass smashed in a desperate effort to stop more bloodshed. It happened on our doorstep, on the threshold of God's house.

And now we're here on this Trinity Sunday, back in this sacred place, which is still sacred. The risen body of Jesus bears the marks of the nails and the spear and Jesus shows his hands and his side to his disciples. The Sacristy door shows the marks of the baton rounds fired at it to break open the door and allow the police access. We bear on our body the marks of suffering that so many bear in their flesh and in their soul and spirit.

St Matthew places the final encounter of the disciples with the risen Jesus not on the Mount of Olives, just outside the city of Jerusalem, but back in Galilee, the place where they started, the place of call and from that place of call he sends them out to the nations, to take the Good News, to baptise and teach. But then, before he leaves them he makes a promise, a promise to them and a promise to us.

> *'Remember, I am with you always, to the end of the age'.*
> (Matthew 28.20)

In the horror of the moment it's all too easy to imagine that you're on your own, that you're abandoned to the nightmare, lost in the terror, but Jesus says 'No; remember, I am with you always, to the end of the age'.

God was not absent on that Saturday night; God is never absent. The Psalmist knows it to be true when they say

> *Where can I go then from your spirit?*
> *Or where can I flee from your presence?*
> *If I climb up to heaven, you are there;*
> *if I make the grave my bed, you are there also.*
> (Psalm 139.7–8)

We are not abandoned by the Spirit, we are not abandoned by the Father, we are not abandoned by the Son for we have this promise 'I am with you always.'

On Friday I was invited to go to our local mosque by the Imam. I went with other clergy from here and we were welcomed with open arms. I'd been invited to speak to a packed congregation. The Imam preached about our shared humanity and our shared heritage through Adam and I was able to respond to that, taking your greetings to our brothers and sisters, telling them that we do not hold the Muslim community to blame, telling them that we recognise that we share so much, praying, peace upon you, greeting them as Paul greets the Christians in the multi-cultural, multi-faith, complex and exciting city of Corinth

> *'Live in peace; and the God of love and peace will be with you'.*
> (2 Corinthians 13.11)

That is what we have to do. What we share is what God has given, a shared heritage, a shared humanity, not just with the Muslim community but with all people, all men and women, regardless of anything that others might identify as difference. Difference does not mean division unless we chose to make it so, and we chose to make difference a blessing and an enrichment to our community which is why we celebrate who you are, who we are, male and female, young and old, black and white, rich and poor, gay and straight – and I will say that again and again and again from this pulpit until it is deep in all our hearts, to the very core of our being.

The great metaphysical poet and Dean of St Paul's, John Donne, famously wrote a poem, so well known.

No man is an island,
Entire of itself,
Every man is a piece of the continent,
A part of the main.
If a clod be washed away by the sea,
Europe is the less.
As well as if a promontory were.
As well as if a manor of thy friend's
Or of thine own were:
Any man's death diminishes me,
Because I am involved in mankind,
And therefore never send to know for whom the bell tolls;
It tolls for thee.

'Any man's death diminishes me', which is what the Quran teaches, that killing one life is killing all life. We have all been scarred by what happened last Saturday on our doorstep and we will bear those scars. But they will not make us bitter but make us stronger.

'*The only thing necessary for the triumph of evil is for good men to do nothing*' said Edmund Burke. We will not do nothing. We will rebuild with the community what good things we have, we will rebuild the joy and diversity, the confidence, the acceptance, the inclusive, radically beautiful nature of this community that has been built over centuries and millennia. The roots go deep and cannot be destroyed by evil men and we will not allow it but will confront that evil with love.

We bear on our body the marks of Jesus.

The Feast of the Holy Trinity is the feast of relationship, that beautiful relationship of diversity in the very Godhead, the Perichoresis, the divine dance into which we're drawn. And we're drawn and invited to this altar, through the Spirit, by the Father, to share in what the Son gives to us. With scarred hands he gives his broken body to us, gives his shed blood to us, and he asks us to eat and drink so that through his death we may have life. He is always with us, always, at the altar, in the world, walking through the dangerous places and showing his scarred self to a scarred world and making it, ultimately, beautiful.

Loving God, when terror came to our doorstep and stalked our streets you were there with us in the fear and agony. Remain with us and with all those caught up in the horror of these events, the injured and distressed, those who died, and all who seek your peace which passes understanding. Amen.

Appendix 2

Extracts from *CRUX*, the magazine of the diocese of Manchester, July 2017[2]

Reflection: a force for Good
The Bishop of Manchester

In the wake of the Manchester Arena bomb, a group of religious leaders, representing most of the major world faiths, met in the Regimental Chapel at the Cathedral to share our thoughts with a visiting government minister.

On one of the walls of the chapel a series of photographs depicts the scene from 1940, when much of that part of the building was destroyed by a previous bomb. Then, as after the 1996 IRA blast, the people of Manchester were not cowed or defeated by such attacks, instead the assault on our people and buildings became the driving force for ever greater efforts to restore and rebuild our city, and to make it stronger than before.

I have seen that same spirit at work over these last few weeks. Manchester has shown its defiance through a great outpouring of love. The challenge now is to sustain that effort. Churches and their members will have important roles to play: supporting the injured; comforting the bereaved; strengthening local links with other faith groups. We will also be called upon to join with wider civil society in the task of making an ever better city. And as we do so we will find ourselves being renewed and reformed into a church more fit for mission in a post-bomb Manchester.

Lots of tears and lots of hugs: Churchwarden, Liz Agbettoh, reflects on the role St Ann's played in supporting people in the city after the attack

St Ann's Church became a focal point for many people who needed to pray, to talk and to seek solace. In the immediate aftermath of the blast, our priority was to comfort the throngs of visitors pouring through our doors. We laid aside our own feelings of grief and disbelief in order to support others.

People have queued quietly and patiently to sign the Book of Condolence (there are now 12 books). A child's simple message, "I am so sorry we could

2 Reproduced with the kind permission of the Diocese of Manchester.

not save you" reflects our city's sorrow and its sadness. The grief is heartfelt and palpable. There have been lots of tears and lots of hugs.

The eyes of the world have been on St Ann's (literally). News teams from across the globe have been camped outside our church, recording Manchester's reaction to this horrendous event. The city has responded with great courage, dignity and unity. Some people have resented the intrusion of what they see as a media circus, others have welcomed an opportunity to show the people of Manchester at their very best.

We have been humbled by the random acts of kindness and selflessness, such as Tommy, a homeless member of our congregation who had been given a fiver by a passerby, and chose to buy a bunch of flowers to lay at the shrine in St Ann's Square, rather than buying a meal; Or the Sikh taxi driver who, following the explosion, ferried people to where they needed to be, and the following day took food to people in hospital and gave flowers to mourners visiting the Square.

Our clergy were asked to prepare a special service for Radio 4's Sunday morning worship. On the Monday we came together with other churches for Manchester's annual Whit Walk. Our Walk of faith and witness had a particular poignancy and significance this year, but we were encouraged and uplifted by the hundreds of Mancunians who lined the streets to cheer us on. As the weeks and months go by we pray that all who have sought sanctuary in our church will return and that all may come to know the hope that comes through Christ's love and Resurrection.

Faith communities stand together: Canon Steve Williams

Faith communities played an important role in the immediate response to the attack on Manchester Arena. Gurdwaras (Sikh Temples) were open immediately offering food and shelter. Jewish and Muslim charity workers collected food to distribute to the injured. Churches were focal points of prayer and meeting. Many thousands attended a rapidly organised Vigil in the city's Albert Square the day after the attack. The visible demonstration of Faith Leaders standing together silently declared to the world that the bomber's agenda would be defied. The Muslim community, in particular, demonstrated its rejection of the bomber's ideology. 30 of the UK's most senior Muslim scholars and representatives of the region's mosques laid floral tributes in St Ann's Square, and faith leaders stood together in solidarity with the bereaved and injured at vigils as far apart as Victoria Gardens in Bury and the Jain Temple in Longsight. The Bishop of Manchester said: "This has been a week like no other in our lives." Beyond words, it was a time for standing together – and being seen to stand together.

Appendix 3

Prayers as the floral tributes and messages are removed from London Bridge[3]

The Dean explains what is going to happen. Others may speak and then the Dean leads this prayer.

Like a flower we blossom and then wither;
like a shadow we flee and never stay.

Loving God,
each bloom here represents life
each message, hope
each gift, love.
As you hold us in life as in death,
as we blossom as flowers
and fall as the leaves
as prayers rise before you
and hope never fails
use these gifts to create new life
that your creation may continue to blossom
and your love never end.
Amen.

3 Reproduced with the kind permission of the Dean of Southwark, the Very Revd Andrew Nunn.

Appendix 4

A celebration of the community life of the city of Salisbury: Sunday 15 April 2018, St Thomas's Church and the Maltings, Salisbury[4]

Welcome

Six weeks ago, on the afternoon of Sunday 4th March, something extraordinary happened in this city. It was my birthday in fact, and having preached on 'living life in its fullness', I was eating out with my family. We sat at a table with a view across the market square, and watched people picking their way through the slush on this snow-thawy sort of day.

As we got on with our lives and others with theirs, someone carried out what has been well described as a brazen and reckless crime. Thankfully no-one lost their life, but it could have been very different. And the effect on the city has been profound. It felt that our normal peace and prosperity had been violated.

We gather today partly to remember those who are suffering as a result of that crime – physically, mentally, economically, financially. We are mindful of those whose normal lives have been much disrupted, not least the shopworkers and stall holders who living with great anxiety now and are anxious for the future.

But we gather also to celebrate our community life. When our city is attacked – and we are so mindful that other places have seen much worse – when our city is attacked, we begin to find out what our people are really made of. And by and large, it's a story of resilience, good humour, imagination, and a slightly grumbly determination not to let the 'bad guys' win.

Our firm response to the criminal act is evident in that each of you has chosen to be here today. I welcome you all to this celebration of our community life.

If I highlight certain individuals and representatives, it is simply because their presence is significant.

> I welcome:
> the Lord Lieutenant,
> the High Sheriff,

4 This 'cleansing ritual' followed a liturgy held at St Thomas's Church. It is reproduced here with the kind permission of the Rector of St. Thomas's Church, the Revd Kelvin Inglis.

our Member of Parliament
the Mayor of Salisbury
the leader of Wiltshire Council
and past and present elected representatives

Your presence signifies our shared values – democracy, accountability and the rule of law.

I welcome members of the emergency services who continue to be most closely involved. I shall return to this later.

I welcome people from the commercial life of the city, including the chamber of commerce and Salisbury Business Improvement District. And I am very pleased to welcome staff and managers from some of the businesses that have most closely felt the impact of recent weeks. We can assure them that they are very much in our thoughts and prayers.

At the end of this service, I hope many of you will join a procession which will go out to the Maltings opposite. There – subject of course to the cordons which still have to be in place – we shall ceremonially reclaim our city for the common good. For *goodness* is what we are about.

One way we can proclaim our shared values is by affirming all that is beautiful in this world. It is in that spirit that we shall now hear the Lord's Prayer in the version written by Nikolai Rimsky-Korsakov.

[anthem]

Opening prayer

Let us pray:
Majestic and gracious God
more awesome than the agents of war
more powerful than the wrath of nations
restrain the violent urges of your peoples
and give us the grace to respond to evil
with acts of love and humility,
obedience and thanksgiving,
discipline, gentleness and peace.
Amen.

First address

When Jesus told the Parable of the Good Samaritan, he wasn't answering the question: 'What are nice people like?' . . . although of course the Good Samaritan is a perfect example of a decent and generous person. I think it's always been pretty clear that – if you're faced with someone in trouble – the right response is to stop and help; the wrong response is to ignore the situation and walk away.

Jesus was asked 'What must I do to inherit eternal life?', and this by someone who claimed already to follow the rules for good living. The question was about something much more profound than just being nice – rather it was about 'how can we live as God wants us to live'. How can we use what God gives us not to exist but to flourish. What is it to be fully human?

One theme of the Christian tradition which comes directly from Jesus's teaching is that true service is not reciprocal. Don't treat people who you know will treat you back, he taught. Rather be like the Good Samaritan, who treats a complete stranger.

When we sing 'when I needed a neighbour were you there'; or hear a story of Jesus about judgement when the sheep are divided from the goats; we meditate on the sure teaching that to live humanity to its fullest, we must drop what we are doing and feed the hungry, clothe the poor, visit the sick.

Today gives an opportunity for the people of this city to say thank you to those who dropped what they were doing and came to our assistance. And so, on their behalf, I say thank you:

- to the staff of the National Health Service – paramedics, air ambulance, ICU, all those at Salisbury District Hospital – who have dealt with so much that has been challenging on 4 March and since then too;
- to the army and security units, fire and rescue service personnel, scientists and researchers who have been dealing with the substance released into our community;
- to the local government officers in Salisbury and at Wiltshire Council dealing with all the complexities of the situation;
- to the police – officers from the county of Wiltshire – but supported by colleagues drawn from Cornwall to Northumberland, from North Wales to London. They have provided a constant, reassuring presence on our streets in all weathers. And they've impressed us all with their capacity to drink multiple coffees and stay on the line.

To all these I offer heartfelt thanks from the people of this city. They have been – and continue to be – models of public service. They can walk tall among us.

Prayers

We give thanks for the professionalism and commitment of the men and women of our public and emergency services:

> those working to ensure the safety of the local community;
> those investigating the crime;
> and the ambulance and hospital staff who have cared for and treated those made ill.

We pray for healing and recovery:

> for those who have suffered physically, most particularly Sergei Skripal, Yulia Skripal and Detective Sergeant Nick Bailey;

for those who are anxious and any others who have been affected in any way;
for shops, stalls, businesses that have suffered, and particularly for workers on low incomes.

We pray for peace and new opportunities for:

the diplomats and their families of any country, who have been uprooted from their homes in the places they love, and whose work has been disrupted.

We pray for the recovery effort in the city:

for those who are working to revive the economy, bring in visitors and plan for the future.

Finally we give thanks for all the good things that have flowed from the challenge of the last six weeks:

for our sense of community and its resilience in difficult times;
for the good humour and wisdom of so many of our people;
for acts of generosity;
for the visitors who have continued to come to Salisbury.

And we ask you Lord God to bless this city in the coming weeks and months, in the name of Jesus Christ our Lord.

Amen.

We seek this day to reclaim our city for the common good.
That Salisbury may once more be a byword – around the world – for the values we cherish.

[At this point those gathered will move in procession from the Church to the Maltings Shopping Centre, the point closest to the police cordon, where the Celebration will continue.]

Here in the Maltings
we name all that has been visited upon us

- violation of our peace and prosperity
- injury inflicted on individuals
- fear and anxiety
- disruption of normal lives
- economic and financial uncertainty

With this water of new life,
I symbolically cleanse our city . . .

May it be vibrant, lively, alert, prosperous.

May our businesses prosper,
our visitors be welcomed,
our art and culture flourish,
our vulnerable be cared for,
our past valued,
our future embraced,
and may all be people be treated alike
with dignity, respect and generosity.
May God bless this fine city of Salisbury
today and always.
Amen.

Appendix 5

The following is an extract from an email received by the Tragedy and Congregations project from a participant at one of the workshops held by the team as part of the project activities. The author of the email is the priest in an Anglican parish in the London area.

After the Tragedy and Congregations workshop I decided that it was time to reframe the story of St [XXX] Church. I had previously reframed the story a number of times, but each time key members of the congregation had been missing so I decided to use the first Sunday of Advent, when most of the regulars turn up, to reframe the story in the context of trauma.

The gospel of the day was Luke 21:25–36.

I told the congregation the history of the parish through the four churches that had been built from 1870 onwards.

I made it clear that the amount of trauma that the church had been though from the 1990s onwards was really unusual. I identified four key trauma events, although there have been more than this.

My sermon became a litany that used the refrain 'Jesus said "There will be signs in the sun, the moon, and the stars, and on the earth distress among nations"' before and after the story of each trauma.

After the litany of trauma and the 'Jesus said' refrain, I talked about responses to trauma, such as denial, anger, depression and asked the congregation about the responses they recognised in the life of the parish.

I then used the parable of the fig tree and the motif of the signs of the kingdom to prompt individuals in the congregation to tell the rest of the congregation what signs of new life they recognised in the parish. I used the phrase 'and yet this congregation is faithful and prayerful' a number of times. The congregation is used to me using this phrase as I have been telling them they are worthy for a couple of years now, but this was the first time they had heard the phrase 'and yet we are faithful and prayerful' in the context of trauma.

I invited the congregation to light a candle for each of the traumatic events. Each candle was an old candle that had been cut down (as candles have a tendency to 'tunnel' when not burned for very long). With the bits that I cut down from the candle I made a new one which was smaller but very pretty as it had gold bits in it.

I told the congregation that the candles represented:

1 Loss of the church hall <white candle>
2 Loss of identity and vocation and faith during the anti-women priest years <purple candle>
3 Closure of our sister Church St [YYY] <gold candle>
4 Loss of hopes and dreams, however they are expressed <pink candle>
5 'And yet this congregation is faithful and prayerful' <recycled candle>

I was very surprised to see how keen people were to light candles. One lady told me the next day at the PCC[5] meeting that she was surprised that she offered to do this as well.

I ended the sermon with a simple repeat of the gospel:

> Jesus tells a parable: 'Look at the fig tree and all the trees; as soon as they sprout leaves you can see for yourselves and know that summer is already near. So also, when you see these things taking place, you know that the kingdom of God is near.'
>
> The Kingdom of God is near. Amen

It felt as if it was a huge risk to reframe the story, yet the next day the PCC meeting was much lighter and positive in tone than it usually is. There was a lot of laughter and people who don't usually speak up said their bit and good decisions were made.

Something has shifted.

5 Parochial Church Council.

Appendix 6

Grenfell Tower National Memorial Service Remembrance, Community and Hope, Thursday 24 December 2017, St Paul's Cathedral[6]

The congregation is asked to join in all texts printed in bold.
Music before the service

Before the service, music is provided by the Salvation Army Band of North London, the Ebony Steel Band and Nicholas Freestone, Organ Scholar of St Paul's Cathedral.

At 10.50am, remain seated as the Lord Mayor is received at the Great West Door.
At 10.55 am, Their Royal Highnesses The Prince of Wales and The Duchess of Cornwall,
The Duke and Duchess of Cambridge, and Prince Henry of Wales are received at the
Great West Door. Please stand as they are escorted to their seats.

Processional Hymn

during which a banner with a large green heart and 'Grenfell' written across it is
carried in from the Great West Door by a representative of the Al-Manaar Mosque
and a local Roman Catholic priest and placed at the front of the Cathedral under the
Dome.

Be still, my soul: the Lord is on your side
Words: Katharina Amalia Dorothea von Schlegel (1697–1768), trans. Jane Laurie Borthwick (1813–97)
Tune: Finlandia – after Jean Sibelius (1865–1957)

6 This slightly abridged Order of Service is reproduced here with the kind permission of the Dean of St. Paul's and the Precentor of St. Paul's Cathedral.

Welcome

given by
The Very Reverend Dr David Ison, Dean of St Paul's

On behalf of this Cathedral in London, I welcome each one of you to this National Memorial Service of Remembrance, Community and Hope. Among us are survivors of the fire in Grenfell Tower exactly six months ago; those who have lost members of their families, or their friends; those who live or work in North Kensington as neighbours and members of the local community; those who served others as front-line responders or volunteers, or who assisted with the immediate tasks of coping with the losses of lives, homes and livelihoods; and there are representatives of our national life, because this is a nation that grieves at the unspeakable tragedy, loss and hurt of that June day.

The welcome also includes all of you watching on national television, among whom are those painfully affected who could not face such a public event, those who would have liked to have been here in solidarity, those whose hearts go out to the many whose lives have been lost or changed forever.

In this service we come together as people of different faiths and none, as we remember with love before God those whose lives were lost, and pray for them to be at peace; as we are alongside brothers and sisters who have lost their homes and their community and those they love; as we commit ourselves to care for each other and to be united in the face of suffering and sorrow; as we seek each other's help and resolve to build on our hopes for a future in which the tragedy that struck the peoples of Grenfell Tower will never happen again.

So now, together, we remember and reflect.

Anthem

The Choir of St Paul's Cathedral sings
The souls of the righteous are in the hand of God
Words: Wisdom 3:1–2
Music: Stanley Marchant (1883–1949), Organist of St Paul's (1927–36)

Reading

read by The Reverend Canon Tricia Hillas, Canon Pastor
Matthew 5:1–12

Voices from Grenfell

An oud sounds as a prelude to the following sound montage.
A sound montage of voices from Grenfell, expressing the different emotions experienced during the tragedy and since, is played.
The oud sounds again.

Song

The Al-Sadiq and Al-Zahra Schools Girls Choir sings
Every time you feel like you cannot go on

Address

given by The Right Reverend Graham Tomlin, Bishop of Kensington

Hymn

For the healing of the nations
Words: Fred Kaan (1929–2009)
Tune: Alleluia Dulce Carmen, Essay on the Church Plain Chant (London, 1782)

Commemoration

led by The Dean

Let us remember those who died in the tragedy of the Grenfell Tower fire.
Let us remember and not forget.
Let us remember, united in grief and hope and love.

Silence is kept.

The souls of the righteous are in the hand of God,
and there shall no torment touch them.
They are at peace.

Anthem

The Choir of St Paul's Cathedral sings
And I saw a new heaven and a new earth
Words: Revelation 21:1–4
Music: Edgar Bainton (1880–1956)

The Prayers

led by
The Reverend James Milne, Minor Canon and Sacrist
The Reverend Rosemary Morton, Minor Canon and Succentor
Jackie Blanchflower, Church Leader, Latymer Community Church
The Reverend Dr Alan Everett, Vicar, St Clement and St James, North Kensington
Pastor Derrick Wilson, Chairman, Tabernacle Christian School
The Reverend Jacqueline Brown, Senior Minister, Lighthouse Community Fellowship
The Reverend Mike Long, Minister, Notting Hill Methodist Church
Major Dawn Scott, Church Leader, The Salvation Army, Notting Hill

United in grief and hope and love,
let us pray for each other,
and for the world in which we live.

Kyrie eleison.

We pray for the families and friends
of those who died in the Grenfell Tower fire,
for all who mourn the loss of a loved one.
May we be comforted in our time of grief.
Lord, hear our prayer,

Kyrie eleison.

We pray for those who survived this tragedy,
for all who are scarred by the horrors of that fateful night.
May all our memories be healed.

Lord, hear our prayer,
Kyrie eleison.

We pray for those who rushed to rescue,
for the members of our emergency services.
May we be saved from all that threatens us.

Lord, hear our prayer,
Kyrie eleison.

We pray for those who have offered their support,
for all who sustain us with their care and friendship.
May we grow through the love of others.

Lord, hear our prayer,
Kyrie eleison.

We pray for those in authority,
for all who will learn from this disaster.
May we live to see a better world.

Lord, hear our prayer,
Kyrie eleison.

We pray for the communities of which we are part,
for those alongside whom we live.
May our shared sorrows bring us closer together.

Lord, hear our prayer,
Kyrie eleison.

God our maker,
You know our hearts and share our sorrows.

We are wounded by the tragedy that has befallen us
and by our parting from those we loved:
when we are angry at the loss we have sustained,
when we long for words of comfort,
yet find them hard to hear,
turn our grief to truer living,
our affliction to firmer hope,
and our sorrow to deeper joy.
Amen.

let us pray in faith and trust:
Our Father, . . .

Music

The Ebony Steel Band plays
Hallelujah
Words and Music: Leonard Cohen (1934–2016)

Poem

read by a bereaved daughter
I will be with you in the grave
Jalal ad-Dın Muhammad Rumı (1207–73), trans. Jonathan Star

Act of commitment

The ministers representing different world faiths speak together the following words
We resolve to continue working together
to make our local community a place where everyone is valued,
where everyone has the opportunity to live free from fear
to become what they can be and to live peacefully with all.
May we be given vision, compassion and patience
as we resolve to work together. So be it.

The people respond
We will work with you as we stand together
in the quest for justice and peace,
remembering those who have died,
and committing ourselves to the future good of our community
in hope and love and peace.

Music

The Choir of St Paul's Cathedral sings
during which local school children bring forward small green hearts which they have made at school and scatter them across the front of the Dome dais to remember those who died.

There's a place for us
Words: Stephen Sondheim (b.1930)
Music: from West Side Story – Leonard Bernstein (1918–90), arr. William Stickles (1882–1971)

The blessing

given by
The Most Reverend and Right Honourable Justin Welby, Archbishop of Canterbury

Hymn

O God, our help in ages past,
Words: Isaac Watts (1674–1748), based on Psalm 90
Tune: St Anne, attrib. William Croft (1678–1727)

The bereaved and survivors, carrying photographs of their loved ones and white roses, follow the Grenfell banner and leave together in silence through the Great West Door. The banner will be taken to the Grenfell Tower area after the service and be carried in this evening's silent march.

Select bibliography

Abbott, Roger, P. *Sit on Our Hands, or Stand on Our Feet?: Exploring a Practical Theology of Major Incidence Response for the Evangelical Catholic Christian Community in the UK*. Eugene, OR: Wipf and Stock, 2013.

Ackermann, Denise M. '"A Voice Was Heard in Ramah": A Feminist Theology of Praxis for Healing in South Africa'. In *Liberating Faith Practices: Feminist Practical Theologies in Context*, ed. Denise M. Ackermann and M. Bons-Storm. Leuven: Peeters, 1998.

Ackermann, Denise M. *After the Locusts: Letters From a Landscape of Faith*. Grand Rapids, MI: Eerdmans, 2003.

Alexander, Jeffrey C. *Trauma: A Social Theory*. Cambridge: Polity, 2012.

Allain-Chapman, Justine. *Resilient Pastors: The Role of Adversity in Healing and Growth*. London: SPCK, 2012.

Althaus-Reid, Marcella. *Indecent Theology: Theological Perversions in Sex, Gender and Politics*. Abingdon/New York: Routledge, 2000.

Althaus-Reid, Marcella, ed. *Liberation Theology and Sexuality*. Aldershot/Burlington, VT: Ashgate, 2006.

American Psychiatric Association. *Diagnostic and Statistical Manual of Psychiatric Disorders (DSM-III)*. Vol. 3. Washington, DC: American Psychiatric Association, 1980.

Anderson, Ray S. *The Shape of Practical Theology: Empowering Ministry With Theological Praxis*. Downer's Grove: InterVarsity, 2001.

Arel, Stephanie N. and Shelly Rambo, eds. *Post-Traumatic Public Theology*. London: Palgrave Macmillan, 2016.

Baldwin, Jennifer. *Trauma-Sensitive Theology: Thinking Theologically in the Era of Trauma*. Eugene, OR: Cascade Books, 2018.

Ballard, Paul and John Pritchard. *Practical Theology in Action: Christian Thinking in the Service of Church and Society*. London: SPCK, 1996.

Barnes, Sandra L. 'Black Church Culture and Community Action'. *Social Forces* 84, no. 2 (2005): 267–994.

Barron Ausbrooks, Carrie Y., Edith J. Barrett, and Maria Martinez-Cosio. 'Ethical Issues in Disaster Research: Lessons From Hurricane Katrina'. *Population Research and Policy Review* 28, no. 1 (2009): 93–106.

Baumgartner, Lisa M. 'Mezirow's Theory of Transformative Learning From 1975 to Present'. In *The Handbook of Transformative Learning: Theory, Research, and Practice*, ed. Edward W. Taylor, Patricia Cranton and Associates. San Francisco: Jossey-Bass, 2012, 99–115.

Begrich, Joachim. 'Das priesterliche Heilsorakel'. *ZAW* 52 (1934): 81–92.

Benyei, Candace R. *Understanding Clergy Misconduct in Religious Systems: Scapegoating, Family Secrets, and the Abuse of Power*. New York/London: Haworth Pastoral, 1998.

Berkouwer, Gerrit Cornelis. *The Providence of God*. Grand Rapids, MI: William B. Eerdmans, 1972.

Billman, Kathleen D. and Daniel L. Migliore. *Rachel's Cry: Prayer of Lament and Rebirth of Hope*. Eugene, OR: Wipf & Stock, 1999.

Bledsoe, T. Scott, Kimberly Setterlund, Christopher J. Adams, Alice Fok-Trela and Melissa Connolly. 'Addressing Pastoral Knowledge and Attitudes About Clergy/Mental Health Practitioner Collaboration'. *Social Work & Christianity* 40, no. 1 (2013): 23–45.

Blumenthal, David R. *Facing the Abusing God: A Theology of Protest*. Louisville, KY: Westminster John Knox, 1993.

Boase, Elizabeth and Christopher Frechette. *Bible Through the Lens of Trauma*. Semeia Studies 86; Atlanta: SBL, 2016.

Bosher, Lee. *Social and Institutional Elements of Disaster Vulnerability: The Case of South India*. Bethesda, MD: Academic, 2007.

Bowie, Fiona. *The Anthropology of Religion: An Introduction*. Oxford: Blackwell Publishing, 2006.

Brett, Mark G. *Decolonizing God: The Bible in the Tides of Empire*. Sheffield: Sheffield Phoenix, 2008.

Brett, Mark G. *Political Trauma and Healing: Biblical Ethics for a Postcolonial World*. Grand Rapids: Eerdmans, 2016.

Brett, Mark G. and Jakob Wöhrle, eds. *The Politics of the Ancestors*. FAT 124. Tübingen: Mohr Siebeck, 2018.

Brooks, Ann K. and Kathleen Edwards. 'Narratives of Women's Sexual Identity Development: A Collaborative Inquiry With Implications for Rewriting Transformative Learning Theory'. *Adult Education Research Conference*. Stillwater, OK: New Prairie, 1997.

Browning, Robert. 'Pippa's Song'. In *The Oxford Book of English Verse*, ed. Arthur Quiller-Couch, 2nd ed. Oxford: Clarendon, 1939, 869.

Bruce, Steve and David Boas. 'Vicarious Religion: An Examination and Critique'. *Journal of Contemporary Religion* 25, no. 2 (2010): 243–259.

Brueggemann, Walter. *The Message of the Psalms: A Theological Commentary*. Minneapolis, MN: Fortress, 1985.

Brumberg-Kraus, Jonathan. 'Contemporary Jewish Theologies: An Essay Review'. *The Reconstructionist* (1994): 86–94.

Burns, Charlene P.E. 'Honesty About God: Theological Reflections on Violence in an Evolutionary Universe'. *Theology and Science* 4, no. 3 (2006): 279–290.

Calvin, John. *Institutes of the Christian Religion*. Ed. John T. McNeill; Trans. Ford Lewis Battles. Philadelphia: Westminster, 1967.

Carr, David M. *The Formation of the Hebrew Bible: A New Construction*. New York: Oxford University Press, 2011.

Carr, David M. *Holy Resilience: The Bible's Traumatic Origins*. New Haven: Yale University Press, 2014.

Carroll, B. Jill. *The Savage Side: Reclaiming Violent Models of God*. Lanham, MD/Oxford: Rowman and Littlefield, 2001.

Carroll R., M. Daniel, and J. Blair Wilgus, eds. *Wrestling With the Violence of God: Soundings in the Old Testament*. Winona Lake, IN: Eisenbrauns, 2015.

Cavanaugh, William T. *Torture and Eucharist: Theology, Politics and the Body of Christ*. Oxford: Blackwell, 1998.

Chadwick, Owen. *The Victorian Church: Part One 1829–1859*, 3rd ed. London: SCM, 1971.

Chalke, Steve, Ian Sansbury and Gareth Streeter. *In the Name of Love: The Church, Exclusion and LGB Mental Health Issues*. London: The Oasis Foundation, 2017.

Charry, Ellen T. 'Experience'. In *The Oxford Handbook of Systematic Theology*, ed. John Webster, Kathryn Tanner and Iain Torrance. Oxford: Oxford University Press, 2007, 413–431.

Chauvet, Louis-Marie. *Symbol and Sacrament: A Sacramental Reinterpretation of Christian Existence*. Trans. Patrick Madigan and Madeleine Beaumont. Collegeville, MN: Liturgical, 1995.

Chester, David K. 'Theology and Disaster Studies: The Need for Dialogue'. *Journal of Volcanology and Geothermal Research* 146 (2005): 319–328.

Churches Together in Britain and Ireland. *Time for Action: Sexual Abuse, the Churches and a New Dawn for Survivors*. London: CTBI, 2002.

Clark, M. Carolyn. 'Narrative Learning: Its Contours and Its Possibilities'. *New Directions for Adult and Continuing Education* 126 (2010): 3–11.

Clark, M. Carolyn. 'Transformation as Embodied Narrative'. In *The Handbook of Transformative Learning: Theory, Research, and Practice*, ed. Edward W. Taylor, Patricia Cranton and Associates. San Francisco: Jossey-Bass, 2012, 425–438.

Clayton, Philip. *In Quest of Freedom: The Emergence of Spirit in the Natural World: Frankfurt Templeton Lectures 2006*. Ed. M.G. Parker and T.M. Schmidt. Göttingen: Vandenhoeck and Ruprecht, 2009.

Cone, James H. *A Black Theology of Liberation*. Maryknoll, NY: Orbis, 2010.

Cooper-White, Pamela. *Shared Wisdom*. Minneapolis, MN: Fortress, 2004.

Covey, Steven. *Speed of Trust*. New York: Free, 2006.

Creegan, Nicola Hoggard. 'Theodicy: A Response to Christopher Southgate'. *Zygon: Journal of Religion and Science* 53 (2018): 808–820.

Crites, Stephen. 'The Narrative Quality of Experience'. *Journal of the American Academy of Religion* 39, no. 3 (1971): 291–311.

Damasio, Antonio. *The Feeling of What Happens: Body, Emotion and the Making of Consciousness*. London: Vintage, 2000.

Davie, Grace. *Religion in Britain, a Persistent Paradox*, 2nd ed. Chichester: Wiley Blackwell, 2015.

Davies, Oliver. *A Theology of Compassion: Metaphysics of Difference and the Renewal of Tradition*. London: SCM, 2001.

Deane-Drummond, Celia. 'Perceiving Natural Evil Through the Lens of Divine Glory? A Conversation With Christopher Southgate'. *Zygon: Journal of Religion and Science* 53 (2018): 792–807.

Dillistone, Frederick W. *The Christian Understanding of Atonement*. Welwyn, UK: Nisbet, 1968.

Dunne, Edward, John L. Mackintosh and Karen Dunne-Maxim. *Suicide and Its Aftermath: Understanding and Counseling the Survivors*. New York: Norton, 1987.

Dynes, Russell R. 'Noah and Disaster Planning: The Cultural Significance of the Flood Story'. *Preliminary Paper 265*, University of Delaware Disaster Research Centre, 1998.

Dyson, Michael Eric. *Come Hell or High Water*. New York: Basic Civitas, 2006.

Eliot, T.S. *Complete Poems and Plays*. London: Faber and Faber, 1969.

Erikson, Kai. *A New Species of Trouble: Explorations in Disaster, Trauma, and Community*. New York: Norton, 1994.

Everett, Alan. *After the Fire: Finding Words for Grenfell*. London: Canterbury, 2018.

Exline, Julie J., Kalman J. Kaplan and Joshua B. Grubbs. 'Anger, Exit and Assertion: Do People See Protest Toward God as Morally Acceptable?'. *Psychology and Religion and Spirituality* 4, no. 4 (2012): 264–277.

Eyre, Anne. 'In Remembrance: Post-disaster Rituals and Symbols'. *The Australian Journal of Emergency Management* 14, no. 3 (1999): 23–29.

Farley, Edward. *The Fragility of Knowledge: Theological Education in the Church and the University*. Philadelphia: Fortress, 1988.

Felitti, Vincent J. et al. 'Relationship of Childhood Abuse and Household Dysfunction to Many of the Leading Causes of Death in Adults. The Adverse Childhood Experiences (ACE) Study'. *American Journal of Preventive Medicine* 14, no. 4 (1998): 245–258.

Felitti, Vincent J. and Robert F. Anda. 'The Relationship of Adverse Childhood Experiences to Adult Medical Disease, Psychiatric Disorders and Sexual Behavior: Implications for Healthcare'. In *The Impact of Early Life Trauma on Health and Disease*, ed. Lanius et al. Cambridge: Cambridge University Press, 2010.

Figley, Charles R. *Compassion Fatigue: Coping With Secondary Traumatic Stress Disorder in Those Who Treat the Traumatized*. London: Routledge, 1995.

Fogler, Jason M., Jillian C. Shipherd, Stephanie Clarke, Jennifer Jensen and Erin Rowe. 'The Impact of Clergy-Perpetrated Sexual Abuse: The Role of Gender, Development, and Posttraumatic Stress'. *Journal of Child Sexual Abuse* 17, nos. 3–4 (2008): 329–358.

Fogler, Jason M., Jillian C. Shipherd, Erin Rowe, Jennifer Jensen and Stephanie Clarke. 'A Theoretical Foundation for Understanding Clergy-Perpetrated Sexual Abuse'. *Journal of Child Sexual Abuse* 17, nos. 3–4 (2008): 301–328.

Fonagy, Peter. 'The Transgenerational Transmission of Holocaust Trauma'. *Attachment and Human Development* (1999): 92–114.

Forsyth, Peter Taylor. *The Justification of God: Lectures for War-Time*. London: Duckworth, 1916.

Fortune, Marie M. *Is Nothing Sacred? When Sex Invades the Pastoral Relationship*. San Francisco: Harper, 1992.

Friberg, Nils C. and Mark R. Laaser. *Before the Fall: Preventing Pastoral Sexual Abuse*. Collegeville, MN: Liturgical, 1998.

Frye, Northrop. *The Anatomy of Criticism*. Princeton, NJ: Princeton University Press, 1957.

Fulkerson, Mary McClintock and Sheila Briggs, eds. *The Oxford Handbook of Feminist Theology*. Oxford: Oxford University Press, 2012.

Gaede, Beth Ann, ed. *When a Congregation Is Betrayed: Responding to Clergy Misconduct*. Herndon, VA: The Alban Institute, 2006.

Ganzevoort, R. Ruard. 'Religious Coping Reconsidered, Part One: An Integrated Approach'. *Journal of Psychology and Theology* 26, no. 3 (1998): 260–275.

Ganzevoort, R. Ruard. 'Religious Coping Reconsidered, Part Two: A Narrative Reformulation'. *Journal of Psychology and Theology* 26 no. 3 (1998): 276–286.

Ganzevoort, R. Ruard. 'Coping With Tragedy and Malice'. In *Coping With Evil in Religion and Culture*, ed. N. van Doorn-Harder and L. Minnema. Amsterdam: Rodopi, 2008, 247–260.

Ganzevoort, R. Ruard. 'Scars and Stigmata: Trauma, Identity and Theology'. *Practical Theology* 1, no. 1 (2008): 19–31.

Ganzevoort, R. Ruard. 'Narrative Approaches'. In *The Wiley-Blackwell Companion to Practical Theology*, ed. Bonnie J. Miller-McLemore. Oxford: Blackwell, 2012, 214–223.

Garber, David G., Jr. 'Trauma Theory'. In *The Oxford Encyclopaedia of Biblical Interpretation*, ed. Steven L. McKenzie. Oxford: Oxford University Press, 2013, 421–428.

Garrett, Stephen L. *God's Beauty-in-Act: Participation in God's Suffering Glory*. Eugene, OR: Pickwick, 2013.

Gerstenberger, Erhard S. *Der bittende Mensch*. WMANT 51. Neukirchen-Vluyn: Neukirchener, 1980.

Gertz, Jan Christian, et al. *T&T Clark Handbook of the Old Testament: An Introduction to the Literature, Religion and History of the Old Testament*. London/New York: T&T Clark, 2012.

Goldingay, John. *After Eating the Apricot: (Inside Out Meditation)*. Carlisle: Solway, 1996.

Goleman, Larry A., ed. *Finding Our Story: Narrative Leadership and Congregational Change*. Lanham, MD: Rowman and Littlefield, 2010.

Gooder, Paula. *Body: Biblical Spirituality for the Whole Person*. London: SPCK, 2016.

Graham, Elaine, Heather Walton and Frances Ward. *Theological Reflection: Methods*, 2nd ed. London: SCM Press, 2019.

Green, Joel B. 'Three Exegetical Forays Into the Body-Soul Discussion'. *Criswell Theological Review* 7, no. 2 (January 1, 2010): 3–18.

Grenz, Stanley J. and Roy D. Bell. *Betrayal of Trust: Confronting and Preventing Clergy Sexual Misconduct*, 2nd ed. Grand Rapids, MI: Baker, 2001.

Grumett, David. *Material Eucharist*. Oxford: Oxford University Press, 2016.

Guinness, Os. *Unspeakable: Facing Up to the Challenge of Evil*. New York: Harper San Fransisco, 2006.

Gula, S.S. Richard M. *Ethics in Pastoral Ministry*. New York/Mahwah, NJ: Paulist Press, 1996.

Habel, Norman C. *The Land Is Mine: Six Biblical Land Ideologies*. Minneapolis: Fortress, 1995.

Haines, Steve. *Trauma Is Really Strange*. London: Jessica Kingsley, 2016.

Hammeal-Urban, Robin. *Wholeness After Betrayal: Restoring Trust in the Wake of Misconduct*. New York: Morehouse, 2015.

Harris, Frederick C. 'Black Churches and Civic Traditions: Outreach, Activism, and the Politics of Public Funding of Faith-Based Ministries'. www.trincoll.edu/depts/csrpl/Charitable%20Choice%20book/Harris.pdf. Accessed July 2018.

Hart, David Bentley. *The Doors of the Sea: Where Was God in the Tsunami*? Grand Rapids, MI: Eerdmans, 2005.

Hauerwas, Stanley and David Burrell. 'From System to Story: An Alternative Pattern for Rationality in Ethics'. In *Why Narrative?*, ed. Stanley Hauerwas and L. Gregory Jones. Grand Rapids, MI: Eerdmans, 1989, 158–190.

Hays, Rebecca W. Poe. 'Trauma, Remembrance and Healing: The Meeting of Wisdom and History in Psalm 78'. *JSOT* 41 (2016): 183–204.

Heiler, Friederich. *Das Gebet: Eine Religionsgeschichtliche und Religionspsychologische Untersuchung*. München: Ernst Reinhardt, 1921.

Helm, Paul. *The Providence of God*. Leicester: InterVarsity, 1993.

Henry, Carl F.H. *God Who Stands and Stays*. Carlisle: Paternoster, 1999.

Herman, Judith. *Trauma and Recovery: The Aftermath of Violence From Domestic Abuse to Political Terror*. New York: Basic, 1997.

Hinton, Boyd. 'The Role of Providence in Evangelical Social Thought'. In *History, Society and The Churches: Essays in Honour of Owen Chadwick*, ed. Derek Beales and Geoffrey Best. Cambridge: Cambridge University Press, 1985, 215–233.

Hopewell, James F. *Congregation: Stories and Structures*, ed. Barbara G. Wheeler. Philadelphia: Fortress, 1987.

Hopkins, Nancy Myer. 'Congregational Intervention When the Pastor Has Committed Sexual Misconduct'. *Pastoral Psychology* 39 no. 4 (1991): 247–255.

Hopkins, Nancy Myer. *The Congregational Response to Clergy Betrayals of Trust*. Collegeville, MN: Liturgical, 1998.

Hopkins, Nancy Myer. 'The Uses and Limitations of Various Models for Understanding Clergy Sexual Misconduct: The Impact on the Congregation'. *Journal of Sex Education and Therapy* 24 no. 4 (1999): 268–276.

Hopkins, Nancy Myer and Mark Laaser, eds. *Restoring the Soul of a Church: Healing Congregations Wounded by Clergy Sexual Misconduct*. Collegeville, MN: Liturgical, 1995.

Hudson, Jill. *Congregational Trauma*. New York: Rowman & Littlefield, 1998.

Janoff-Bulman, Ronnie. *Shattered Assumptions: Towards a New Psychology of Trauma*. New York: Free, 1992.

Johnson, Luke Timothy. *The Revelatory Body: Theology as Inductive Art*. Grand Rapids, MI/Cambridge, UK: William B. Eerdmans, 2015.

Jonas, Hans. *Morality and Morality: A Search for the Good after Auschwitz – A (Posthumous) Collection of Essays edited by Lawrence Vogel*. Evanston, IL: Northwestern University Press, 1996.

Jones, Serene. *Trauma and Grace: Theology in a Ruptured World*. Louisville, KY: Westminster John Knox, 2009.

Karkkainen, Veli-Matti. 'Evil, Love and the Left Hand of God: The Contribution of Luther's Theology of the Cross to an Evangelical Theology of Evil'. *Evangelical Quarterly* 74, no. 3 (2002): 215–234.

Kauffman, Jeffrey, ed. *Loss of the Assumptive World: A Theory of Traumatic Loss*. New York: Brunner-Routledge, 2002.

Kavanagh, Aidan. 'The Role of Ritual in Personal Development'. In *The Roots of Ritual*, ed. James Shaughnessy. Grand Rapids, MI: William B. Eerdmans Publishing Co., 1973, 145–160.

Kay, William K. *Pentecostals in Britain*. Carlisle: Paternoster, 2000.

Kennerley, Helen. *Overcoming Childhood Trauma*. London: Robinson, 2009.

Kettler, Christian D. 'He Takes Back the Ticket . . . For Us: Providence, Evil, Suffering, and the Vicarious Humanity of Christ'. *Journal of Christian Theological Research* 8 (2003): 32–57.

Kline, Paul M., Robert McMackin and Edna Lezotte. 'The Impact of the Clergy Abuse Scandal on Parish Communities'. *Journal of Child Sexual Abuse* 17, nos. 3–4 (2008): 290–300.

Kolpacoff Deane, Jennifer. *A History of Medieval Heresy and Inquisition*. Plymouth: Rowman and Littlefield, 2011.

Kraus, Laurie, David Holyan, and Bruce Wismer. *Re-covering From Un-natural Disasters: A Guide for Pastors and Congregations After Violence and Trauma*. Louisville, KY: Westminster John Knox, 2017.

Lago, Colin. *Race, Culture and Counselling*, 2nd ed. Berkshire: Open University Press, 2006.

Larsen, Brian. *Archetypes in the Fourth Gospel: Literature and Theology in Conversation*. London: T&T Clark, 2018.

Layzell, Ruth. 'A Case of the Baby and the Bathwater'. *Practical Theology* 4, no. 1 (2011): 97–116.

Lebacqz, Karen and Ronald G. Barton. *Sex in the Parish*. Louisville, KY: Westminster John Knox, 1991.

Lee, Nancy C. *Lyrics of Lament: From Tragedy to Transformation*. Minneapolis, MN: Fortress, 2010.

Levine, Peter A. *Waking the Tiger: Healing Trauma*. Berkeley: North Atlantic, 1997.

Levine, Peter A. *In an Unspoken Voice: How the Body Releases Trauma and Restores Goodness*. Berkeley: North Atlantic, 2010.

Levinson, Bernard M. *Legal Revision and Religious Renewal in Ancient Israel*. New York: Cambridge University Press, 2008.

Lloyd, Michael. 'The Fallenness of Nature: Three Nonhuman Suspects'. In *Finding Ourselves After Darwin*, ed. Stanley P. Rosenberg et al. Grand Rapids, MI: Baker Academic, 2018, 262–279.

Lohr, Kathy D. 'Tapping Autobiographical Narratives to Illuminate Resilience: A Transformative Learning Tool for Adult Educators'. *Educational Gerontology* 44, nos. 2–3 (2018): 163–170.

MacIntyre, Alasdair. *After Virtue*, 3rd ed. London: Gerald Duckworth, 2007.

Mällki, Kaisu. 'Rethinking Disorienting Dilemmas Within Real-Life Crises: The Role of Reflection in Negotiating Emotionally Chaotic Experiences'. *Adult Education Quarterly* 62, no. 3 (2012): 207–229.

Marshal, Michael P., et al. 'Suicidality and Depression Disparities Between Sexual Minority and Heterosexual Youth: A Meta-Analytic Review'. *Journal of Adolescent Health* 49 (2011): 115–123.

McCann, J. Clinton. *A Theological Introduction to the Book of Psalms: The Psalms as Torah*. Nashville: Abingdon, 1993.

McClung, Emily, et al. 'Collaborating With Chaplains to Meet Spiritual Needs'. *Medsurg Nursing* 15, no. 3 (2006): 147–155.

McWhinney, Will and Laura Markos. 'Transformative Education: Across the Threshold'. *Journal of Transformative Education* 1, no. 1 (January 2003): 16–37.

Melinda. 'A Bent-Over Woman Stands Up'. In *Victim to Survivor: Women Recovering From Clergy Sexual Abuse*, ed. Nancy Werking Poling. Cleveland: United Church, 1999, 1–21.

Messer, Neil. 'Evolution and Theodicy: How (Not) to Do Science and Theology'. *Zygon: Journal of Religion and Science* 53 (2018): 821–835.

Mezirow, Jack. *Education for Perspective Transformation: Women Re-entry Programs in Community College*. New York: Columbia University Press, 1978.

Moltmann, Jürgen. *The Crucified God: The Cross of Christ as the Foundation and Criticism of Christian Theology*. Trans. R.A. Wilson and J. Bowden. London: SCM, 1974.

Mosgofian, Peter and George Ohlschlager. *Sexual Misconduct in Counseling and Ministry*. Eugene, OR: Wipf & Stock, 1995.

Murphy, Francesca Aran and Philip G. Ziegler. *The Providence of God*. London: T&T Clark, 2009.

National Cancer Services. *Manual for Cancer Services: Psychological Support Measures Version 1.0*, NHS Crown Communications, April 2011.

National Child Traumatic Stress Network, The. 'Psychological First Aid'. www.nctsn.org, home/treatmentsandpractices/psychologicalfirstaidandSPR/aboutPFA. Accessed 17 September 2018.

Nichols, Ryan. 'Re-evaluating the Effects of the 1755 Lisbon Earthquake on Eighteenth-Century Minds: How Cognitive Science of Religion Improves Intellectual History With Hypothesis Testing Methods'. *Journal of the American Academy of Religion* 82, no. 4 (2014): 970–1009.

Norris, Kathleen. *The Cloister Walk*. New York: Riverhead, 1996.

O'Connor, Kathleen. *Lamentations: The Tears of the World*. Maryknoll, NY: Orbis, 2002.

O'Donnell, Karen. *Broken Bodies: The Eucharist, Mary and the Body in Trauma Theology*. London: SCM Press, 2018.

Ollenburger, Ben C., ed. *Old Testament Theology: Flowering and Future*. Winona Lake, IN: Eisenbrauns, 2004.

Olonfinjana, Israel. 'The History of Black Majority Churches in London (ND)'. www.open.ac.uk/arts/research/religion-in-london/sites/www.open.ac.uk.arts.research.religion-in-london/files/files/ecms/arts-rl-pr/web-content/Black-Majority-Churches-in-London.pdf. Accessed July 2018.

O'Sullivan, Barry. *The Burden of Betrayal: Non-offending Priests and the Clergy Child Sexual Abuse Scandals*. Leominster: Gracewing, 2018.

Pannenberg, Wolfhart. *What Is Man? Contemporary Anthropology in Theological Perspective*. Philadelphia: Fortress, 1970.

Pargament, Kenneth I., Nichole A. Murray-Swank and Annette Mahoney. 'Problem and Solution: The Spiritual Dimension of Clergy Sexual Abuse and Its Impact on Survivors'. *Journal of Child Sexual Abuse* 17, nos. 3–4 (2008): 397–420.

Park, Crystal L. 'Making Sense of the Meaning Literature: An Integrative Review of Meaning Making and Its Effects on Adjustment to Stressful Life Events'. *Psychological Bulletin* 136 (2010): 257–301.

Parry, Sarah. *Effective Self-care and Resilience in Clinical Practice*. London: Jessica Kingsley Publishers, 2017.

Pearsall, Judy, ed. *The New Oxford Dictionary of English*. Oxford/New York: Oxford University Press, 1998.

Pellauer, Mary D., Barbara Chester and Jane Boyajian, eds. *Sexual Assault and Abuse: A Handbook for Clergy and Religious Professionals*. San Francisco: Harper, 1987.

Pennebaker, James, W. *Opening Up: The Healing Power of Expressing Emotions*, Rev. ed. New York: Guilford, 1997.

Peyton, Sarah. *Your Resonant Self: Guided Meditations and Exercises to Engage Your Brain's Capacity for Healing*. London: W.W. Norton, 2017.

Phillips, Dewi Zephaniah. *The Problem of Evil and the Problem of God*. London: SCM, 2004.

Phillips, Mike and Trevor Phillips. *Windrush: The Irresistible Rise of Multi-Racial Britain*. London: Harper Collins, 1998.

Piper, John. 'Are There Two Wills in God?'. In *Still Sovereign: Contemporary Perspectives on Election, Foreknowledge and Grace*, ed. Thomas R. Schreiner and Bruce R. Ware. Grand Rapids: Baker, 2000, 107–131.

Plantinga, Alvin. *God, Freedom and Evil*. Grand Rapids, MI: Eerdmans, 1977.

Plantinga, Cornelius. *Not the Way It's Supposed to Be: A Breviary of Sin*. Grand Rapids, MI: Eerdmans, 1996.

Poling, James. *The Abuse of Power: A Theological Problem*. Nashville, TN: Abingdon, 1991.

Purves, Andrew. *Search for Compassion: Spirituality and Mission*. Louisville, KY: John Knox, 1989.

Rambo, Shelly. 'Haunted (by the) Gospel: Theology, Trauma and Literary Theory in the Twenty-first Century'. *PMLA* 125, no. 4 (2010): 936–941.

Rambo, Shelly. *Spirit and Trauma: A Theology of Remaining*. Louisville, KY: WJK, 2010.

Rambo, Shelly. *Resurrecting Wounds: Living in the Aftermath of Trauma*. Waco, TX: Baylor University Press, 2017.

Randall, William L. 'The Importance of Being Ironic: Narrative Openness and Personal Resilience in Later Life'. *The Gerontologist* 53 (2013): 9–16.

Rawlings, Helen. *The Spanish Inquisition*. Oxford: Blackwell, 2006.

Ricœur, Paul. 'Life: A Story in Search of a Narrator'. In *A Ricœur Reader: Reflection and Imagination*, ed. Mario J. Valdés. Toronto: University of Toronto, 1991, 425–437.

Roberts, Vaughan S. and David Sims. *Leading by Story: Rethinking Church Leadership*. London: SCM Press, 2017.

Rohr, Richard. *The Divine Dance: The Trinity and Your Transformation*. London: SPCK, 2016.

Rose, Marika. *A Theology of Failure: Žižek Against Christian Innocence*. New York: Fordham University Press, 2019.

Ruether, Rosemary Radford. 'Feminist Theology: Methodology, Sources and Norms'. In *Theological Reflection: Sources*, ed. Elaine Graham, Heather Walton and Frances Ward. London: SCM, 2007, 294–302.

Ruppert, Franz. *Trauma, Fear & Love: How the Constellation of the Intention Supports Healthy Autonomy*. London: Green Balloon, 2014.

Sands, Diana and Mark Tennant. 'Transformative Learning in the Context of Suicide Bereavement'. *Adult Education Quarterly* 60, no. 2 (2010): 99–121.

Saul, Jack. *Collective Trauma and Collective Healing*. New York: Routledge, 2014.

Schmid, Konrad. *The Old Testament: A Literary History*. Minneapolis: Fortress, 2012.

Senn, Frank C. *Christian Liturgy: Catholic and Evangelical*. Minneapolis: Fortress, 1997.

Shay, Jonathan. *Odysseus in America: Combat Trauma and the Trials of Homecoming*. New York: Scribner, 2002.

Shay, Jonathan. *Achilles in Vietnam: Combat Trauma and the Undoing of Character*. New York: Simon and Schuster, 2010.

Smellick, Klaas A.D. *Etty: The Letters and Diaries of Etty Hillesum 1941–1943*. Trans. Arnold J. Pomerans. Grand Rapids, MI/Cambridge, UK: William B. Eerdmans, 1986.

Southgate, Christopher. *The Groaning of Creation: God, Evolution and the Problem of Evil*. Louisville, KY: Westminster John Knox, 2008.

Southgate, Christopher. 'Cosmic Evolution and Evil'. In *The Cambridge Companion to the Problem of Evil*, ed. C. Meister and P.K. Moser. Cambridge: Cambridge University Press, 2017, 147–164.

Southgate, Christopher. '"Free-Process" and "Only-Way" Arguments'. In *Finding Ourselves after Darwin: Conversations on the Image of God, Original Sin, and the Problem of Evil*, ed. Stanley P. Rosenberg, Michael Burdett, Michael Lloyd, and Benno van den Toren. Grand Rapids, MI: Baker Academic, 2018, 293–305.

Southgate, Christopher. 'Response With a Select Bibliography'. *Zygon: Journal of Religion and Science* 53 (2018): 909–930.

Southgate, Christopher. *Theology in a Suffering World: Glory and Longing*. Cambridge: Cambridge University Press, 2018.

Staudacher, Carol. *Beyond Grief: A Guide for Recovering from the Death of a Loved One*. London: Souvenir, 1988.

Stephens, Darryl W. 'Fiduciary Duty and Sacred Trust'. In *Professional Sexual Ethics: A Holistic Ministry Approach*, ed. Patricia Beattie Jung and Darryl W. Stephens. Minneapolis: Fortress, 2013, 23–33.

Stolorow, Robert. 'Phenomenological-Contextualism in Trauma'. In *Trauma and Transcendence*, ed. Eric Boynton and Peter Capretto. New York: Fordham University Press, 2018, 53–69.

Surin, Kenneth. *Theology and the Problem of Evil*. Oxford: Basil Blackwell, 1986, 161–162.

Sweeney, Marvin A. *Reading the Hebrew Bible After the Shoah: Engaging Holocaust Theology*. Minneapolis: Fortress, 2008.

Swinburne, Richard. *Providence and the Problem of Evil*. Oxford: Oxford University Press, 1998.

Swinton, John. *Raging With Compassion: Pastoral Responses to the Problem of Evil*. Grand Rapids, MI/Cambridge: Wm B. Eerdmans, 2007.

Taylor, Antony James William. 'Value Conflict Arising From a Disaster'. *Australasian Journal of Disaster and Trauma Studies* 3, no. 2 (1999).

Taylor, Edward W. 'An Update of Transformative Learning Theory: A Critical Review of the Empirical Research (1999–2005)'. *International Journal of Lifelong Education* 26, no. 2 (2007): 173–191.

Terrien, Samuel. *The Elusive Presence: Toward a New Biblical Theology*. Eugene, OR: Wipf and Stock, 2005.

Terry, Karen J. 'Stained Glass: The Nature and Scope of Child Sexual Abuse in the Catholic Church'. *Criminal Justice and Behaviour* 35, no. 5 (2008): 549–569.

Thatcher, Adrian. 'Introduction'. In *The Oxford Handbook of Theology, Sexuality, and Gender*, ed. Adrian Thatcher. Oxford: Oxford University Press, 2015, 1–17.

Thiselton, Anthony C. *New Horizons in Hermeneutics: The Theory and Practice of Transforming Biblical Reading*. Grand Rapids, MI: Zondervan, 1997.

Thompson, Deanna A. *Glimpsing Resurrection: Cancer, Trauma and Ministry*. Louisville, KY: Westminster John Knox, 2018.

Thompson, Judith with Stephen Pattison and Ross Thompson. *Theological Reflection*. London: SCM, 2008.

Tilley, Terrence. *The Evils of Theodicy*. Georgetown, VA: Georgetown University Press, 1991.

Timmerman, Joan. *Sexuality and Spiritual Growth*. New York: Crossroad, 1993.

Tollerton, David. 'Reconfiguring the Theodicy-Antitheodicy Boundary Between Responses to the Holocaust'. *Journal of Jewish Thought and Philosophy* 26 (2018): 278–292.

Turner, Victor. *The Ritual Process: Structure and Anti-Structure*. London: Aldine Transaction, 2008.

Valdés, Mario J. *A Ricœur Reader: Reflection and Imagination*. Toronto: University of Toronto, 1991.

Van der Kolk, Bessel. 'The Body Keeps the Score: Memory and the Evolving Psychobiology of Post-Traumatic Stress'. *Harvard Review of Psychiatry* 1, no. 5 (1994): 253–265.

Van der Kolk, Bessel. *The Body Keeps the Score: Brain, Mind and Body in the Healing of Trauma*. New York: Viking, 2014.

Van Gennep, Arnold. *The Rites of Passage*. Trans. Monika B. Vizedom and Gabrielle L. Caffe. Chicago: University of Chicago, 1960.

Vanstone, William Hubert. *The Stature of Waiting*. London: Darton, Longman and Todd, 1982.

Vanstone, William Hubert. *Farewell in Christ*. London: Darton, Longman and Todd, 2007.

Villanueva, Frederico G. *The Uncertainty of a Hearing: A Study of the Sudden Change of Mood in the Psalms of Lament*. VTSupp 121. Leiden: Brill, 2008.

Vincent, Thomas. *God's Terrible Voice in the City*. London: George Calvert, 1667; Reprinted Morgan, PA: Soli Deo Gloris, 1997.

Volf, Miroslav. *After Our Likeness: The Church as the Image of the Trinity*. Cambridge: Wm. B. Eerdmans, 1998.

Wall, John. *Moral Creativity: Paul Ricœur and the Poetics of Possibility*. Oxford: Oxford University Press, 2005.

Wallace, Howard Neil. *Words to God, Word From God: The Psalms in the Prayer and Preaching in the Church*. Aldershot, UK and Burlington, VT: Ashgate, 2005.

Warner, Megan. *Abraham: A Journey Through Lent*. London: SPCK, 2015.

Warner, Megan. *Re-Imagining Abraham: A Re-assessment of the Influence of Deuteronomism in Genesis*. OTS 72. Leiden/Boston: Brill, 2018.

Waterstradt, Carolyn. *Fighting the Good Fight: Healing and Advocacy After Clergy Sexual Assault*. splatteredinkpress.com, 2012.

Webster, John. 'The Self-Organizing Power'. *International Journal of Systematic Theology* 3 (2001): 69–82.

Wells, Ken. 'A Needs Assessment Regarding the Nature and Impact of Clergy Sexual Abuse Conducted by the Interfaith Sexual Trauma Institute'. *Sexual Addiction and Compulsivity* 10 (2003): 201–217.

Wells, Ken, Ralph H. Earle and Marcus R. Earle. 'Outpatient and Inpatient Intensive Treatment Models'. In *Clergy Sexual Misconduct: A Systems Approach to Prevention, Intervention and Oversight*, ed. John Thoburn, Rob Baker and Maria Dal Maso. Carefree, AZ: Gentle Path, 2011.

Westermann, Claus. 'The Role of Lament in the Theology of the Old Testament'. *Interpretation* 28 (1974): 20–38.

White, Robert S. *Who Is to Blame: Disasters, Nature and Acts of God*. Oxford: Monarch, 2014.

Whitefield, George. *Whitefield at Lisbon: Being a Detailed Account of the Blasphemy and Idolatry of Popery . . . With Mr. Whitefield's Remarks Thereon*. London: R. Groombridge and Sons, 1851.

Whittington, John. *Systemic Coaching & Constellations: The Principles, Practices and Application for Individuals, Teams and Groups*, 2nd ed. London/Philadelphia: Kogan Page, 2016.

Wiesel, Elie. *Night*. Trans. Stella Rodway. New York: Bantam, 1982.

Wildman, Wesley J. *In Our Own Image: Anthropomorphism, Apophaticism and Ultimacy*. Oxford: Oxford University Press, 2017.

Willard, W.C. Ashley and Stephen B. Roberts, eds. *Disaster Spiritual Care*, 2nd ed. Nashville, TN: SkyLight Paths, 2017.

Williams, Rowan. *Writing in the Dust: Reflection on 11th September and Its Aftermath*. London: Hodder and Stoughton, 2002.

Williams, Rowan. 'Trinity and Revelation'. In *Theological Reflection: Sources*, ed. Elaine Graham, Heather Walton and Frances Ward. London: SCM, 2007, 23–31.

Williamson, Hugh G.M. 'Reading the Lament Psalms Backwards'. In *A God So Near: Essays on Old Testament Theology in Honor of Patrick D. Miller*, ed. Brent A. Strawn and Nancy R. Bowen. Winona Lake, IN: Eisenbrauns, 2003.

Wiman, Christian. *My Bright Abyss: Meditations of a Modern Believer*. New York: Farrer, Strauss and Giroux, 2013.

Winnicott, Donald Woods. 'Transitional Objects and Transitional Phenomena – A Study of the First Not-Me Possession'. *International Journal of Psycho-Analysis* 34 (1953): 89–97.

Winnicott, Donald Woods. *Playing and Reality*. London/New York: Routledge Classics, 2005.

Wollaston, Isabel. 'The Possibility and Plausibility of Divine Abusiveness or Sadism as the Premise for a Religious Response to the Holocaust'. *Journal Religion and Society* 2 (2000): 1–15.

Woodhead, Linda, Mathew Guest and Karen Tusting. 'Congregational Studies: Taking Stock'. In *Congregational Studies in the UK: Christianity in a Post-Christian Context*, ed. Matthew Guest, Karen Trusting and Linda Woodhead. Aldershot: Ashgate, 2004, 1–23.

Woodhouse, Patrick. *Etty Hillesum: A Life Transformed*. London: Bloomsbury, 2009.

Wright, Nicholas Thomas. *Evil and the Justice of God*. London: SPCK, 2006.

Young, Frances. *God's Presence: A Contemporary Recapitulation of Early Christianity*. Cambridge: Cambridge University Press, 2013.

Young, Wm. Paul. *The Shack*. London: Hodder & Stoughton, 2008.

Index

For Product Safety Concerns and Information please contact our EU representative GPSR@taylorandfrancis.com Taylor & Francis Verlag GmbH, Kaufingerstraße 24, 80331 München, Germany

Printed and bound by CPI Group (UK) Ltd, Croydon, CR0 4YY
08/06/2025
01897001-0018